Breast Imaging Review

Biren A. Shah • Gina M. Fundaro
Sabala R. Mandava

Breast Imaging Review

A Quick Guide to Essential Diagnoses

Second Edition

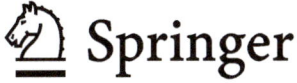 Springer

Biren A. Shah, MD, FACR
Department of Radiology
Henry Ford Hospital
Detroit, MI
USA

Sabala R. Mandava, MD
Department of Radiology
Henry Ford Hospital
Detroit, MI
USA

Gina M. Fundaro, MD
Department of Radiology
Henry Ford Hospital
Detroit, MI
USA

ISBN 978-3-319-07790-1   ISBN 978-3-319-07791-8   (eBook)
DOI 10.1007/978-3-319-07791-8
Springer Cham Heidelberg New York Dordrecht London

Library of Congress Control Number: 2014951344

Printed on acid-free paper

Springer is part of Springer Science+Business Media (www.springer.com)

To my parents, Ashok and Jyoti Shah, who I owe everything I am to them.
I am guided by their strong principles of life and work ethic that they
instilled in me.
To my sister, Dr. Binita Shah Ashar, for her sound advice and constant
encouragement.
To my wife, Dharmishtha Shah, for her endless support and love.
To my two sons, Aren and Deven, who make life all worthwhile.

Biren A. Shah

To my mother and father, Jacqueline and William,
for their guidance, teaching, and unconditional love.
To my brother, Bill, for his encouragement, friendship,
and innate ability to always make me laugh.
To my grandparents, Irene and William Fundaro, for all
of the sacrifices they made to provide me with a college education.
To my godfather, Thomas Capraro, and my grandma, Alyce Jarvis,
for never giving up once they were diagnosed. They remind
me daily to fight for my patients.
Ryan, my love and best friend, words cannot express my gratitude.
Thank you for committing to our journey with an open heart.
I would not be who I am today without your love and constant
unwavering support.
Asher Thomas and Arden Joy, my sunshine and butterfly,
you have inspired me to put my best efforts forward with this project.
My hope is to pave the way for you, so that your lives are full
of opportunities and rich experiences. You are the loves of my life,
and every day I am so grateful that you are my children.

Gina M. Fundaro

To my parents, Vasu and Saranya, for their guidance and
unconditional love and support.
To my sister, Amulya, for always being there for me.
To my children, Milind and Ariana, for the joy and laughter
they have brought into all our lives.
To my husband, Rajesh, for his love and tireless belief in me.
I wouldn't be here without him.

Sabala Mandava

Foreword

I am frequently asked by radiologists to offer advice on cases involving breast imaging diagnosis. This may include a rare presentation of a common disease versus a more typical presentation of a relatively common disease. Radiologists from all different experience levels, whether those who practice breast imaging relatively infrequently to radiologists in training, such as residents, will have moments of wondering whether they are interpreting the mammogram accurately or performing the most effective follow-up evaluation. Breast imaging has evolved to include multiple modalities such as mammography, ultrasound and MRI, and newer types of imaging such as molecular imaging, along with multimodality biopsy techniques. With the ever-changing field of breast imaging, radiologists find themselves wishing they had previously seen a case similar to the one they are working on, to guide them through the workup to the final diagnosis.

Breast Imaging Review: A Quick Guide to Essential Diagnoses is an exciting collaboration of multiple case studies, with beautiful didactic images. The workup evaluation and captions are included with every set of images, offering detailed explanation. In addition, references are given for the reader who may wish to seek additional information on each topic. The book has so many wonderful case studies, which include cases seen frequently in routine daily practice by the radiologist on the breast rotation, as well as the resident or fellow rotating through the breast imaging section. The cases are well organized and facilitate a quick review of one specific disease or an overall review of many disease processes.

The book is a helpful tool for the more senior resident preparing for their board exam or in preparation for rotating through the breast imaging section. Each case shown is followed by multiple sets of images with all the modalities utilized for diagnosis of each specific patient and each unique condition. Each case study is different and includes many of the imaging studies each patient may undergo as part of their workup. Each study is identified and discussed to facilitate accurate diagnosis as well as provide a detailed review.

When Drs. Shah, Fundaro, and Mandava asked me to write this Foreword, I was curious to read the book and identify what I liked about it and whether I found it helpful. I was happy to see that *Breast Imaging Review* is everything its name eludes. The cases are arranged similarly to what a radiologist would experience in our typical clinical workday. Some masses, some microcalcifications, and lots of correlative images with many different modalities are showcased. The interventional section is very helpful, especially for the radiologist just starting to do procedures on his or her own.

Each section of the book has a lot to offer for the trainee or the radiologist out in the clinical arena seeing patients. This is a comprehensive case review book that will be useful as a quick reference for anyone working in the field of breast imaging.

Stamatia V. Destounis, MD, FACR
Elizabeth Wende Breast Care, LLC
Clinical Associate Professor
University of Rochester School of Medicine & Dentistry
Rochester, NY, USA

Preface

The second edition of *Breast Imaging Review* is a new volume with all the pearls of the first edition combined with updated material and improved images. In this edition, most of the images are digital, allowing for better visualization of the findings. There is information pertaining to the recently released BI-RADS, 5th Edition, as well as additional material on many of the cases and the high-yield facts.

Although written primarily as a review for residents and fellows, we hope it will be a useful tool for radiologists out in the real world as well. We have kept the easy-to-follow format of the first edition, with different sections and a case-based approach. Wherever possible, we have tried to include images in multiple modalities for each diagnosis.

The section on interventional procedures gives a step-by-step approach to the common breast interventions. The high-yield facts at the end of the book are just that: an organized review of important points in breast imaging that can serve as a quick reference.

We hope you get as much pleasure in reading through the book as we had writing in it.

Anyone who stops learning is old, whether at twenty or eighty.
Anyone who keeps learning stays young.
The greatest thing in life is to keep your mind young.

Henry Ford

Detroit, MI, USA

Biren A. Shah, MD, FACR
Gina M. Fundaro, MD
Sabala R. Mandava, MD

Acknowledgments

It all started at the tail end of a busy clinic day in breast imaging. Biren mentioned to Gina an idea that he had been mulling over for a while, to write a review book in breast imaging geared toward the oral boards. After hearing the idea, Gina enthusiastically became a part of the project. A few days later, Biren explained the concept to Sabala who also hopped on board the review book bandwagon. And so a book was born.

From then on, it has been a whirlwind of research, writing, deadlines, emails (hundreds of emails), early mornings, and late nights. We were all at once elated, frustrated, overwhelmed, and subdued. As this is a freshman project for all of us, we have learned many things by trial and error. We also found hidden talents in each other, which emerged along the way:

Biren's resourcefulness and quick solutions to roadblocks are belied by his calm and quiet exterior.

Gina, with her attention to detail and task-oriented lists, helped us meet every deadline.

Sabala's natural loquaciousness translated into a flair for sentence structure and layout.

This book would not have been possible without the help of many people:

Dr. Manuel L. Brown, MD, our chairman, who has given us his unconditional support from the beginning.

Dr. Kanwal Merchant, MD, and Dr. John Blasé, MD, our former residents and now fellows, who graciously reviewed our initial efforts and gave us valuable feedback.

Rhonda Pate, R.T.(R)(M); Penny Rizzo, R.T.(R)(M); and Carmen Czajka, R.T.(R)(M), for their help in finding many of our images.

Susie Stephen, radiology support assistant, and Sharnita Powell-Bryson, radiology support assistant leader, who pulled countless folders and digitized images.

Sadie Gomez, our professional assistant, for her hard work and dedication to this project.

Dr. Safwan Halabi, MD, our colleague and friend, who found images when no one else could.

Dr. Stamatia Destounis, MD, who graciously agreed to write the Foreword for this book.

Janet Foltin, Senior Editor, and Margaret Burns, our development editor, for their guidance and support.

Our residents and fellows, who keep our minds sharp and our work environment fun.

To all of you, our heartfelt thanks. We could not have accomplished this without you.

Contents

Mammography and Ultrasound Review

1

B.A. Shah et al., *Breast Imaging Review: A Quick Guide to Essential Diagnoses*,
DOI 10.1007/978-3-319-07791-8_1, © Springer International Publishing Switzerland 2015

Case 1
Mammographic Artifacts

Patient History

Screening mammograms in multiple different patients.

Radiology Findings

Fig. 1.1 (**a**) CC and (**b**) MLO images show a broken ventricular peritoneal shunt catheter in the lower inner right breast at posterior depth.

Fig. 1.2 AP supine view of the chest reveals a broken right ventricular peritoneal shunt catheter and intact left ventricular peritoneal shunt catheter.

Fig. 1.3 Left MLO view demonstrates chin artifact obscuring the superior posterior tissues.

Fig. 1.4 Deodorant artifact. Left MLO view demonstrates (**a**) scattered radiopaque particles in the skinfold and axillary region. (**b**) Scattered radiopaque particles in the skinfold and axillary region are no longer seen on repeat left MLO view following cleansing of the patient's axilla.

Fig. 1.5 Hair artifact. CC view demonstrates curvilinear densities with intervening lucencies at posterior depth laterally.

Fig. 1.6 Motion artifact. Right MLO view demonstrates patient's motion causing blurring of the upper breast tissues.

Diagnosis

Mammographic artifacts

Discussion

- Artifacts are any objects or abnormalities that are not native to the breast.
- May interfere with image interpretation.
- Certain artifacts are typically seen in particular locations:
  - Deodorant: axilla
  - Catheters or pacemakers: close to chest wall
  - Hair: typically inner breast seen on CC view
- Recognition, awareness, and history are important.
- Correct presumed problems and repeat imaging can be done.

References

Berg WA, Birdwell RL, Gombos EC, et al. Diagnostic imaging breast. 1st ed. Salt Lake City: Amirsys; 2006. Section IV-7, p. 10–1.

Hogge JP, Palmer CH, Muller CC, et al. Quality assurance in mammography: artifact analysis. Radiographics. 1999;19:503–22.

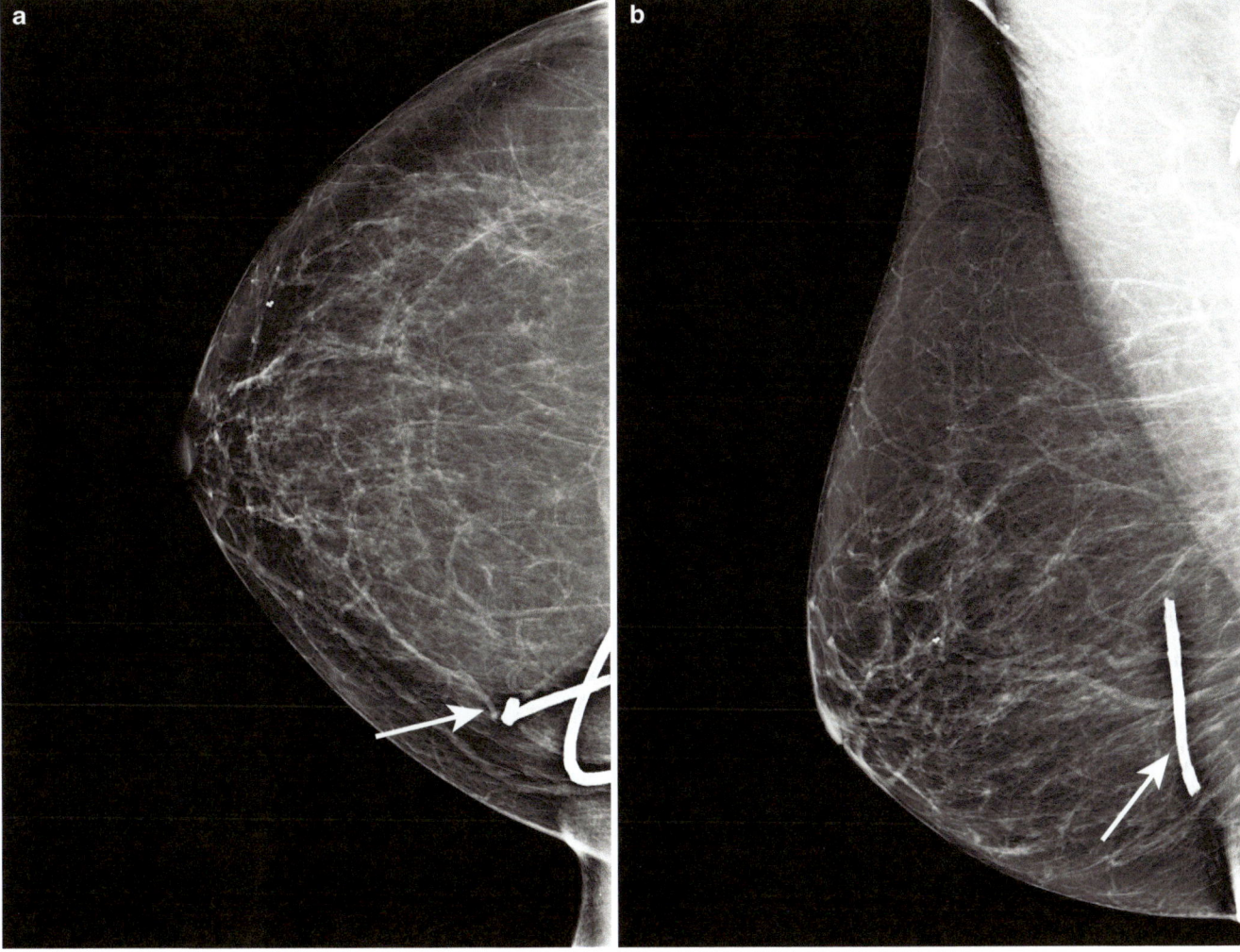

Fig. 1.1

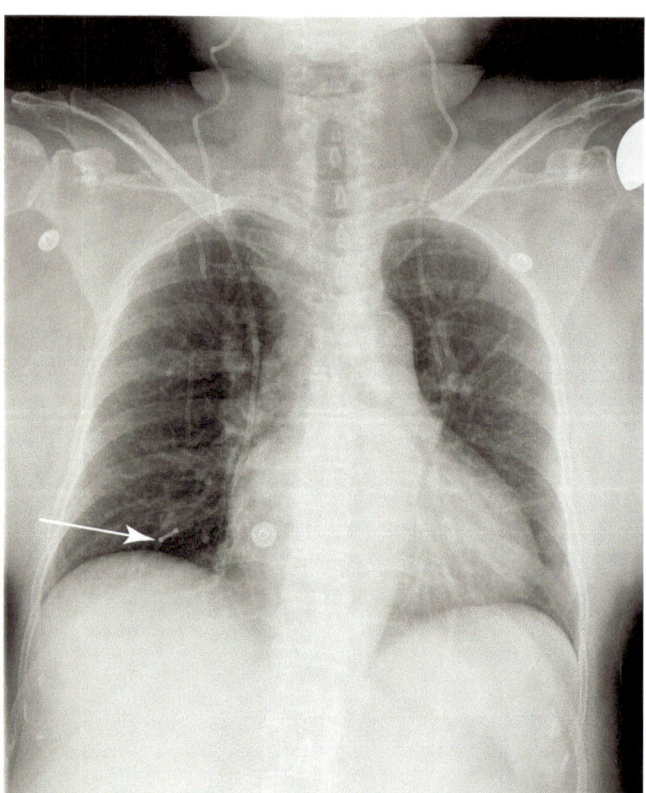

Fig. 1.2

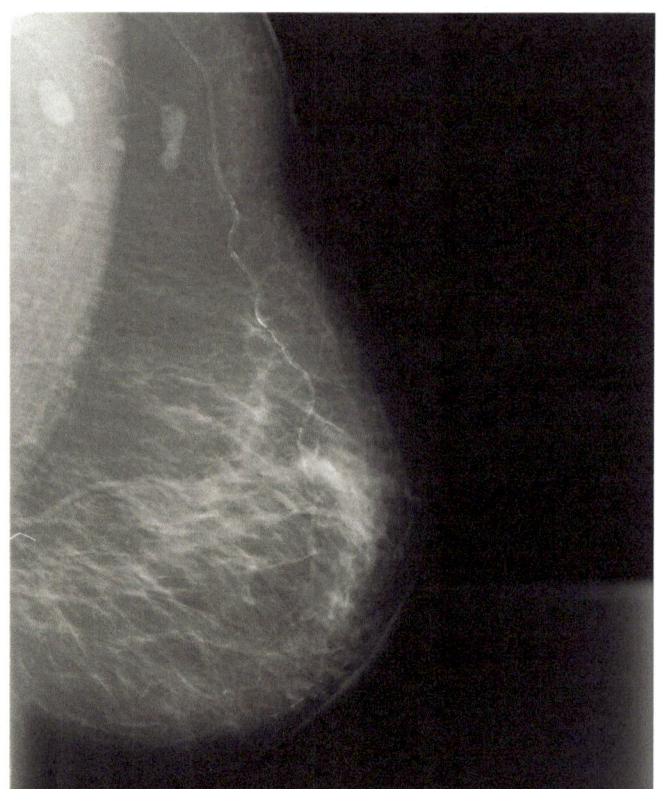

Fig. 1.3

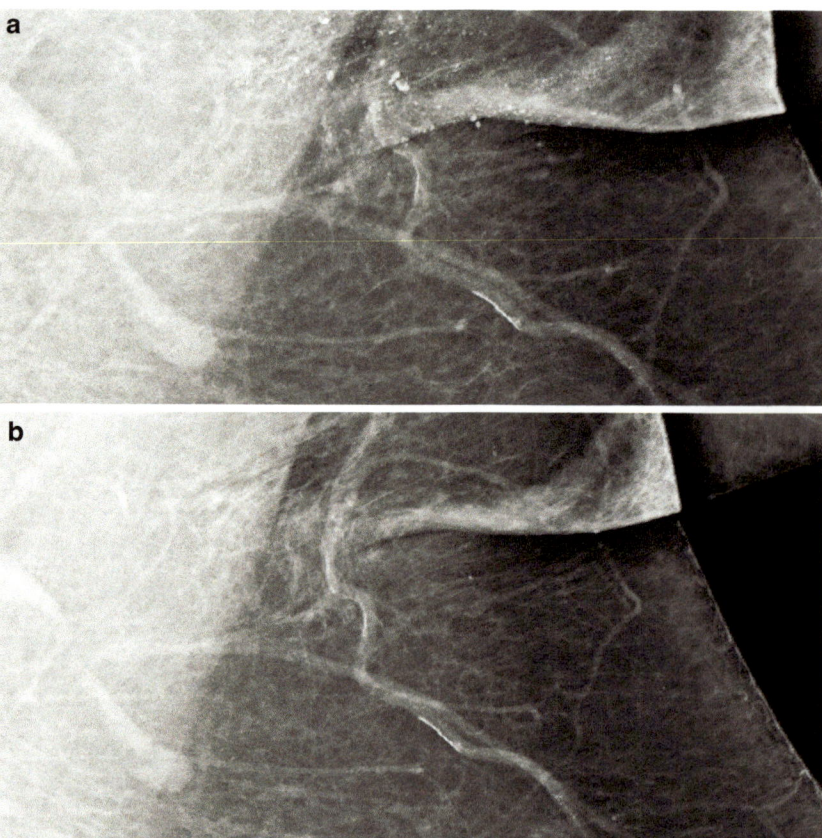

Fig. 1.4

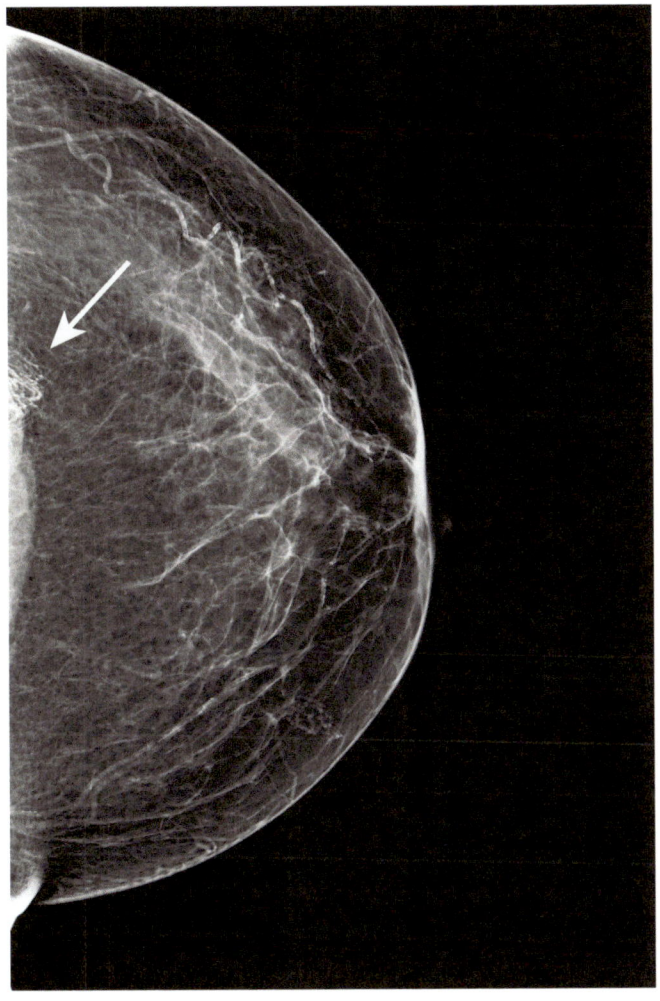

Fig. 1.5

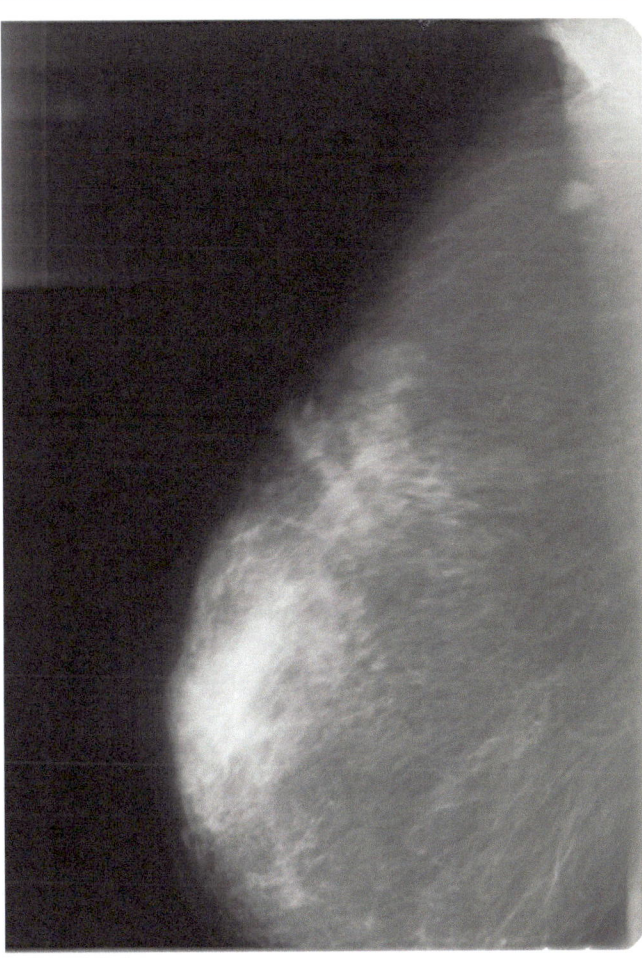

Fig. 1.6

Case 2
Secretory Calcifications

Patient History

A 60-year-old female for bilateral screening mammogram.

Radiology Findings

Fig. 1.1 Bilateral (**a**, **b**) CC and (**c**, **d**) MLO views demonstrate dense, thick, continuous rodlike calcifications in a ductal pattern.

BI-RADS Assessment

BI-RADS 2. Benign finding.

Diagnosis

Secretory calcifications

Discussion

- Secretory calcifications arise from secretions and debris within the ducts, which calcify and cause inflammation.
- Other names include plasma cell mastitis (typically in premenopausal women) and mammary duct ectasia (typically in post menopausal women).
- The calcifications are large and rodlike. Typically radiate from the nipple in a ductal pattern.
- Size of the calcifications is greater than or equal to 1 mm.
- Rarely seen in patients before the age of 60.
- Usually bilateral.
- Asymptomatic.
- No intervention necessary.

References

American College of Radiology (ACR) BI-RADS® Atlas. ACR BI-RADS® atlas-mammography. 5th ed. Reston: American College of Radiology; 2013. p. 44–6.

Bassett LW, Jackson VP, Fu KL, Fu YS. Diagnosis of diseases of the breast. 2nd ed. Philadelphia: Elsevier; 2005. p. 444–5.

Berg WA, Birdwell RL, Gombos EC, et al. Diagnostic imaging breast. 1st ed. Salt Lake City: Amirsys; 2006. Section IV 1, p. 74–5.

Fig. 1.1

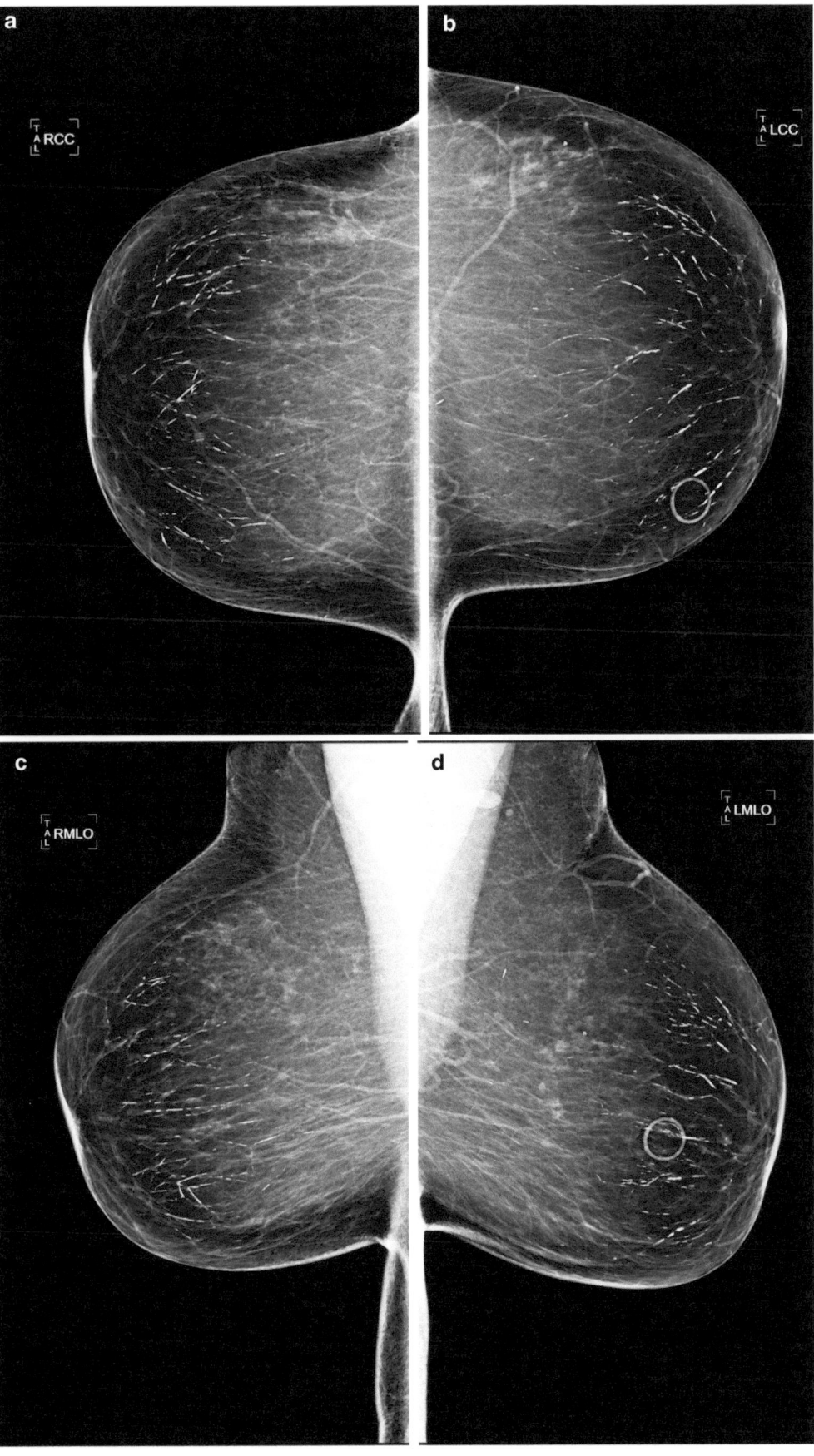

CASE 3
INVASIVE DUCTAL CARCINOMA (IDC)

PATIENT HISTORY

A 55-year-old female for screening mammogram.

RADIOLOGY FINDINGS

Fig. 1.1 (**a**) CC and (**b**) ML images show a mass with spiculated margins at 6 o'clock in the left breast at the anterior depth. Another irregular mass with spiculated margins is seen in the upper outer left breast at posterior depth.

Fig. 1.2 (**a**) Grayscale and (**b**) color Doppler ultrasound images show a hypoechoic mass with spiculated margins and vascular flow.

Fig. 1.3 (**a**) Grayscale and (**b**) color Doppler ultrasound images show an enlarged lymph node with a thickened hypoechoic cortex and a compromised hyperechoic hilum. There is vascular flow within the hilum.

BI-RADS ASSESSMENT

BI-RADS 5. Highly suggestive of malignancy (following diagnostic workup, prior to biopsy).

DIAGNOSIS

Invasive ductal carcinoma (IDC) (not otherwise specified) with axillary lymph node metastasis

DISCUSSION

- Eighty percent of breast cancers are ductal in origin.
- Up to 65 % of breast cancers diagnosed in the USA represent IDC, not otherwise specified.
- IDC forms a desmoplastic reaction with cicatrization and fibrosis, thus commonly seen as a spiculated mass on mammogram.
- Usually seen as a hypoechoic mass with spiculated or ill-defined margins on ultrasound. Posterior acoustic shadowing of the mass can be seen.
- Secondary signs of IDC on imaging include skin thickening, nipple inversion, and lymphadenopathy.

REFERENCES

Kopans DB. Breast imaging. 2nd ed. Philadelphia: Lippincott Williams and Wilkins; 1998. p. 577–81.
Ruhbar G, Sie AC, Hansen GC. Benign versus malignant breast masses: ultrasound differentiation. Radiology. 1999;213:889–94.

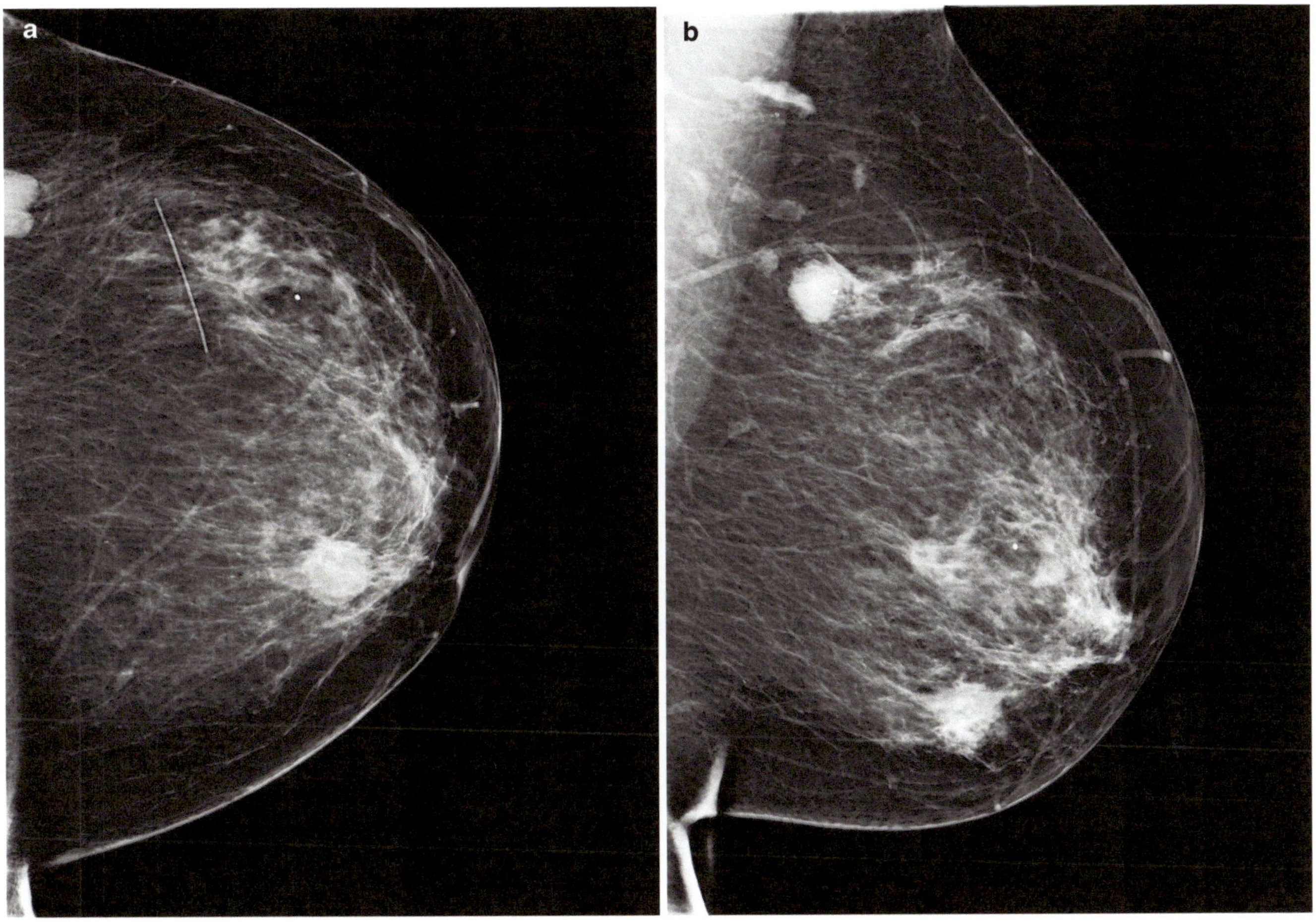

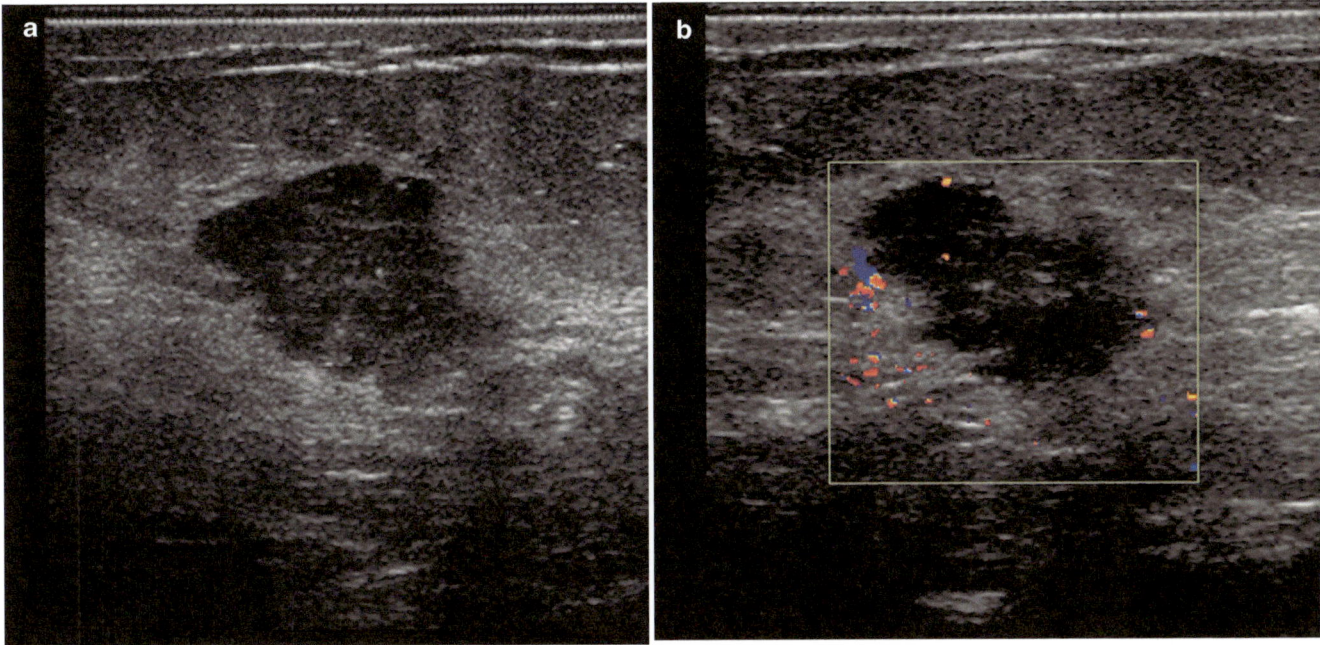

Fig. 1.1

Fig. 1.2

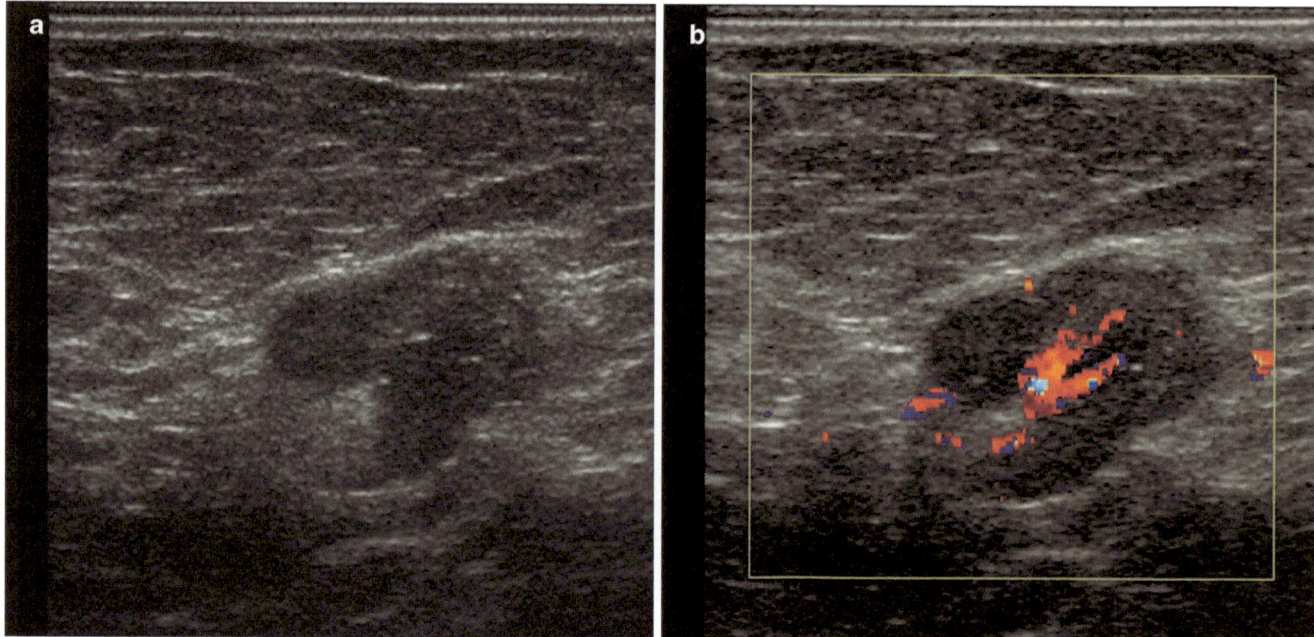

Fig. 1.3

CASE 4
COMPLICATED CYST

PATIENT HISTORY

A 50-year-old female with a palpable mass in the left breast.

RADIOLOGY FINDINGS

Fig. 1.1 (**a**, **b**) Grayscale and (**c**) color Doppler ultrasound images show an avascular oval circumscribed predominately anechoic mass with a dependent layering debris and posterior enhancement.

Fig. 1.2 (**a**) Grayscale, (**b**) color Doppler, and (**c**) grayscale (*left image*) and strain elastogram ultrasound images of a different patient show an avascular oval circumscribed mass that contains homogeneous, low-level echoes and an intermediate pattern on elastography. On the elastogram color scale, red represents soft and blue represents hard. An adjacent benign simple cyst is seen that has a soft pattern and trilaminar appearance on elastography.

DIAGNOSIS

Complicated cyst

DISCUSSION

- A complicated cyst contains:
  - Fluid–debris level or homogeneous, low-level echoes, without a discrete solid component and with an imperceptible wall.
  - Imperceptible wall on ultrasound
  - Mobile debris or homogeneous low-level echoes
  - Complex features, such as thick irregular septations, intracystic mass, or thick cyst wall, are not seen in complicated cysts.
  - Can have simple cysts within the vicinity.
  - Less than two percent risk of malignancy.
  - No further management necessary for an asymptomatic complicated cyst.
  - A complicated cyst on baseline mammogram or incidental finding on ultrasound can be followed at 6 months.
  - Aspiration with possible biopsy can be performed if the following are present:
    - Symptomatic
    - New finding
    - Enlarging complicated cyst

REFERENCES

American College of Radiology (ACR) BI-RADS® Atlas. ACR BI-RADS® atlas-ultrasound. 5th ed. Reston: American College of Radiology; 2013. p. 96–7, 103.

Berg WA, Birdwell RL, Gombos EC, et al. Diagnostic imaging breast. 1st ed. Salt Lake City: Amirsys; 2006. Section IV-1, p. 34–9.

Berg WA, Campassi CI, Ioffe OB. Cystic lesion of the breast: sonographic-pathologic correlation. Radiology. 2003;227:183–91

Mandell J. Core radiology: a visual approach to diagnostic imaging. 1st ed. Cambridge: Cambridge University Press; 2013. p. 629.

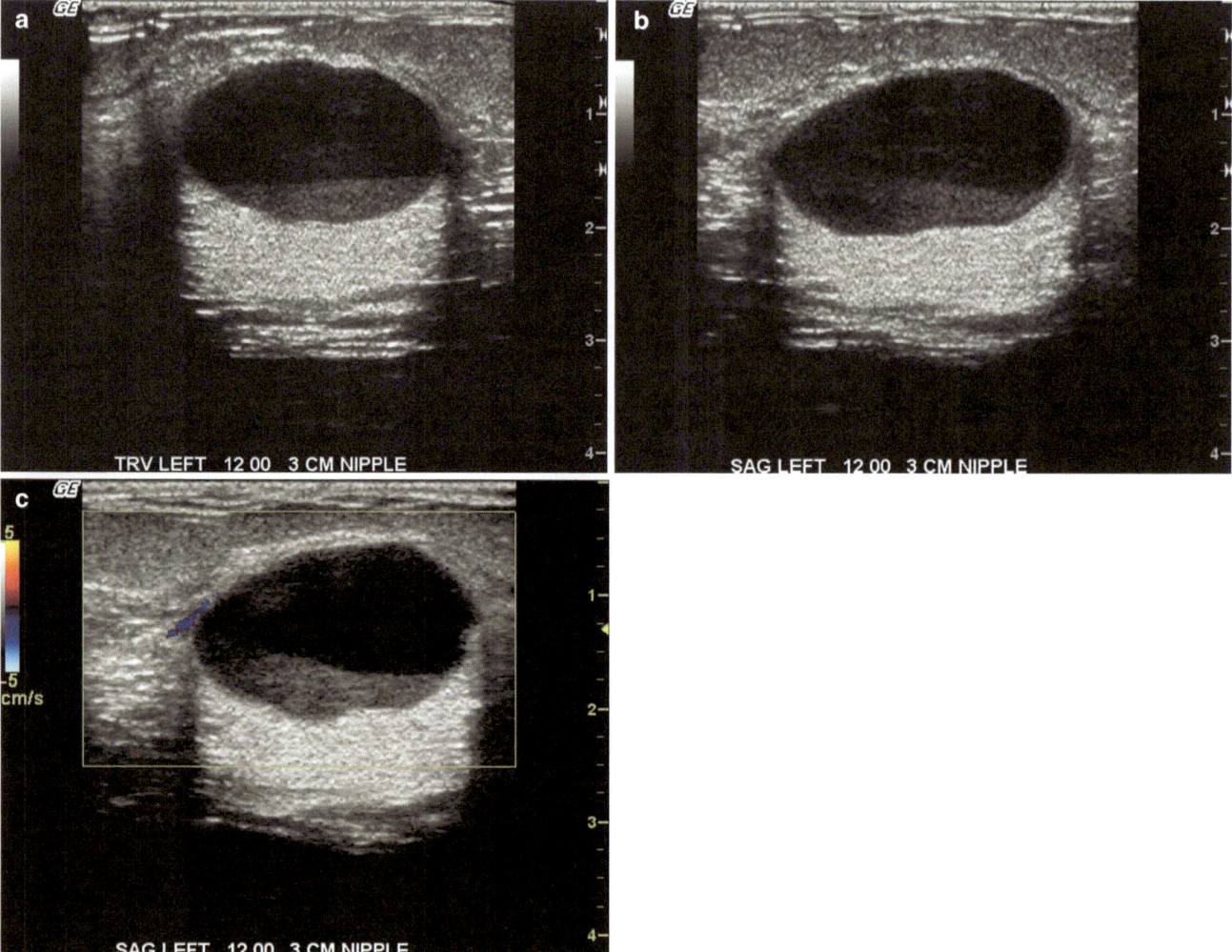

Fig. 1.1

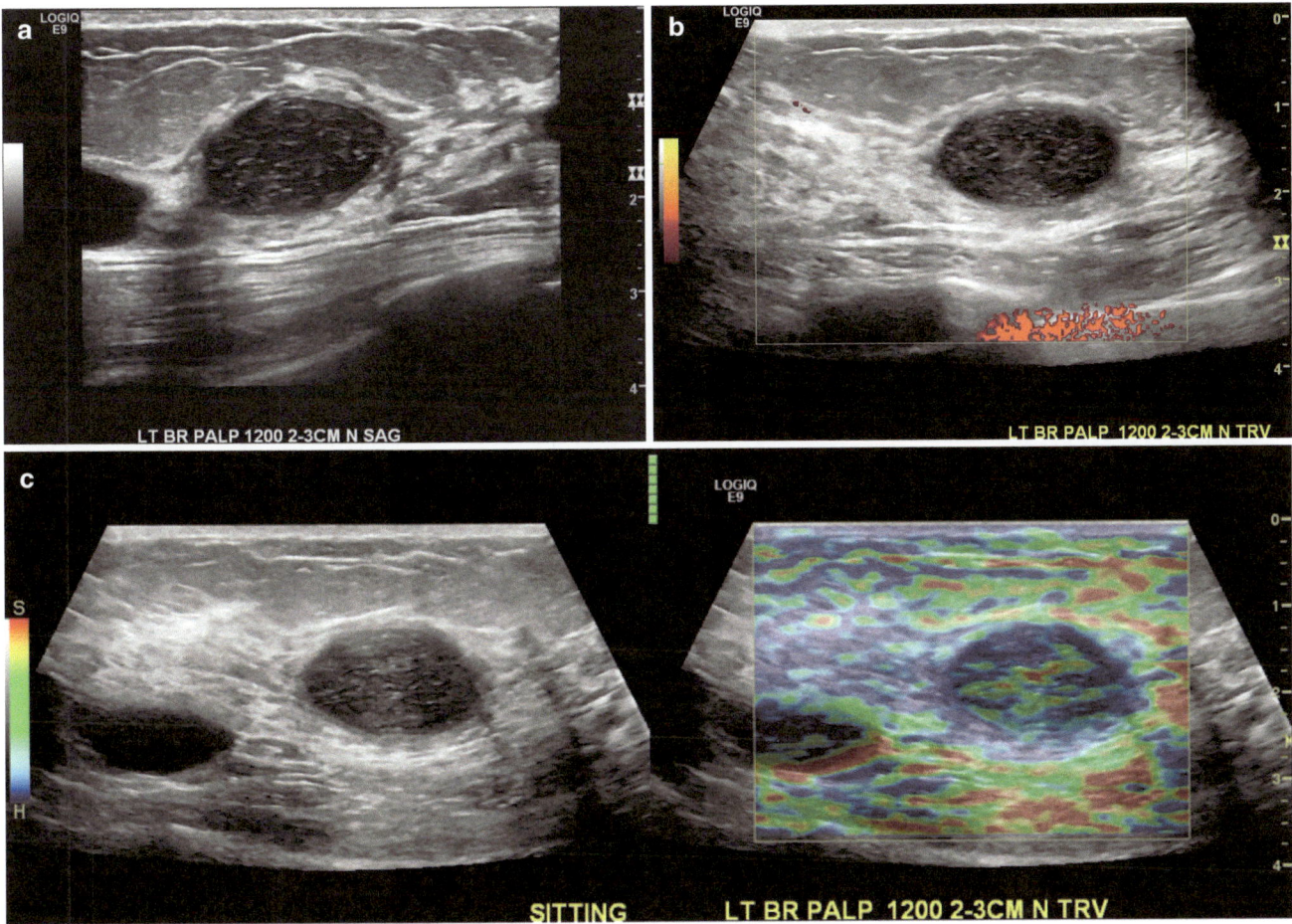

Fig. 1.2

CASE 5
DESMOID TUMOR

PATIENT HISTORY

An 83-year-old female with a palpable mass in the right axilla. History of right breast lumpectomy and radiation therapy for ductal carcinoma in situ (DCIS).

RADIOLOGY FINDINGS

Fig. 1.1 MLO view shows an asymmetry in the right axilla seen only on the MLO view.
Fig. 1.2 (**a**) Grayscale and (**b**) color Doppler images show an irregular spiculated hypoechoic mass that is avascular.

BI-RADS ASSESSMENT

BI-RADS 2. Benign finding (following diagnostic workup and biopsy).

DIAGNOSIS

Desmoid tumor (extra-abdominal desmoid)

DISCUSSION

- Desmoid tumor is an infiltrative, locally aggressive area of fibromatosis that may recur locally.
- May be related to prior trauma or surgery and has been reported in women with saline breast implants.
- Can present as a solitary, hard, painless mass.
- On mammography, a mass with indistinct or spiculated margins can be seen.
- On ultrasound, a hypoechoic mass with posterior acoustic shadowing can be seen.
- Treatment is local surgical excision.

REFERENCES

Cardenosa G. Breast imaging companion. 3rd ed. Philadelphia: Lippincott Williams and Wilkins; 2008. p. 411–2.
Ikeda DM. Breast imaging the requisites. 2nd ed. Philadelphia: Elsevier, Mosby; 2011. p. 401–2.

Fig. 1.1

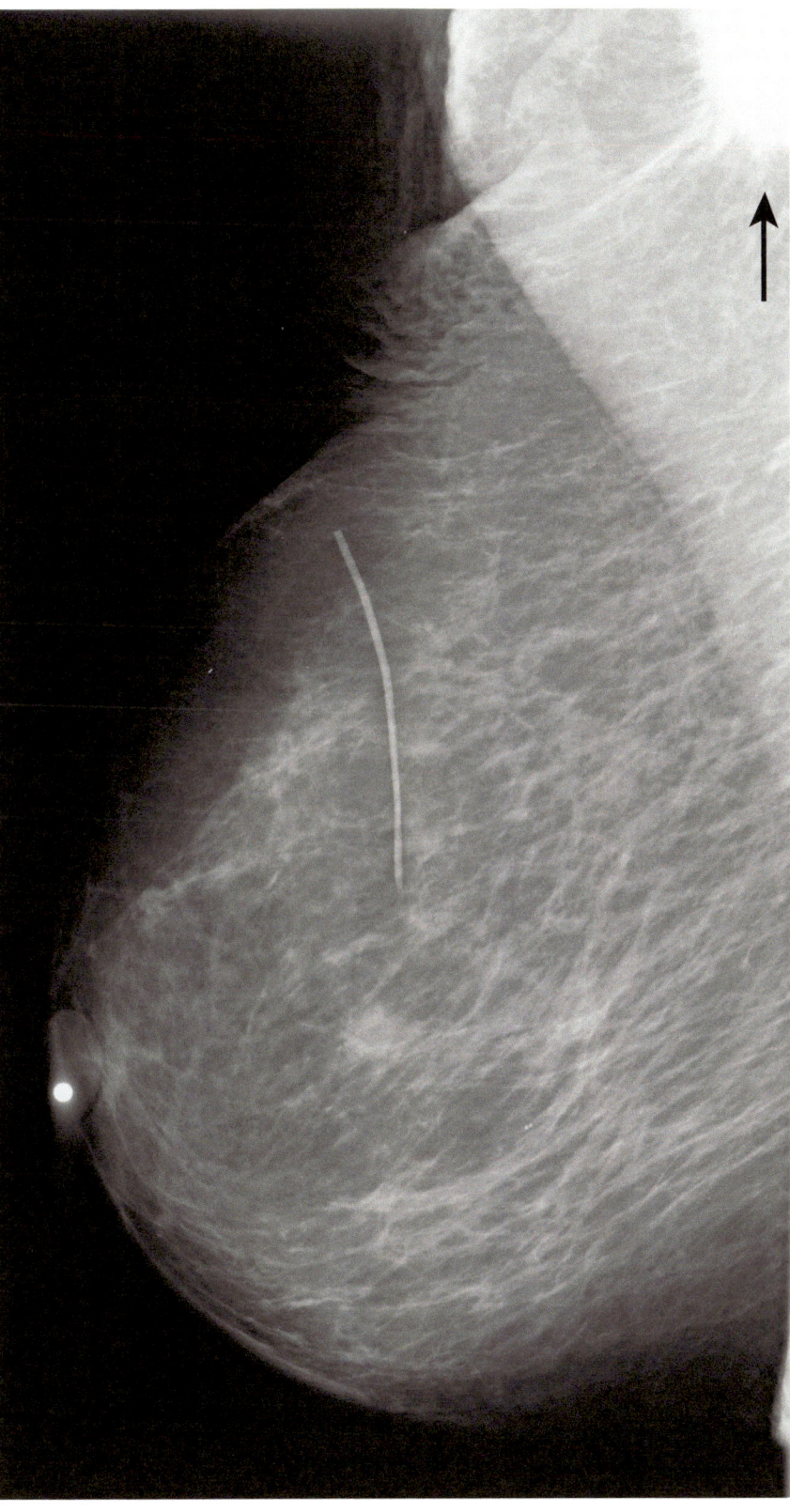

Fig. 1.2

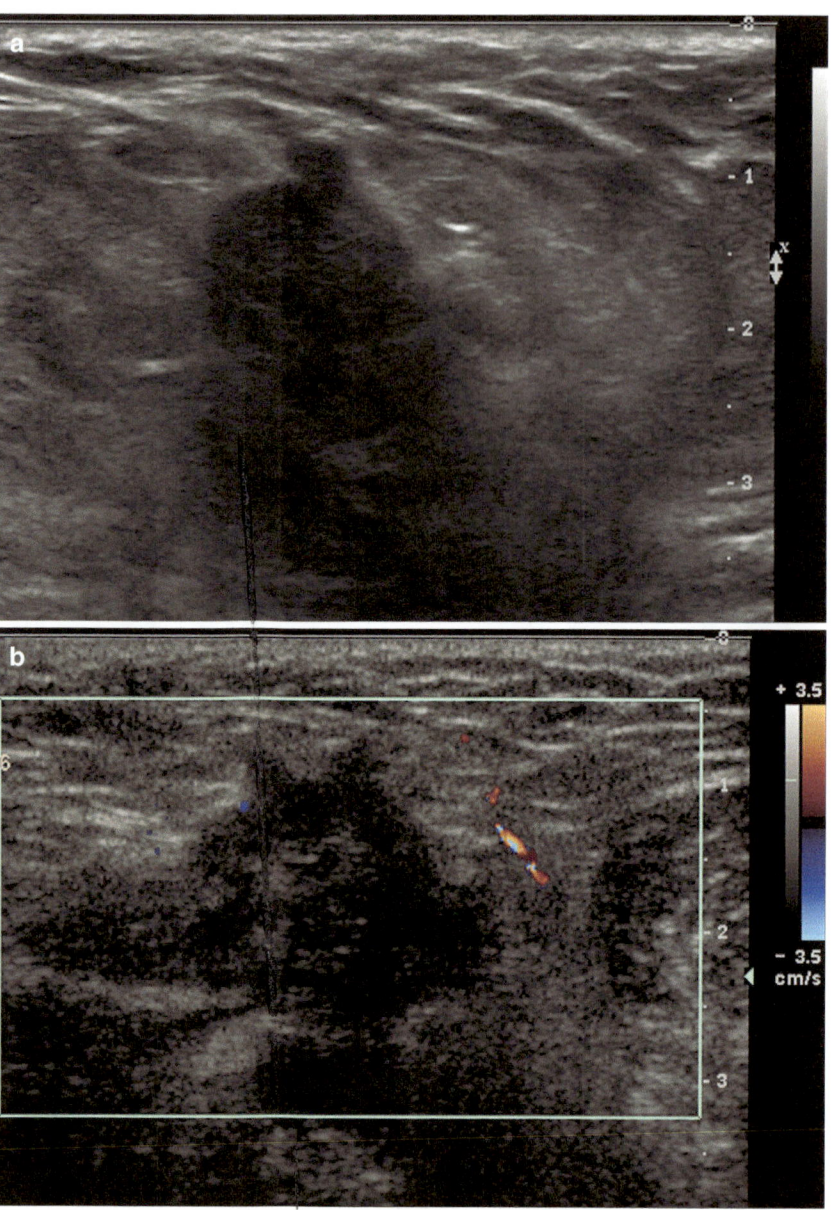

CASE 6
GYNECOMASTIA

PATIENT HISTORY

An 87-year-old male with left breast pain and a palpable mass.

RADIOLOGY FINDINGS

Fig. 1.1 Bilateral (**a, b**) CC and (**c, d**) MLO images show a focal asymmetry in the retroareolar left breast, corresponding to the triangular marker indicating a palpable mass (*circle marker* corresponds to a skin mole). The right breast mammogram is negative.

BI-RADS ASSESSMENT

BI-RADS 2. Benign finding (following diagnostic workup).

DIAGNOSIS

Gynecomastia

DISCUSSION

- Gynecomastia is characterized by hyperplasia of ductal and stromal elements of the male breast.
- Clinically, it may present as pain, breast enlargement, diffuse thickening, or palpable thickening behind the nipple.
- Three patterns of gynecomastia have been described: nodular, dendritic, and diffuse.
- Common mammographic appearance is a triangular- or flame-shaped density present behind the nipple or diffuse-increased density.
- Gynecomastia may be unilateral or bilateral.
- Some causes of gynecomastia include:
  - Idiopathic
  - Drugs: marijuana, thiazides, reserpines, cardiac glycosides, and cimetidine
  - Testicular tumors: embryonal cell carcinoma, seminoma, and choriocarcinoma
  - Klinefelter's disease
  - Chronic hepatic disease
  - Exogenous estrogen administration

REFERENCES

Applebaum AH, Evans GF, Levy KR, Amirkhan RH, Schumpert TD. Mammographic appearance of male breast disease. Radiographics. 1999;19:559–68.

Kopans DB. Breast imaging. 2nd ed. Philadelphia: Lippincott Williams and Wilkins; 1998. p. 497, 501–2.

Mandell J. Core radiology: a visual approach to diagnostic imaging. 1st ed. Cambridge: Cambridge University Press; 2013. p. 651.

Fig. 1.1

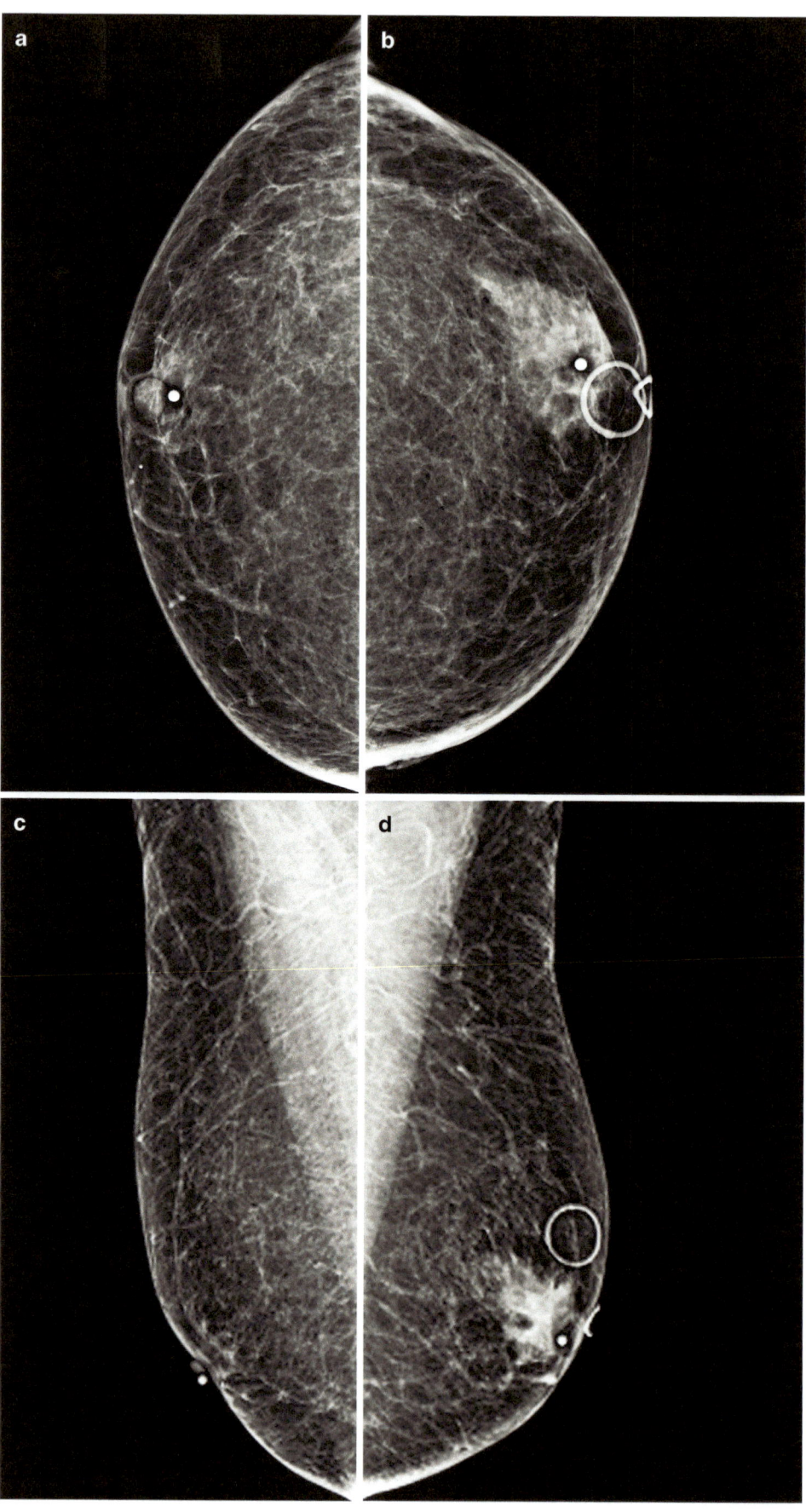

CASE 7
ATYPICAL LOBULAR HYPERPLASIA (ALH)

PATIENT HISTORY

A 49-year-old female for a screening mammogram.

RADIOLOGY FINDINGS

Fig. 1.1 (**a**) Spot-magnification CC and (**b**) spot-magnification LM views demonstrate grouped amorphous and heterogeneous calcifications at 12 o'clock at anterior depth.

ASSESSMENT

High-risk lesion.

DIAGNOSIS

Atypical lobular hyperplasia (ALH)

DISCUSSION

- ALH presents commonly as amorphous calcifications.
- Usually incidentally found at biopsy.
- ALH is a high-risk lesion associated with increased risk of malignancy in either breast.
- Treatment continues to be controversial following diagnosis on core needle biopsy.
- Excision is generally recommended following diagnosis of ALH on core needle biopsy.
- With excision, upgrade rates to malignancy range from 0 to 23 %.

REFERENCES

Berg WA, Birdwell RL, Gombos EC, et al. Diagnostic imaging breast. 1st ed. Salt Lake City: Amirsy; 2006. Section IV-2, p. 74–5.
Foster M, Helvie M, Gregory N, Rebner M, Nees A, Paramagul C. Lobular carcinoma in situ or atypical lobular hyperplasia at core needle biopsy: is excisional biopsy necessary? Radiology. 2004;231:813–9.

Fig. 1.1

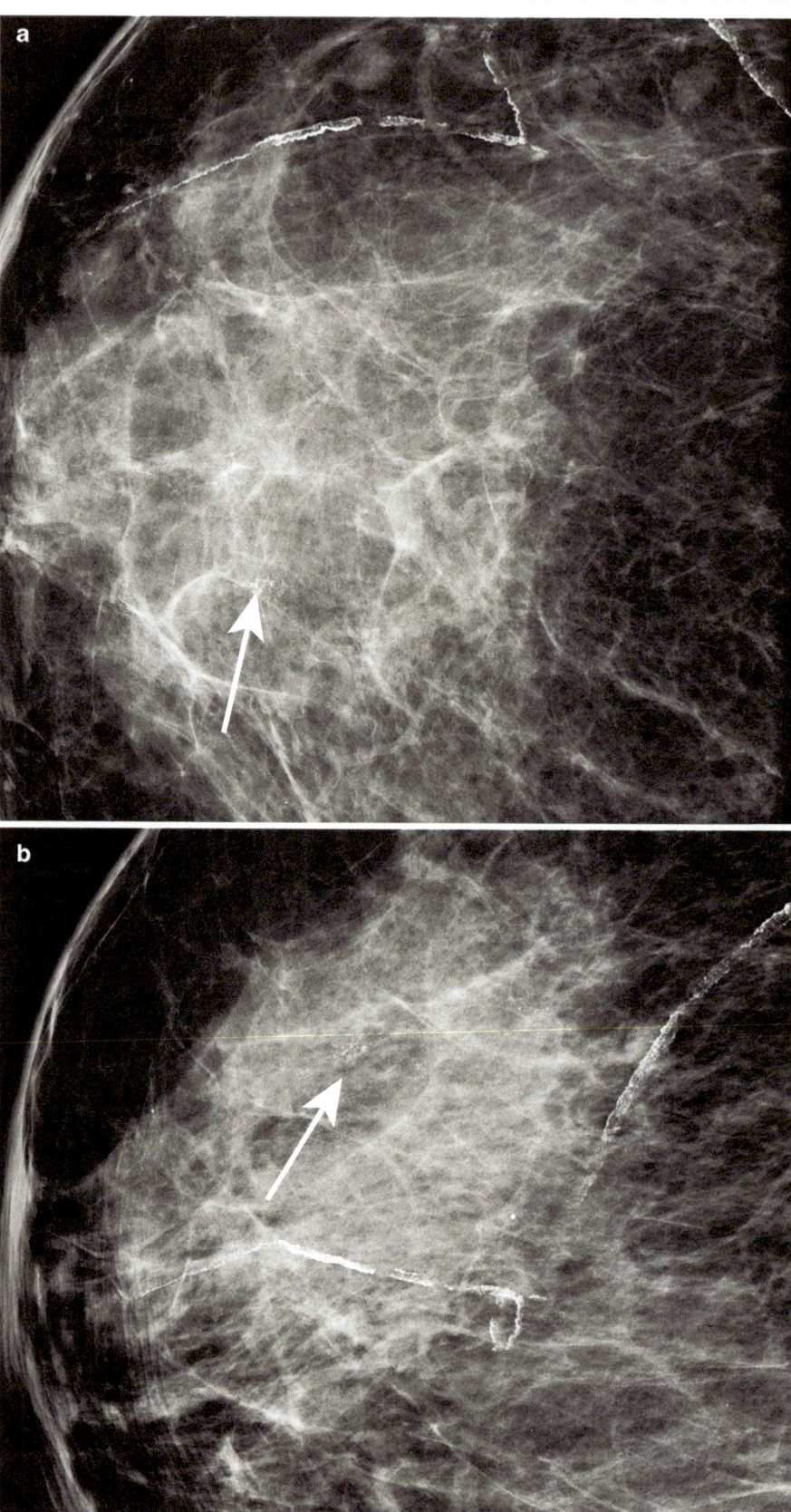

CASE 8
STERNALIS MUSCLE

PATIENT HISTORY

A 40-year-old female for a screening mammogram.

RADIOLOGY FINDINGS

Fig. 1.1 (**a**, **b**) Bilateral CC views demonstrate flame-shaped densities medially.

BI-RADS ASSESSMENT

BI-RADS 1. Negative.

DIAGNOSIS

Sternalis muscle

DISCUSSION

- Sternalis muscle is an anatomic variant of chest wall musculature.
- Location is medial and parasternal.
- It runs parallel to the sternum and perpendicular to the pectoralis muscle.
- Sternalis muscle is seen only on CC views.
- Sternalis muscle is triangular or rounded in shape.
- Found in <10 % of individuals.
- Twice as often unilateral as bilateral.
- Main differential diagnosis is a medially located mass.
- Location, shape, and lack of corresponding density on lateral views suggest the diagnosis.

REFERENCES

Berg WA, Birdwell RL, Gombos EC, et al. Diagnostic imaging breast. 1st ed. Salt Lake City: Amirsys; 2006. Section IV-3, p. 40–1.

Bradley FM, Hoover HC Jr, Hulka CA, et al. The sternalis muscle: an unusual normal finding seen on mammography. AJR. 1996;166:33–6.

Kopans DB. Breast imaging. 2nd ed. Philadelphia: Lippincott Williams and Wilkins; 1998. p. 9–10.

Mandell J. Core radiology: a visual approach to diagnostic imaging. 1st ed. Cambridge: Cambridge University Press; 2013. p. 638.

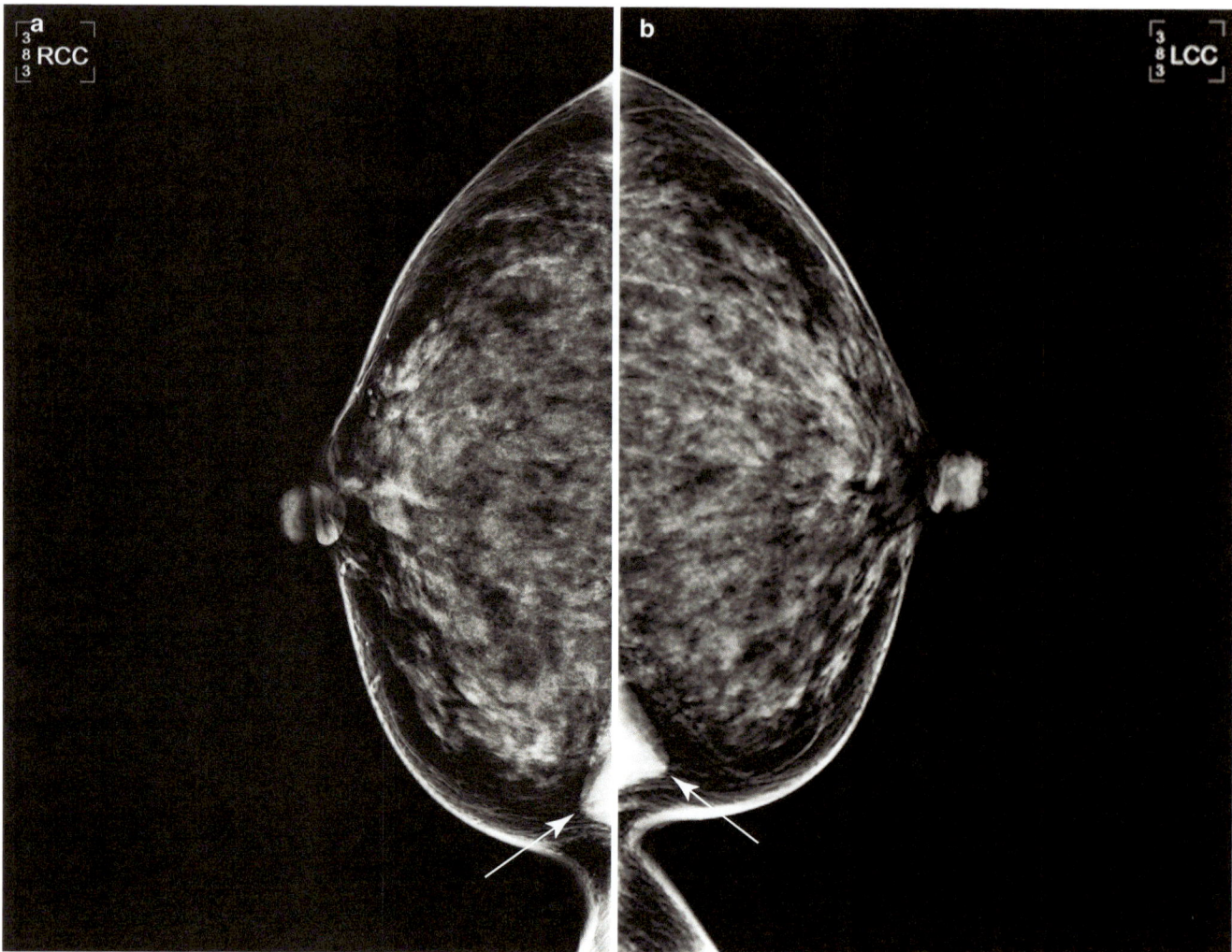

Fig. 1.1

CASE 9
TRANSVERSE RECTUS ABDOMINIS MYOCUTANEOUS (TRAM) FLAP

PATIENT HISTORY

A 62-year-old female with a history of left mastectomy and reconstruction.

RADIOLOGY FINDINGS

Fig. 1.1 MLO view demonstrates the typical appearance of a transverse rectus abdominis myocutaneous (TRAM) flap.

Fig. 1.2 CC view of a different patient demonstrates a large area of heterogeneous calcifications having a mass-like appearance.

Fig. 1.3 Axial nonfat suppressed T1-weighted image demonstrates that the central area of the left breast is isointense to the surrounding fat representing fat necrosis. This corresponds to the mammographic calcifications seen in Fig. 1.2.

BI-RADS ASSESSMENT

BI-RADS 2. Benign finding.

DIAGNOSIS

TRAM flap

DISCUSSION

- A TRAM flap is a means of reconstruction following mastectomy or after implant removal.

- There is a spectrum of myocutaneous flaps including the following:
  - TRAM flap
  - Latissimus dorsi myocutaneous (LDM) flap
  - Deep inferior epigastric perforator (DIEP) flap
- Contraindications include the following:
  - Poor general health
  - Extensive abdominal scarring
  - Vascular disease
  - Locally advanced primary breast malignancy
- Complications include the following:
  - Partial/complete loss of flap
  - Abdominal muscle weakness
  - Fat necrosis
  - Disease recurrence
  - Postreconstruction radiotherapy complications
- Local recurrence rates are similar in patients with mastectomy and TRAM reconstruction vs. mastectomy alone.
- TRAM screening is controversial.
- Fat necrosis in a TRAM may present as a calcified mass.
- Fat necrosis is commonly seen in the upper outer breast owing to decreased vascularity.

REFERENCES

Berg WA, Birdwell RL, Gombos EC, et al. Diagnostic imaging breast. 1st ed. Salt Lake City: Amirsys; 2006. Section V-3, p. 22–5.

Helvie MA, Bailey JE, Roubidoux MA, et al. Mammographic screening of TRAM flap breast reconstructions for detection of nonpalpable recurrent cancer. Radiology. 2002;222:211–6.

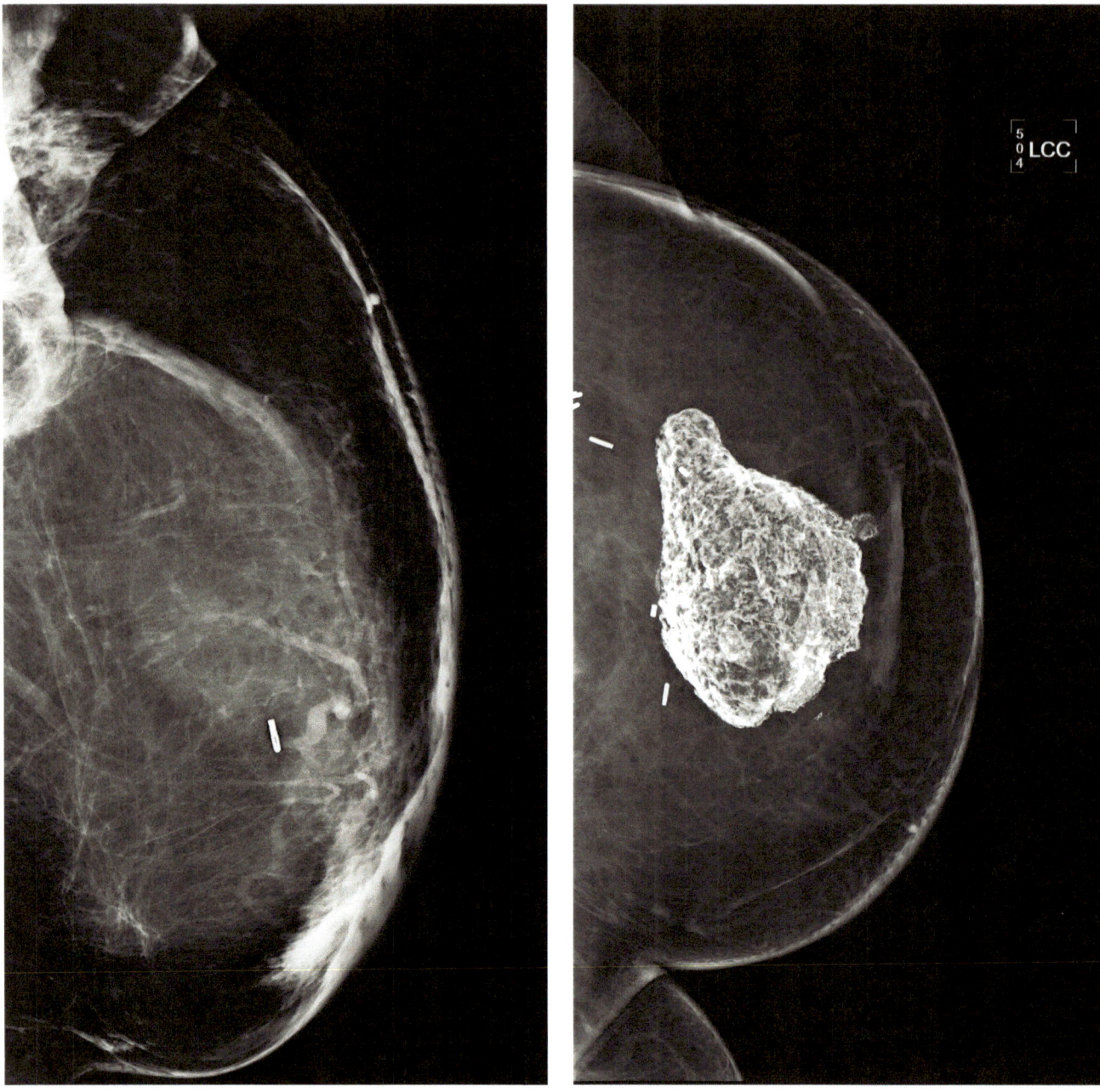

Fig. 1.1   **Fig. 1.2**

Fig. 1.3

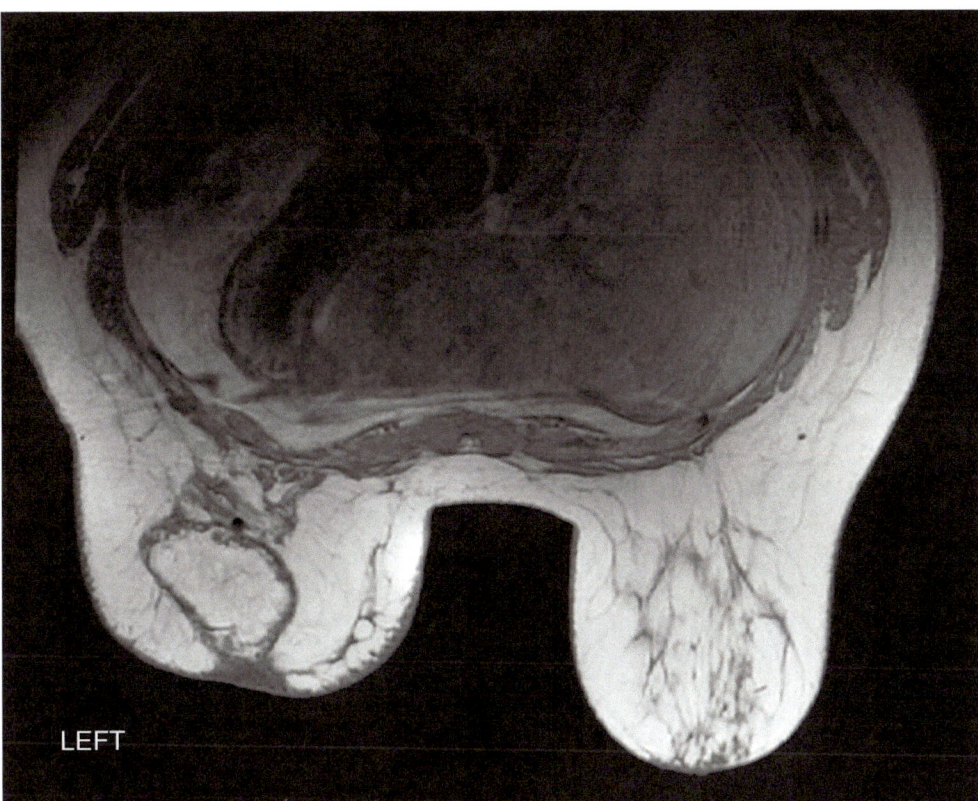

Case 10
Galactocele

Patient History

A 35-year-old female with a palpable mass in the left breast who recently stopped breast feeding.

Radiology Findings

Fig. 1.1 Spot magnification (**a**) CC and (**b**) MLO demonstrate an oval, low-density mass with circumscribed margins in the upper outer left breast at middle depth.

Fig. 1.2 ML view shows a fat–fluid level within the mass in the upper left breast at middle depth.

Fig. 1.3 Grayscale (**a**) transverse, (**b**) sagittal, and (**c**) color Doppler ultrasound images show an oval mass with a fluid–debris level.

BI-RADS Assessment

BI-RADS 2. Benign finding (following diagnostic workup).

Diagnosis

Galactocele

Discussion

- A galactocele is a focal collection of breast milk.
- On mammography, a galactocele presents as a low-density or equal-density mass with a fat–fluid level appreciated on the lateral mammogram.
- On ultrasound, a fluid–debris level in the mass (fat rising to the top of the galactocele and milk/fluid layering dependently below) can be seen.
- Typically seen in a lactating or postlactational woman.
- Usually resolves spontaneously within a few weeks to months.
- Aspiration can be performed for symptomatic relief.

References

Berg WA, Birdwell RL, Gombos EC, et al. Diagnostic imaging breast. 1st ed. Salt Lake City: Amirsys; 2006. Section IV-5, p. 6–9.

Ikeda DM. Breast imaging the requisites. 2nd ed. Philadelphia: Elsevier, Mosby; 2011. p. 379–80.

Mandell J. Core radiology: a visual approach to diagnostic imaging. 1st ed. Cambridge: Cambridge University Press; 2013. p. 623–4.

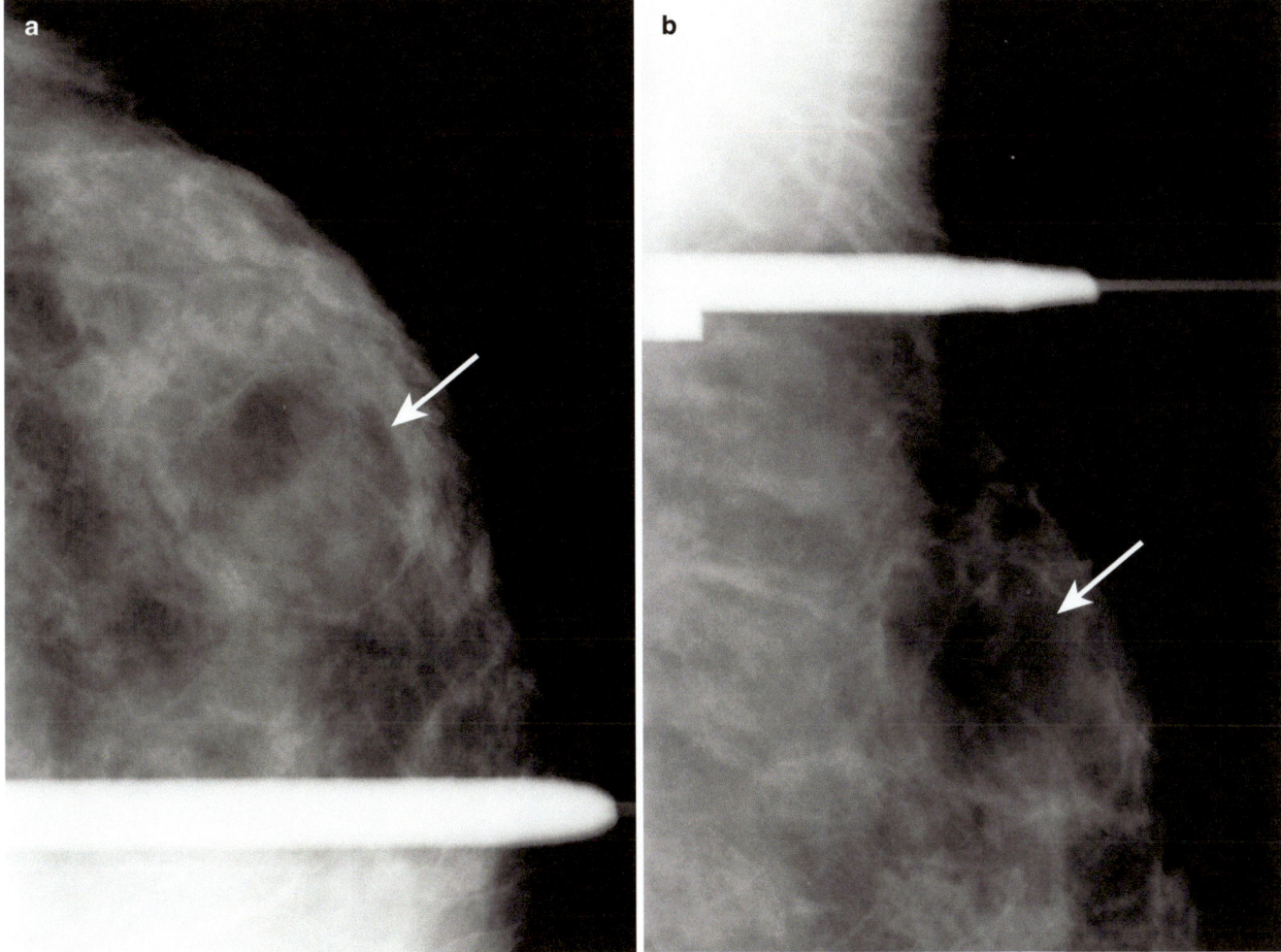

Fig. 1.1

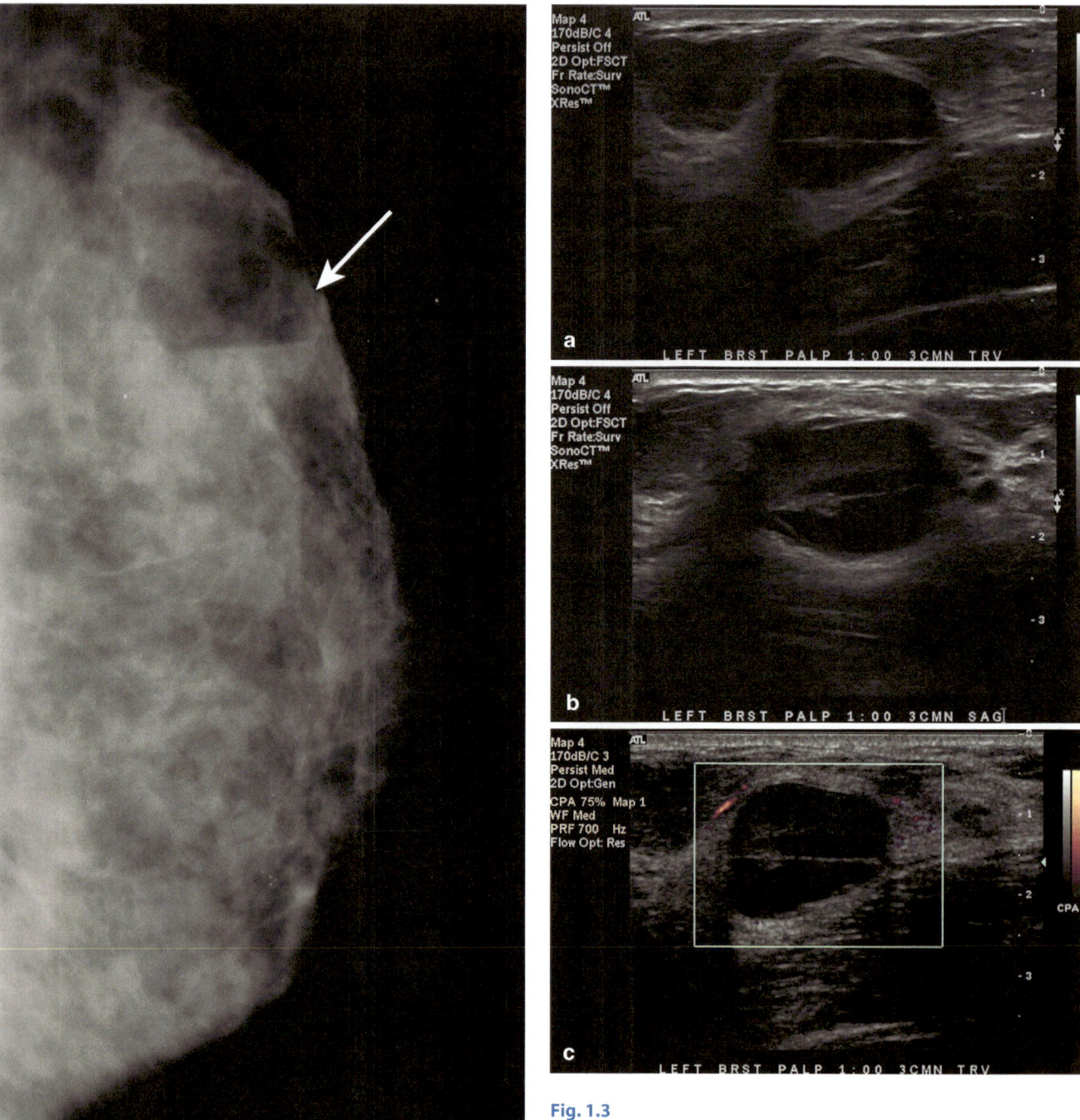

Fig. 1.2

Fig. 1.3

CASE 11
MILK OF CALCIUM

PATIENT HISTORY

A 45-year-old female for a screening mammogram.

RADIOLOGY FINDINGS

Fig. 1.1 (**a**) Spot-magnification CC and (**b**) MLO images show a cluster of round calcifications at 3 o'clock in the left breast at middle depth.

Fig. 1.2 Spot-magnification ML image of the left breast demonstrates the cluster of microcalcifications to have a curvilinear appearance.

BI-RADS ASSESSMENT

BI-RADS 2. Benign findings (following diagnostic workup).

DIAGNOSIS

Milk of calcium

DISCUSSION

- Milk of calcium is sedimented calcium-oxalate calcifications within tiny benign cysts and dilated lobules.
- Key diagnostic clue is the different shapes of calcifications between CC and lateral views.
- Rounded or amorphous ("smudgy") calcifications are seen on the CC view.
- "Teacup," linear, or crescent calcifications are seen on the lateral view.
- Biopsy not warranted.

REFERENCES

American College of Radiology (ACR) BI-RADS® Atlas. ACR BI-RADS® atlas-mammography. 5th ed. Reston: American College of Radiology; 2013. p. 55–7.

Berg WB, Birdwell RB, Gombos EC, et al. Diagnostic imaging: breast. 1st ed. Salt Lake City: Amirsys; 2006. Section IV-1, p. 68–70.

Ikeda DM. Breast imaging the requisites. 2nd ed. Philadelphia: Elsevier, Mosby; 2011. p. 79–81.

Mandell J. Core radiology: a visual approach to diagnostic imaging. 1st ed. Cambridge: Cambridge University Press; 2013. p. 608.

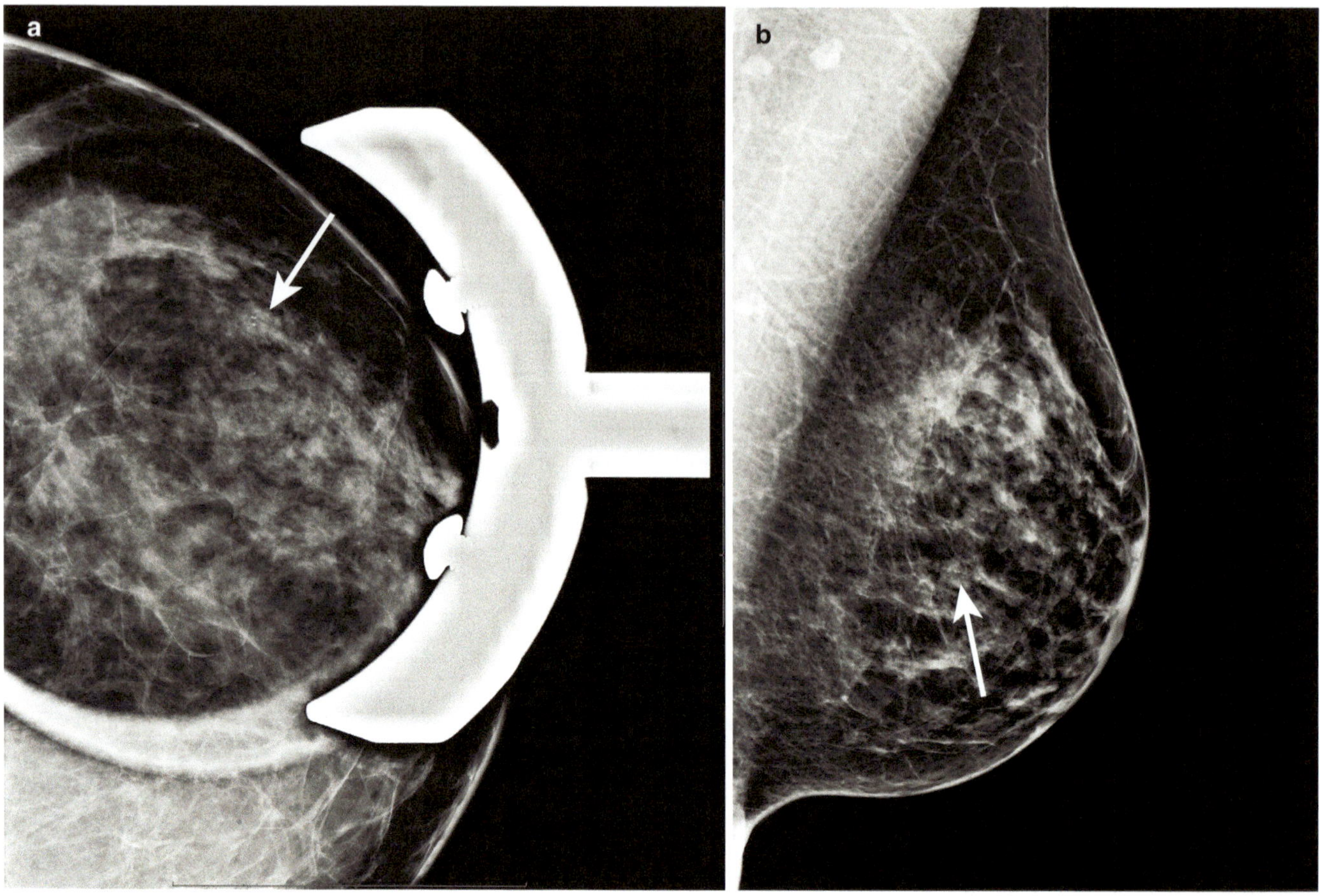

a

b

Fig. 1.1

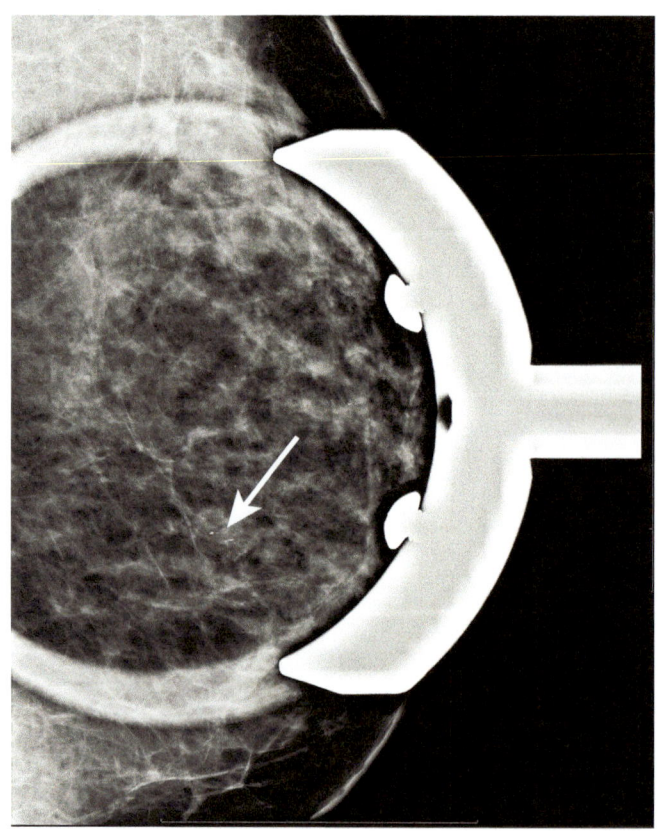

Fig. 1.2

CASE 12
LYMPHOMA

PATIENT HISTORY

A 68-year-old female with an enlarging breast mass.

RADIOLOGY FINDINGS

Fig. 1.1 (**a**) CC and (**b**) MLO images show an irregular mass with spiculated margins at 12 o'clock in the right breast at middle depth.

Fig. 1.2 Grayscale (**a**) transverse and (**b**) sagittal ultrasound images show an irregular hypoechoic mass surrounded by a hyperechoic rim.

Fig. 1.3 Color Doppler ultrasound image shows vascular flow within the mass.

BI-RADS ASSESSMENT

BI-RADS 5. Highly suggestive of malignancy (following diagnostic workup, prior to biopsy).

DIAGNOSIS

Lymphoma

DISCUSSION

- Lymphoma accounts for approximately 0.1–0.2 % of all breast carcinomas.
- Diagnosis of primary breast lymphoma is reserved for patients with no evidence of systemic lymphoma.
- More commonly lymphoma occurs in the breast due to metastasis of extramammary lymphoma.
- Mammographically, lymphoma can be seen as a solitary noncalcified mass, often well marginated and less often irregular.
- A hypoechoic mass with indistinct margins and vascular flow is commonly seen on ultrasound.
- On MRI, lymphoma is often seen as intense heterogeneous enhancement with a washout kinetic curve (type III).

REFERENCES

Feder JM, Shaw de Paredes E, Hogge JP, Wilken JJ. Unusual breast lesions: radiologic-pathologic correlation. Radiographics. 1999;19:S11–26.

Yang WT, Lane DL, Le-Petross HT, Abruzzo LV, Macapinlac HA. Breast lymphoma: imaging findings of 32 tumors in 27 patients. Radiology. 2007;245:692–702.

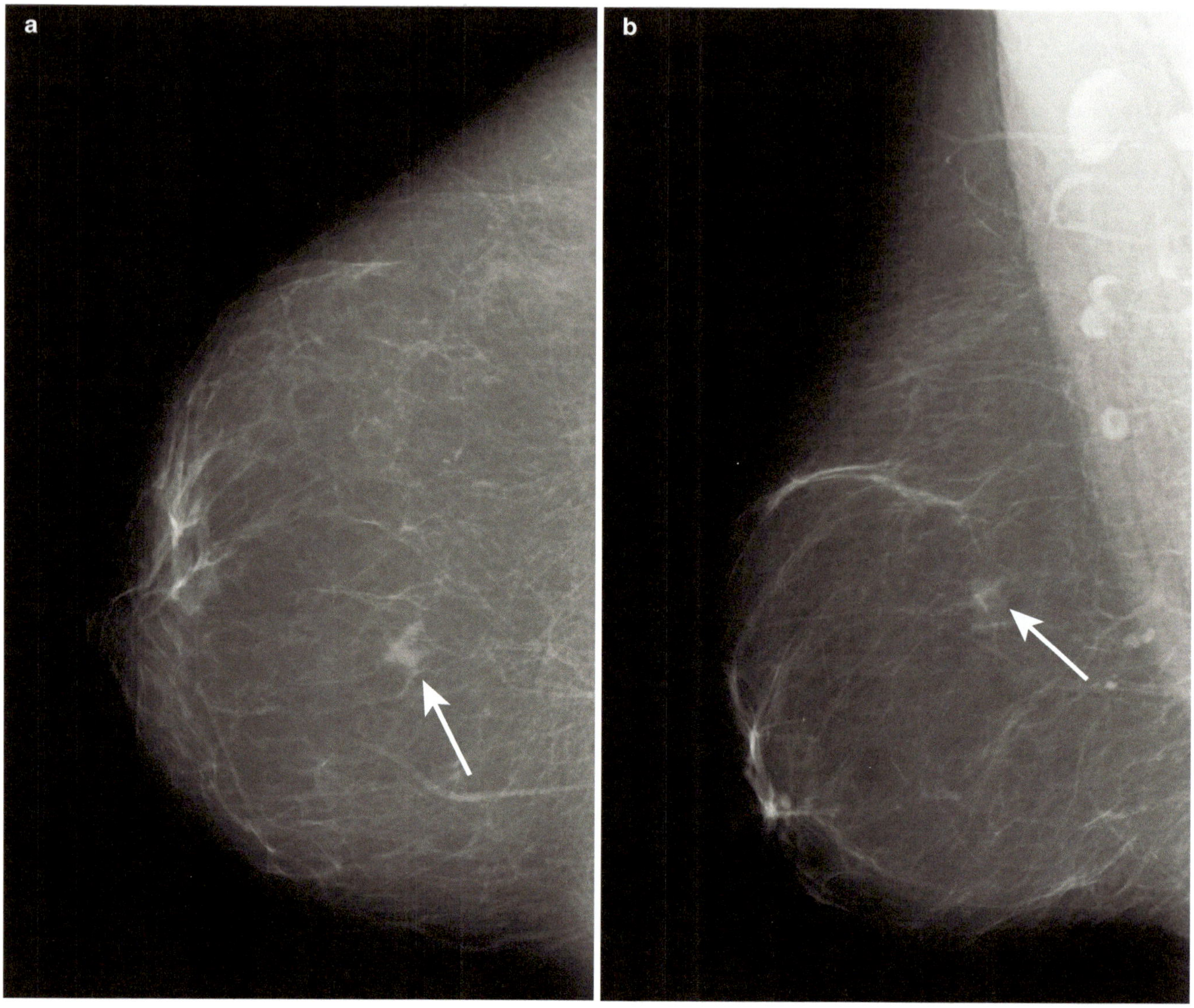

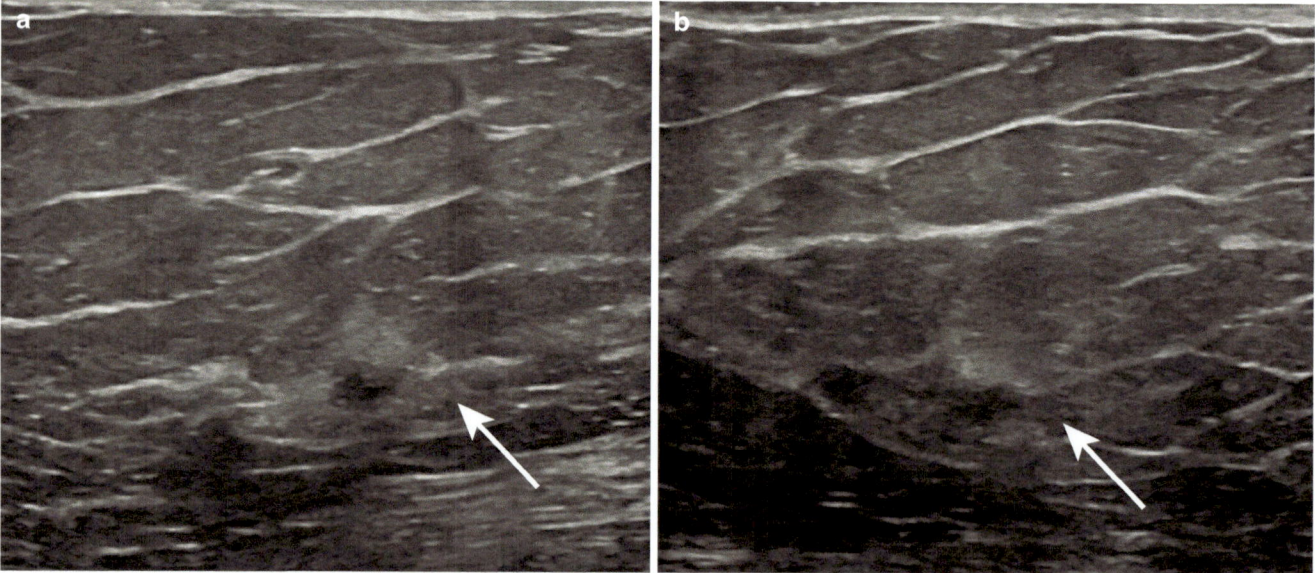

Fig. 1.1

Fig. 1.2

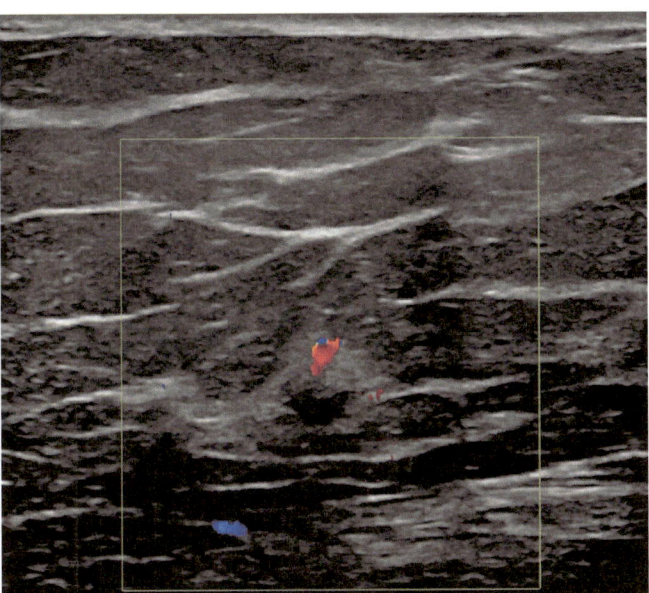

Fig. 1.3

CASE 13
FIBROADENOMA

PATIENT HISTORY

A 29-year-old female with a palpable mass at 12 o'clock in the left breast.

RADIOLOGY FINDINGS

Fig. 1.1 (**a**) Grayscale and (**b**) color Doppler images show an oval circumscribed hypoechoic avascular mass at 12 o'clock, corresponding to the patient's palpable mass.

BI-RADS ASSESSMENT

BI-RADS 2. Benign finding (following diagnostic workup and biopsy).

DIAGNOSIS

Fibroadenoma

DISCUSSION

- Fibroadenoma is a benign fibroepithelial tumor with mixed stromal and epithelial elements.

- Juvenile-type fibroadenoma:
  - Is a "cellular" fibroadenoma
  - Has no leaflike growth pattern on pathology (which is a differentiating factor from phyllodes tumor)
  - Has a uniform stromal hypercellularity
  - Is usually seen between 10 and 20 years of age and rare in >45 years of age
- Adult-type fibroadenoma:
  - Most common type
  - On pathology, has bland, fibroblastic stroma.
  - Is hypocellular to variably hypercellular.
- Most fibroadenomas in teenagers are adult type.
- Most commonly presents as a palpable, painless, mobile, firm mass.
- Biopsy is indicated if it is new, enlarging, and palpable or has suspicious features. Otherwise, clinical and sonographic follow-up may be adequate.
- Cryoablation therapy can be considered as an alternative treatment.

REFERENCES

Berg WA, Birdwell RB, Gombos EC, et al. Diagnostic imaging breast. 1st ed. Salt Lake City: Amirsys; 2006. Section IV-2, p. 32–7.

Cyrlak D, Pahl M, Carpenter SE. Breast imaging case of the day. Radiographics. 1999;19:549–51.

Mandell J. Core radiology: a visual approach to diagnostic imaging. 1st ed. Cambridge: Cambridge University Press; 2013. p. 625.

Fig. 1.1

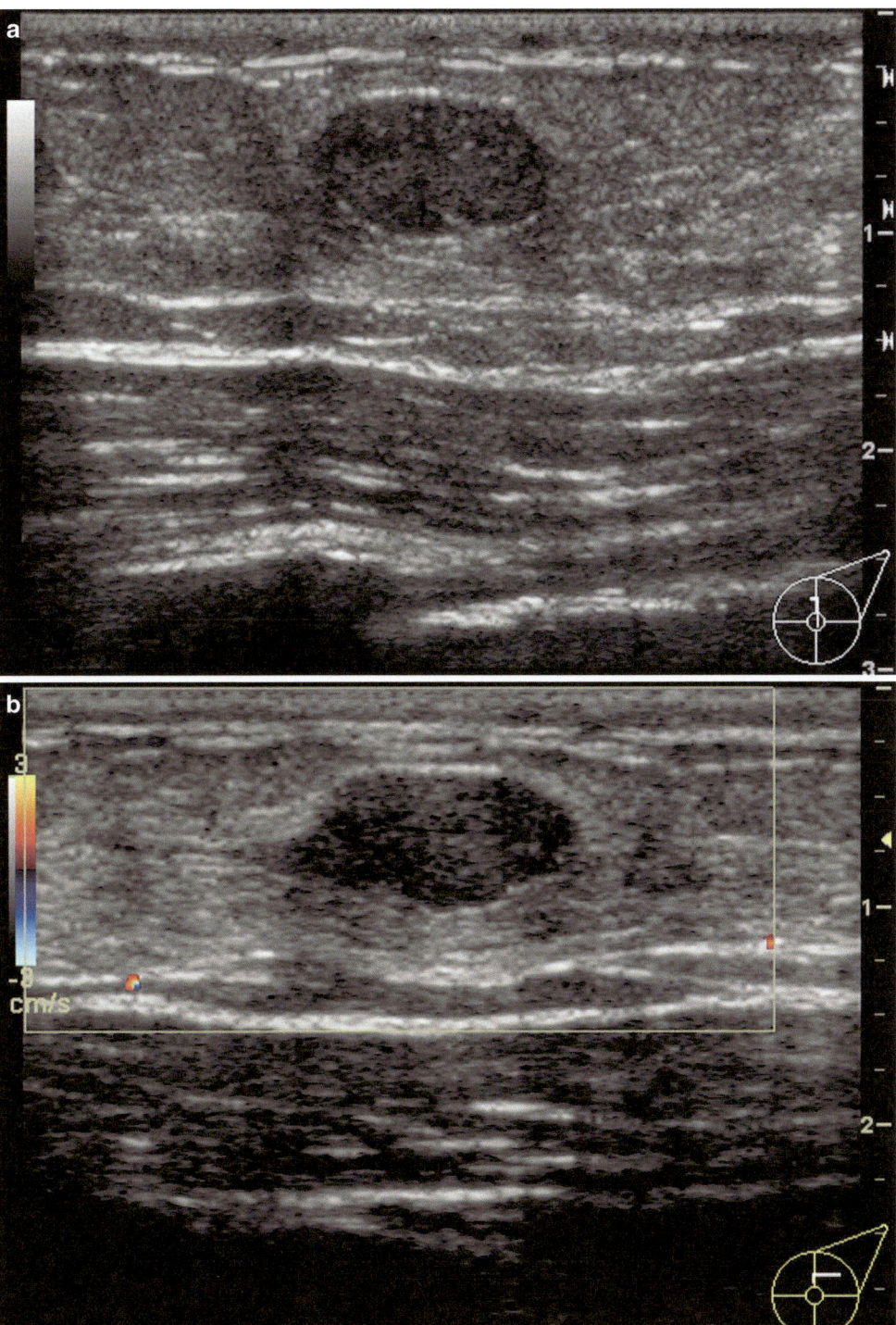

Case 14
Paget's Disease

Patient History

A 58-year-old female with nipple erythema and retraction.

Radiology Findings

Fig. 1.1 (**a**) CC, (**b**) ML, (**c**) spot-magnification CC, and (**d**) spot-magnification MLO images show indistinct calcifications in a linear distribution, extending from the nipple to middle depth in the right breast. The nipple is inverted.

Fig. 1.2 (**a**) Axial subtracted T1-weighted and (**b**) sagittal contrast-enhanced delayed T1-weighted images show non-mass-like enhancement extending from the nipple to the posterior depth of the right breast. There is abnormal enhancement of the nipple–areolar complex.

BI-RADS Assessment

BI-RADS 5. Highly suggestive of malignancy (following diagnostic workup, prior to biopsy).

Diagnosis

Paget's disease

Discussion

- Paget's disease is an extension of carcinoma to the epidermal layers of the nipple.
- Often associated with an underlying DCIS and less commonly with IDC.
- Clinically, Paget's disease presents as scaling, erosions, erythema, or eczematous reaction of the nipple.
- Mammogram can often be negative; however, calcifications or a mass associated with an underlying DCIS or IDC can be seen.
- Skin thickening and heterogeneity of the breast parenchyma can be seen on ultrasound; the same nonspecific changes can be seen with mastitis.
- MRI can be of value when the mammogram is normal, often showing abnormal nipple enhancement, thickening of the nipple–areolar complex, or an enhancing underlying carcinoma.
- Diagnosis can be made by a punch biopsy of the nipple–areolar complex, which will demonstrate cancer cells.
- Paget's disease can be rarely associated with invasive lobular carcinoma.

References

Harvey JA, March DE. Making the diagnosis: a practical guide to breast imaging. Philadelphia: Elsevier; 2013. p. 375.

Kopans DB. Breast imaging. 2nd ed. Philadelphia: Lippincott Williams and Wilkins; 1998. p. 583–4.

Nicholson BT, Harvey JA, Cohen MA. Nipple-areolar complex: normal anatomy and benign and malignant processes. Radiographics. 2009;29:509–23.

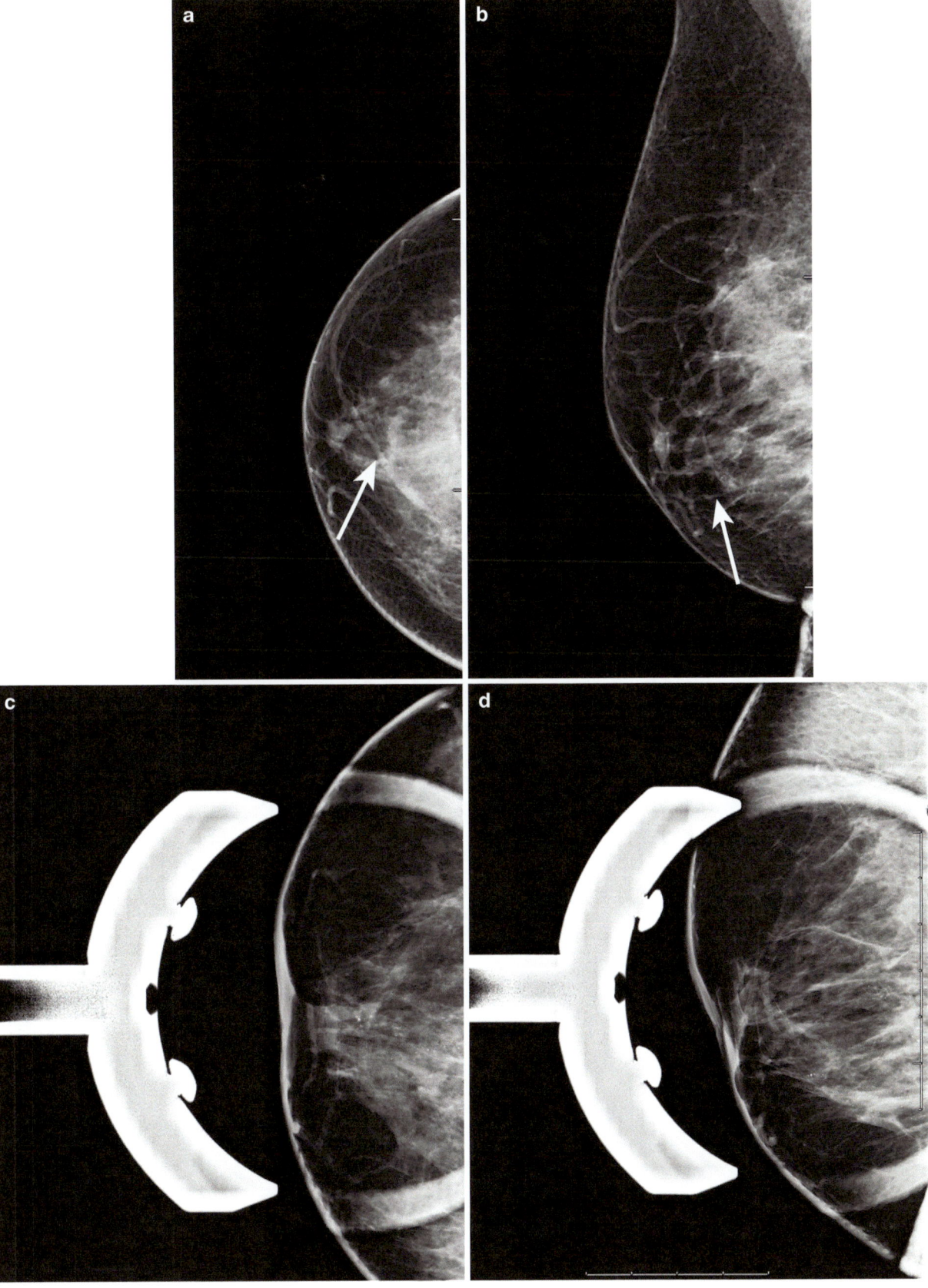

Fig. 1.1

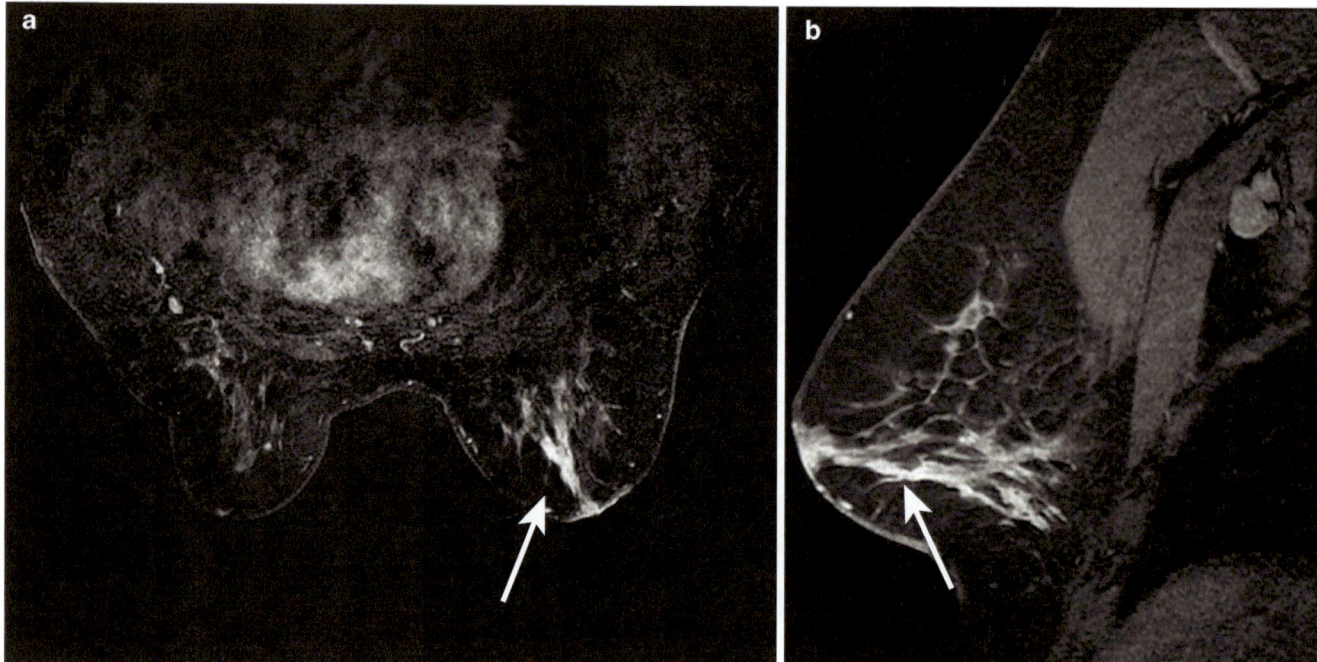

Fig. 1.2

CASE 15
MASTITIS

PATIENT HISTORY

A 51-year-old male with swelling and erythema of the left breast following a human bite to the left breast.

RADIOLOGY FINDINGS

Fig. 1.1 (**a**) CC and (**b**) MLO images show an asymmetry in the central anterior left breast.
Fig. 1.2 (**a, b**) Grayscale and (**c**) color Doppler ultrasound images show skin thickening and edematous tissue.

BI-RADS ASSESSMENT

BI-RADS 2. Benign findings (following diagnostic workup).

DIAGNOSIS

Mastitis

DISCUSSION

- Mastitis can present with pain, skin edema, erythema, and a palpable mass.
- Mammographically, it can be seen as skin thickening and trabecular thickening, with or without an area of asymmetry in the breast.
- Reactive lymphadenopathy can be present.
- Skin thickening, edema, and increased echogenicity of the breast can be seen on ultrasound.
- Most common pathogens are *Staphylococcus aureus* and Streptococcus.
- Puerperal mastitis is most common.
- A skin-punch biopsy is needed to differentiate inflammatory breast cancer from mastitis refractory to treatment.

REFERENCES

Bassett LW, Feig SA, Hendrick RE, Jackson VP, Sickles EA. Breast disease (third series) test and syllabus. Reston: American College of Radiology; 2000. p. 82.
Berg W, Birdwell R, Gombos EC, et al. Diagnostic imaging: breast. 1st ed. Salt Lake City: Amirsys; 2006. Section IV-6, p. 10–2.

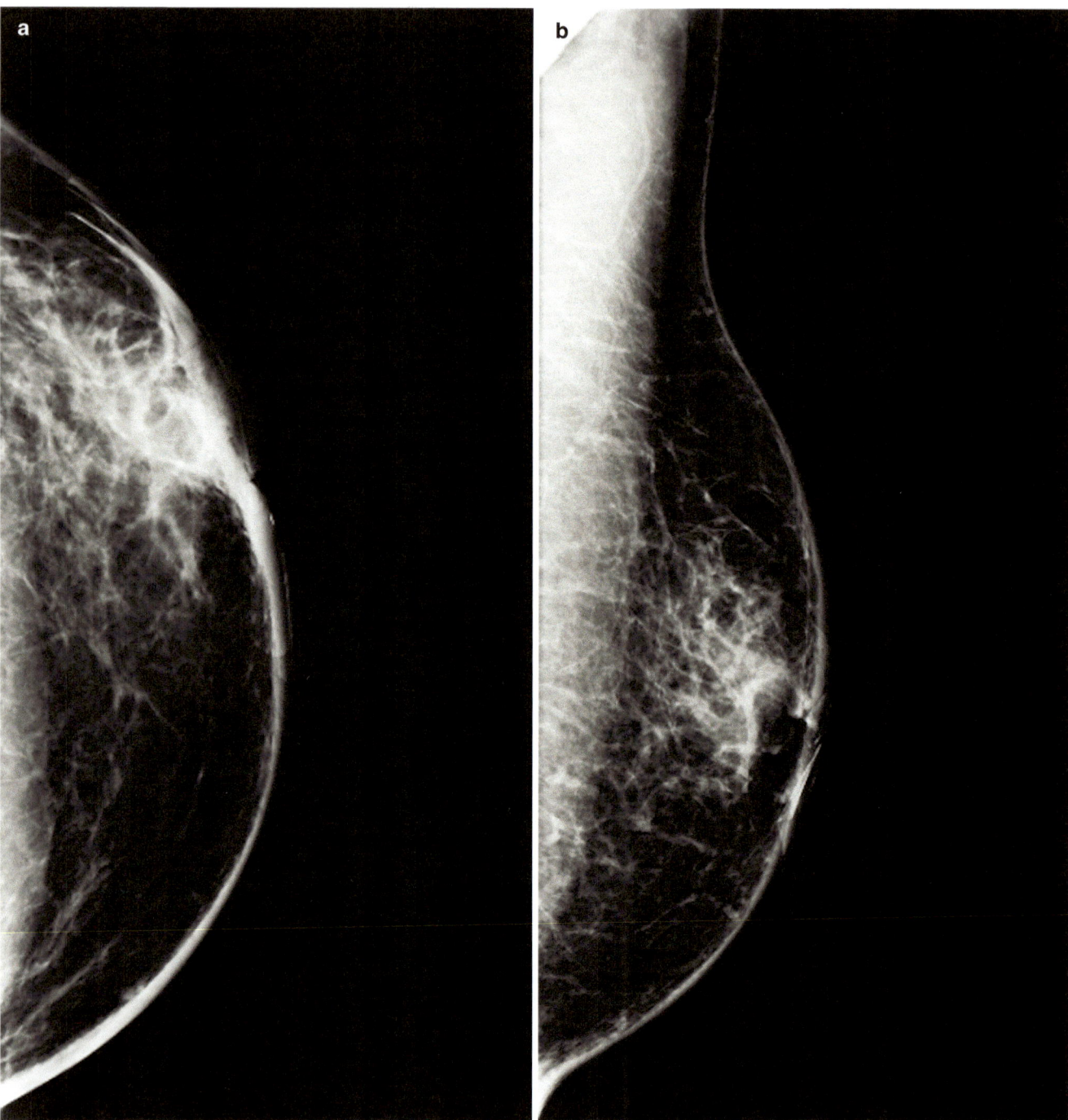

Fig. 1.1

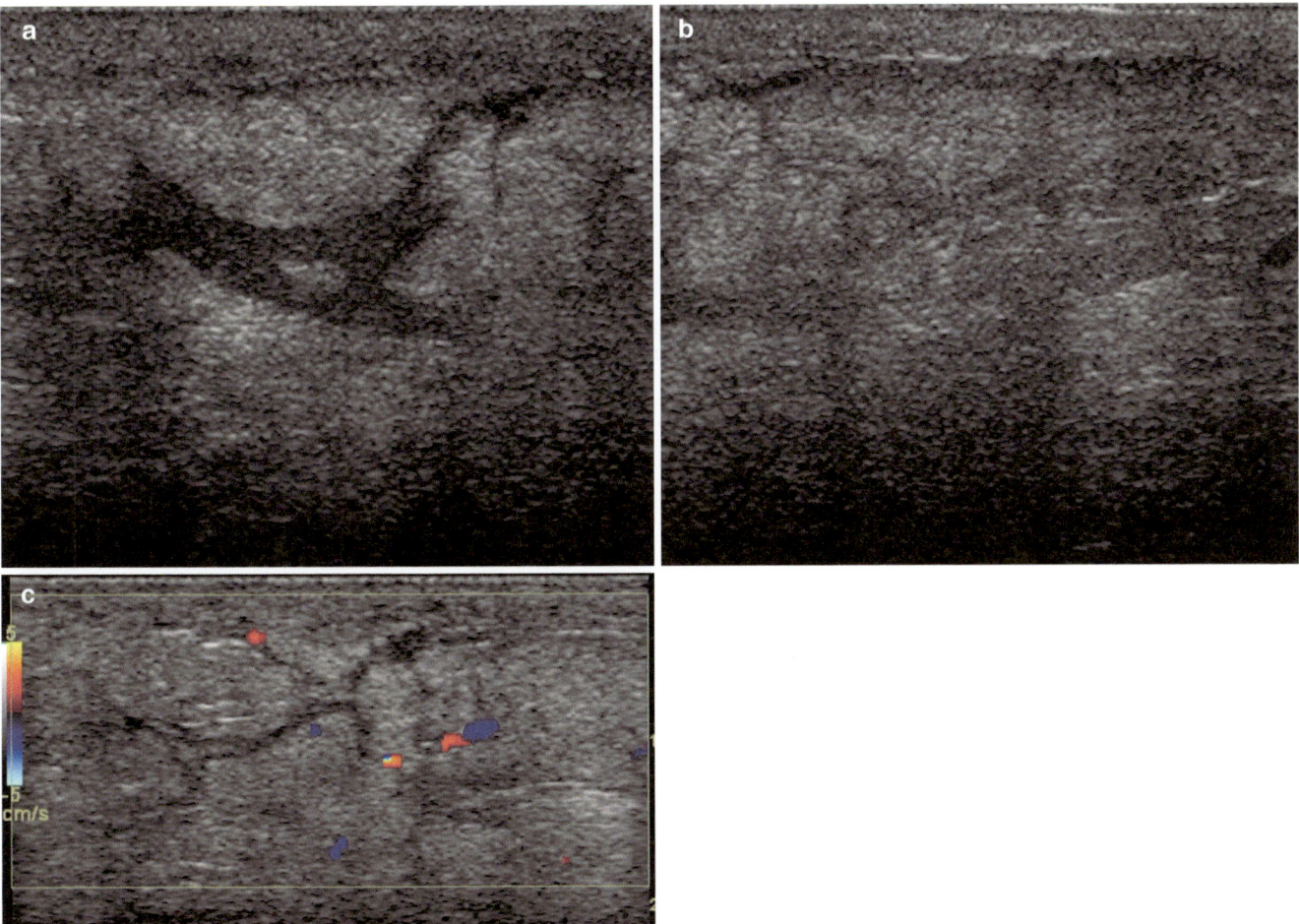

Fig. 1.2

CASE 16
NEUROFIBROMATOSIS TYPE I (NF I)

PATIENT HISTORY

A 52-year-old female with multiple skin lesions for screening mammogram.

RADIOLOGY FINDINGS

Fig. 1.1 (**a**, **b**) CC and (**c**, **d**) MLO views show multiple circumscribed skin masses bilaterally.

BI-RADS ASSESSMENT

BI-RADS 2. Benign findings.

DIAGNOSIS

Neurofibromatosis Type I (NF I)

DISCUSSION

- NF I, also termed as von Recklinghausen's disease, presents initially in children and young adults.
- Classic features of NF I include neurofibromas and cafe au lait spots.
- NF I also has vascular, skeletal, and pulmonary manifestations.
- Associated neoplasms with NF I include meningiomas, optic gliomas, neurofibrosarcomas, and pheochromocytomas.
- Likely associated with an increased risk for breast cancer.
- Neurofibromas can project over the breast and have the appearance of masses within the breast on mammogram.

REFERENCES

Brant WE, Helms CA, editors. Fundamentals of diagnostic radiology. 2nd ed. Philadelphia: Lippincott Williams and Wilkins; 1999. p. 430.
Harvey JA, March DE. Making the diagnosis: a practical guide to breast imaging. Philadelphia: Elsevier; 2013. p. 352.

Fig. 1.1

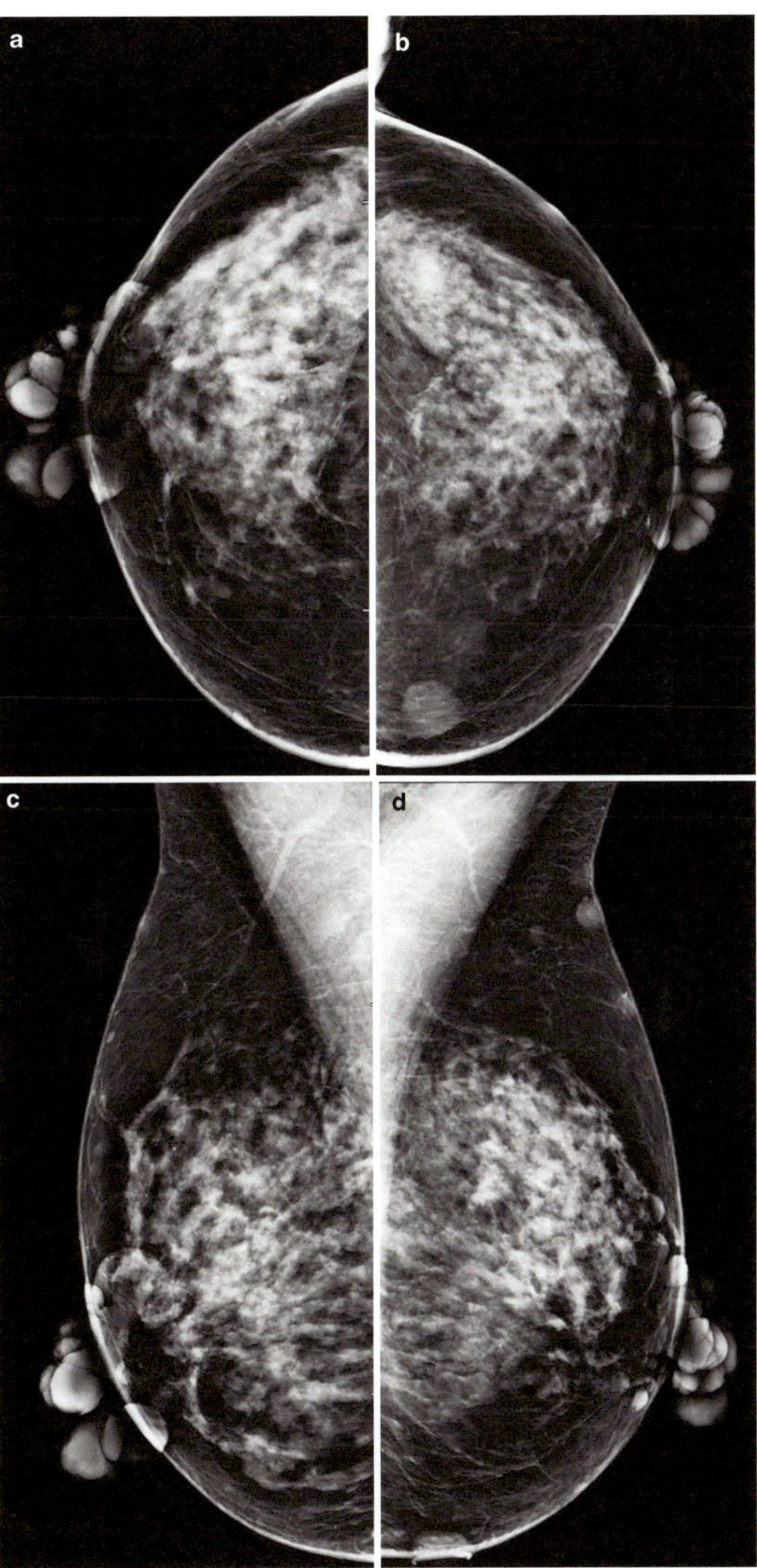

CASE 17
MULTIPLE, BILATERAL CIRCUMSCRIBED MASSES

PATIENT HISTORY

A 42-year-old female for a screening mammogram.

RADIOLOGY FINDINGS

Fig. 1.1 (**a**, **b**) Bilateral CC views demonstrate multiple, bilateral, noncalcified circumscribed masses.

BI-RADS ASSESSMENT

BI-RADS 2. Benign findings.

DIAGNOSIS

Multiple, bilateral circumscribed masses

DISCUSSION

- Multiple, bilateral masses are defined as at least three masses in total with at least one in each breast.
- Multiple masses are seen in 1.7 % of screening mammograms.
- Margins must be 75 % circumscribed and the remainder can be obscured.
- No mass can have spiculated margins.
- Excludes palpable masses and those with suspicious calcifications.
- Interval cancer rate associated with multiple, bilateral masses is 0.14 %.
- Ultrasound is indicated if any mass is palpable, rapidly growing, or has an otherwise suspicious appearance.
- Differential diagnosis includes:
  - Cysts
  - Fibroadenomas
  - Papillomas
  - Oil cysts

REFERENCES

Berg WA, Birdwell RL, Gombos EC, et al. Diagnostic imaging breast. 1st ed. Salt Lake City: Amirsys; 2006. Section IV-5, p. 22–5.

Leung JW, Sickles EA. Multiple bilateral masses detected on screening mammography: assessment of need for recall imaging. AJR. 2000;175:23–9.

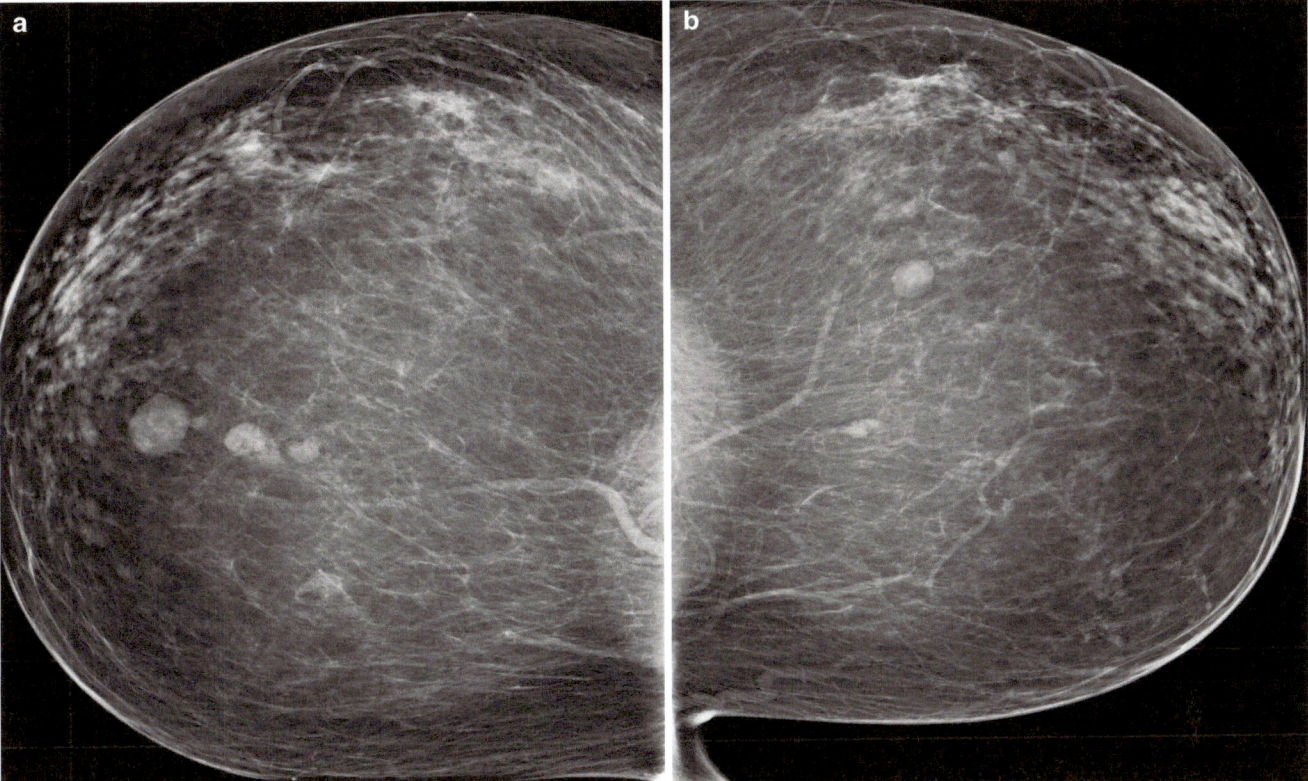

Fig. 1.1

CASE 18
VASCULAR CALCIFICATIONS

PATIENT HISTORY

A 74-year-old female for a screening mammogram.

RADIOLOGY FINDINGS

Fig. 1.1 Bilateral (**a**, **b**) CC and (**c**, **d**) MLO views demonstrate linear, serpiginous, parallel calcifications.

BI-RADS ASSESSMENT

BI-RADS 2. Benign finding.

DIAGNOSIS

Vascular calcifications

DISCUSSION

- Vascular calcifications are calcifications within the media of the arterial wall.

- Classic "tram track" pattern.
- Seen in 8–9 % of all screening mammograms.
- Increased frequency with advancing age.
- Vascular calcifications are more common in women with diabetes and renal dialysis.
- Some studies have shown that breast arterial calcifications are an independent risk factor for cardiovascular mortality.
- Atypical vascular calcifications may mimic malignancy.
- No specific breast-related treatment.
- If not a classic appearance, differential diagnosis includes:
  - DCIS
  - Secretory calcifications
  - Mondor's disease
  - Fat necrosis

REFERENCES

American College of Radiology (ACR) BI-RADS® Atlas. ACR BI-RADS® atlas-mammography. 5th ed. Reston: American College of Radiology; 2013. p. 40–1.

Berg WA, Birdwell RL, Gombos EC, et al. Diagnostic imaging breast. 1st ed. Salt Lake City: Amirsys; 2006. Section IV-1, p. 76–8.

Kemmeren J, Beijerinck D, van Noord PA, et al. Breast arterial calcifications: association with diabetes mellitus and cardiovascular mortality. Work in progress. Radiology. 1996;201:75–8.

Moshyedi AC, Puthawala AH, Kurland RJ, O'Leary DH. Breast arterial calcifications: association with coronary artery disease. Work in progress. Radiology. 1995;194:181–3.

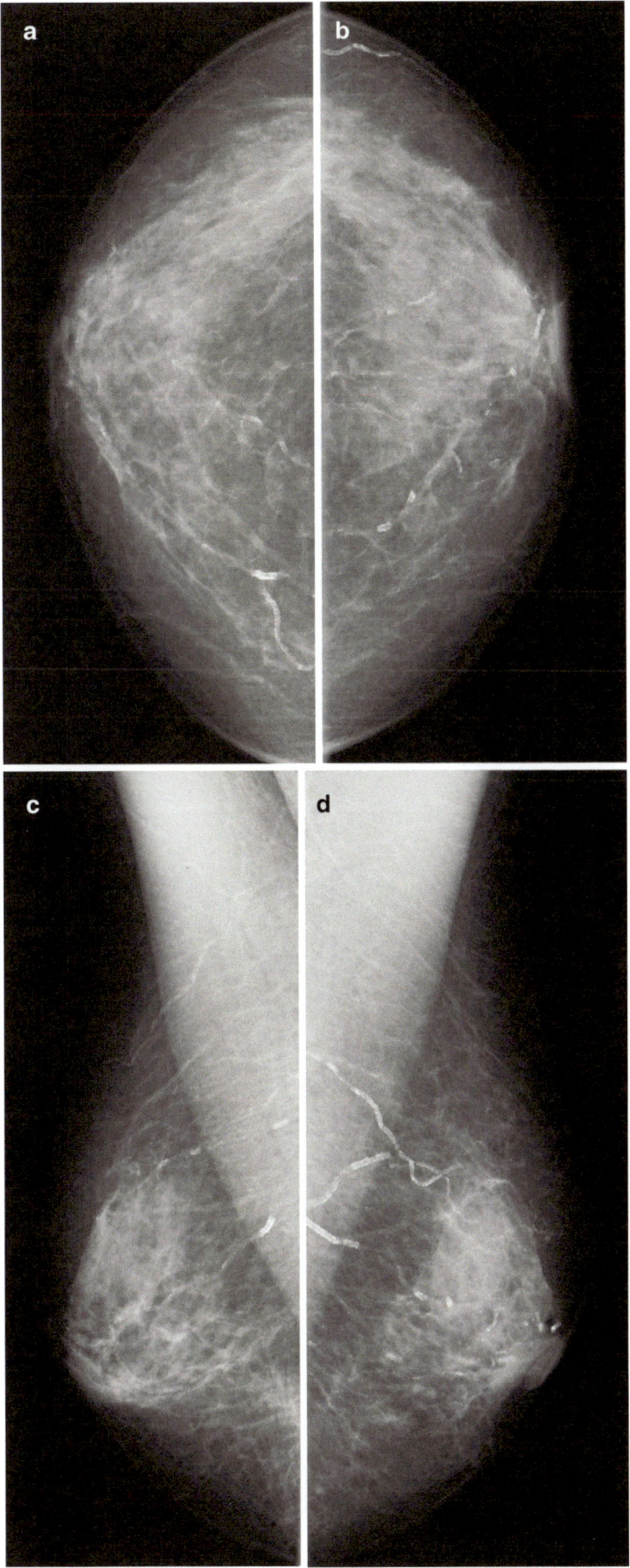

Fig. 1.1

CASE 19
STROMAL FIBROSIS

PATIENT HISTORY

A 60-year-old female for a screening mammogram.

RADIOLOGY FINDINGS

Fig. 1.1 (**a**) CC and (**b**) MLO views demonstrate an oval mass with partly circumscribed and partly ill-defined margins in the lower inner left breast at posterior depth.
Fig. 1.2 Grayscale ultrasound image demonstrates a hypoechoic oval mass with ill-defined margins and posterior acoustic shadowing.

BI-RADS ASSESSMENT

BI-RADS 2. Benign finding (following diagnostic workup and biopsy).

DIAGNOSIS

Stromal fibrosis

DISCUSSION

- Stromal fibrosis may present incidentally on imaging or as a palpable mass.
- Formed by proliferation of collagenized stroma between terminal ductal lobular units.
- On mammography, stromal fibrosis can present as a benign-appearing mass or lesion that has features suggestive of malignancy.
- On ultrasound, stromal fibrosis appears hypoechoic or of mixed echogenicity and is nonvascular.
- No malignant potential and no intervention are necessary.
- It is important to assess radiology/pathology concordance after a diagnosis of stromal fibrosis on core needle biopsy.
  - If concordant, 6-month follow-up may be performed to assess stability.
  - Discordance between imaging features and diagnosis of stromal fibrosis should result in rebiopsy or excision.

REFERENCES

Berg WA, Birdwell RL, Gombos EC, et al. Diagnostic imaging breast. 1st ed. Salt Lake City: Amirsys; 2006. Section IV-2, p. 46–9.
Sklair-Levy M, Samuels TH, Catzavelos C, Hamilton P, Shumak R. Stromal fibrosis of the breast. AJR. 2001;177(3):573–7.

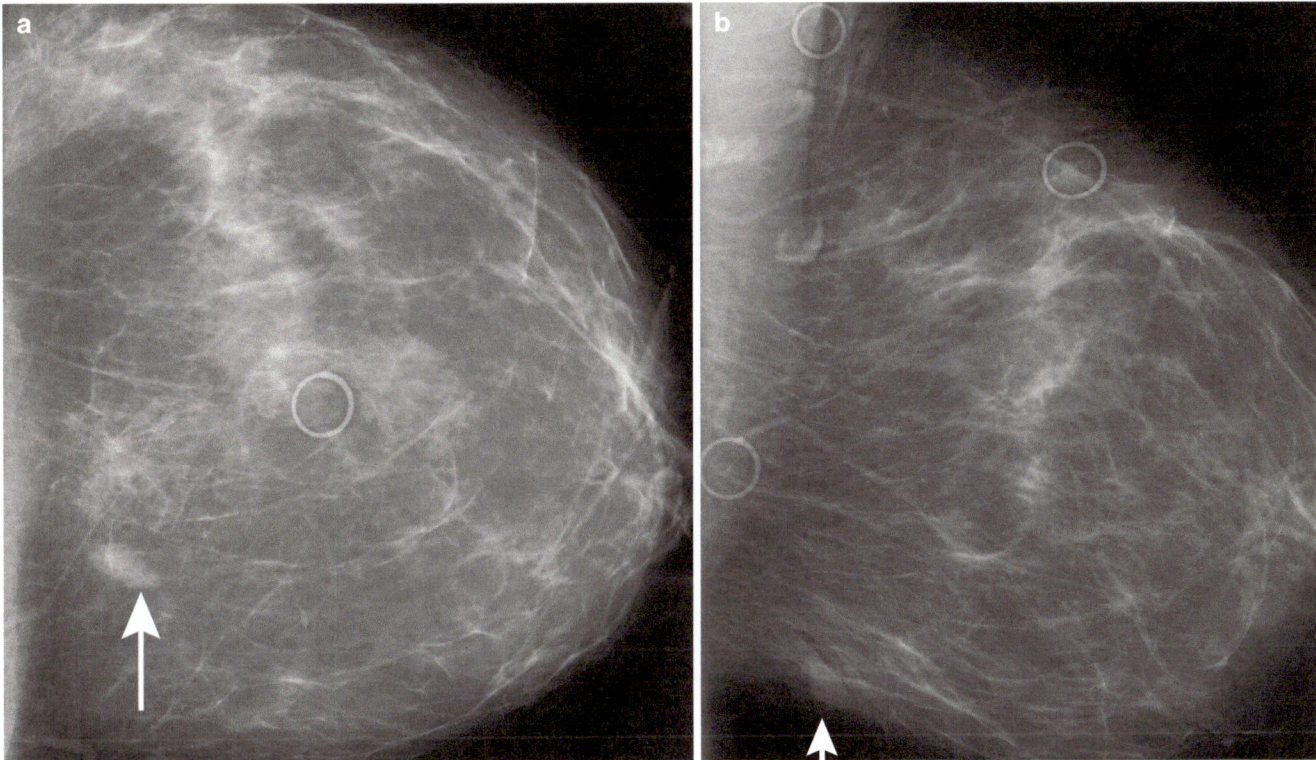

Fig. 1.1

Fig. 1.2

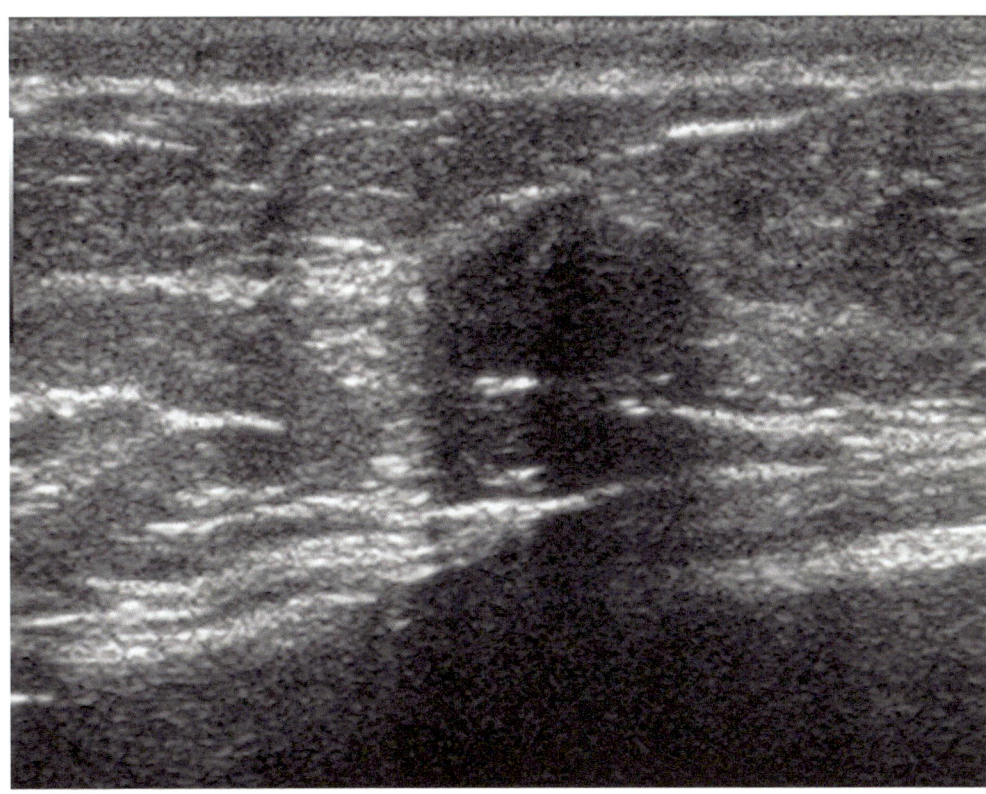

REDUCTION MAMMOPLASTY

PATIENT HISTORY

A 51-year-old female with a history of prior bilateral breast surgery for a screening mammogram.

RADIOLOGY FINDINGS

Fig. 1.1 Bilateral (**a**, **b**) CC and (**c**, **d**) MLO views demonstrate prominent fibroglandular tissue with a swirled pattern of architectural distortion in the lower breast. An oval lucent mass in the lower inner breast represents fat necrosis.

BI-RADS ASSESSMENT

BI-RADS 2. Benign finding.

DIAGNOSIS

Reduction mammoplasty

DISCUSSION

- Reduction mammoplasty is a plastic surgery procedure to decrease the breast size in macromastia, in the setting of contralateral mastectomy or breast conservation surgery, trauma, or congenital asymmetry. A keyhole incision is usually made.
- Characteristic mammographic findings include:
  - Elevation of nipple with more skin inferior than superior.
  - Redistribution of fibroglandular tissue from upper outer quadrant to lower inner quadrant.
  - "Swirled pattern" of fibroglandular tissue in the lower inner quadrant.
  - Dermal calcifications are common in the scar tissue.
  - The breasts appear higher and flatter in contour than normal breasts.
- Associated findings include:
  - Fat necrosis
  - Postsurgical skin thickening
  - Sutural calcifications
  - Retroareolar fibrotic band
- Baseline mammogram is generally performed prior to the surgery to evaluate for any suspicious masses or calcifications.
- Mammogram is recommended 3–6 months postoperatively, which becomes the new baseline.

REFERENCES

Bassett LW, Jackson VP, Fu KL, Fu YS. Diagnosis of diseases of the breast. 2nd ed. Philadelphia: Elsevier; 2005. p. 617–21.
Berg WA, Birdwell RL, Gombos EC, et al. Diagnostic imaging breast. 1st ed. Salt Lake City: Amirsys; 2006. Section IV-4, p. 32–4.
Harvey JA, March DE. Making the diagnosis: a practical guide to breast imaging. Philadelphia: Elsevier; 2013. p. 470–2.

Fig. 1.1

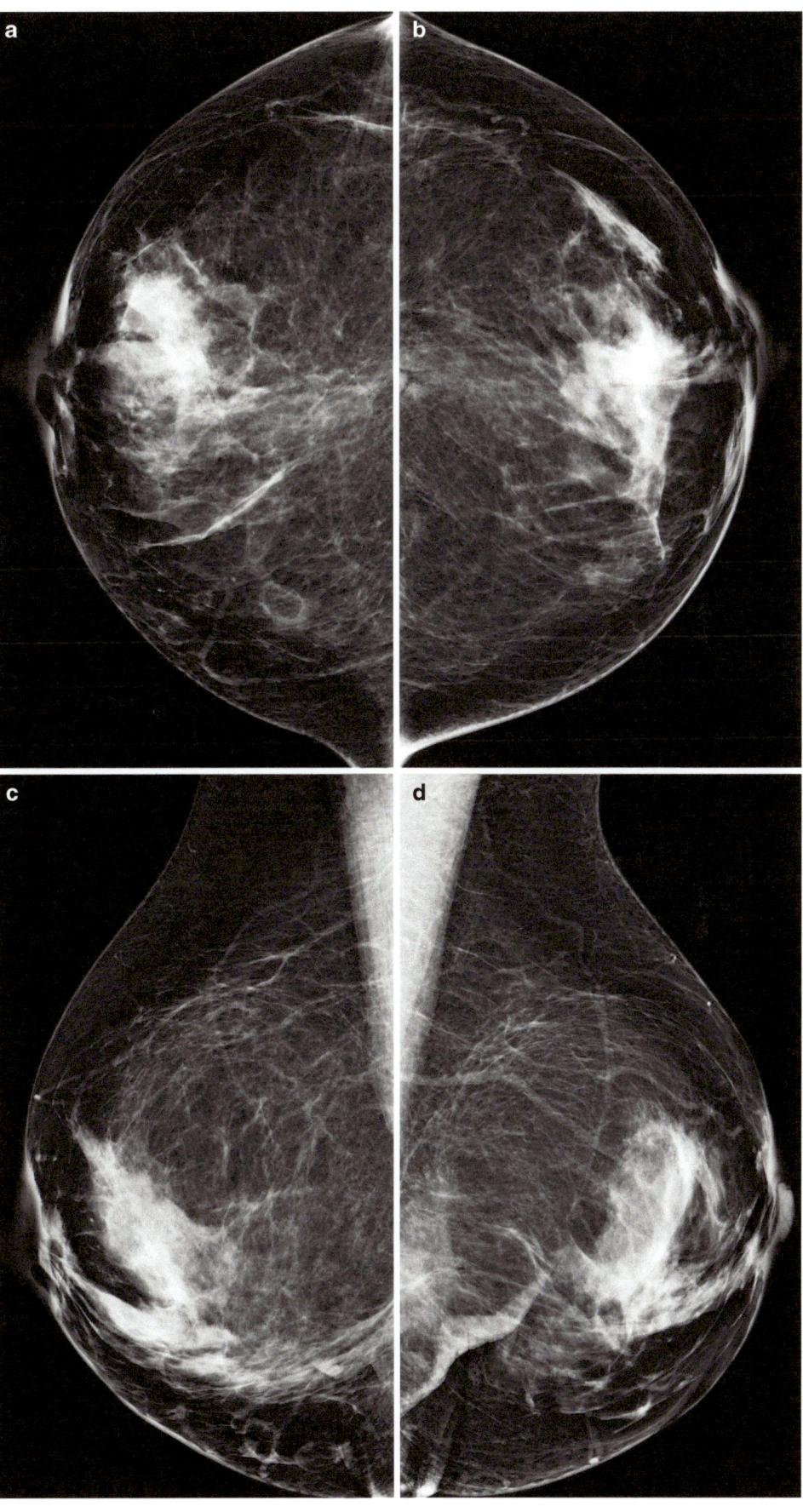

CASE 21
INVASIVE LOBULAR CARCINOMA (ILC)

PATIENT HISTORY

A 66-year-old female for a screening mammogram.

RADIOLOGY FINDINGS

Fig. 1.1 (**a**) CC, (**b**) MLO, and (**c**) LM images show an area of architectural distortion in the upper inner left breast at posterior depth.

Fig. 1.2 (**a**) Grayscale and (**b**) color Doppler ultrasound images show a lobular hypoechoic mass with spiculated margins. There is vascular flow within the mass.

BI-RADS ASSESSMENT

BI-RADS 4. Suspicious abnormality (following diagnostic workup, prior to biopsy).

DIAGNOSIS

Invasive lobular carcinoma (ILC)

DISCUSSION

- ILC arises from the lobular epithelium.
- It is the second most common breast cancer and accounts for 10–15 % of all invasive breast malignancies.
- Malignant cells grow in single file, and therefore, ILC does not evoke a desmoplastic reaction.

- On mammogram, ILC may be difficult to detect due to its growth pattern, decreased likelihood to develop calcifications, and atypical presentation such as a single-view finding of architectural distortion.
- ILC is seen as an ill-defined or spiculated mass on mammogram in 45–65 % of the cases.
- Usually detected at a later stage mammographically and clinically, thus increasing the likelihood of a large primary tumor and positive axillary lymph nodes at the time of diagnosis.
- When ILC is large, the breast may appear smaller on mammogram owing to decreased compressibility of the breast from the sheets of tumor cells, commonly referred to as the "shrinking breast."
- ILC can metastasize to peritoneal surfaces, bladder, stomach, uterus, and ovaries, thus causing presenting symptoms of ascites, pelvic masses, or hydronephrosis.
- A high rate of false-negative findings with PET has been reported with ILC.

REFERENCES

Avril N, Rose CA, Schelling M, et al. Breast imaging with PET and fluorine-18 fluorodeoxyglucose: uses and limitations. J Clin Oncol. 2000;18:3495–502.

Breas RF, Ioffe M, Rapelyea JA, et al. ILC: detecting with mammography, sonography, MRI and breast specific gamma imaging. AJR. 2009;192:379–83.

Harvey JA. Unusual breast cancers: useful clues to expanding the differential diagnosis. Radiology. 2007;242:638–94.

Harvey JA, March DE. Making the diagnosis: a practical guide to breast imaging. Philadelphia: Elsevier; 2013. p. 295.

Lopez JK, Bassett LW. ILC of the breast: spectrum of mammographic, ultrasound and MRI imaging findings. Radiographics. 2009;29:165–76.

Sickles EA. The subtle and atypical mammographic features of invasive lobular carcinoma. Radiology. 1991;178:25–6.

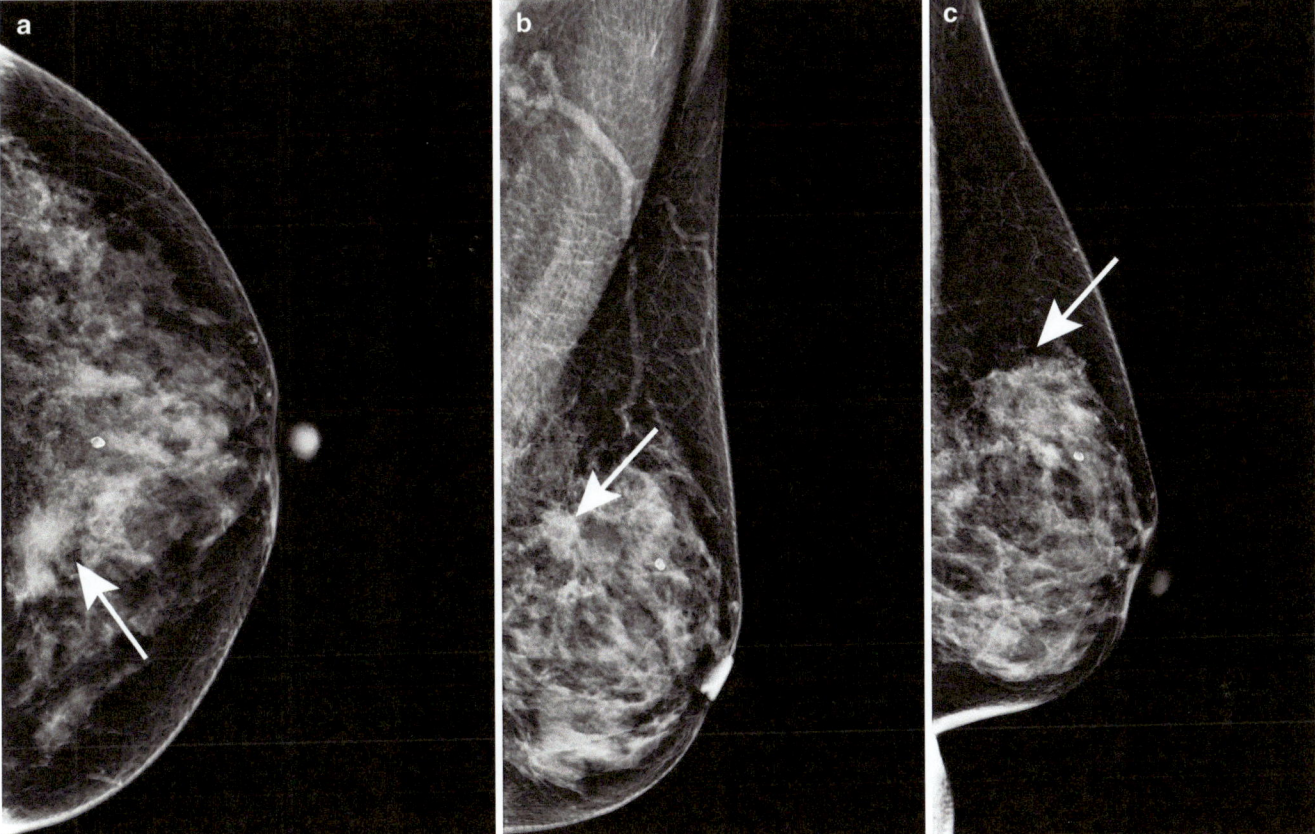

Fig. 1.1

Fig. 1.2

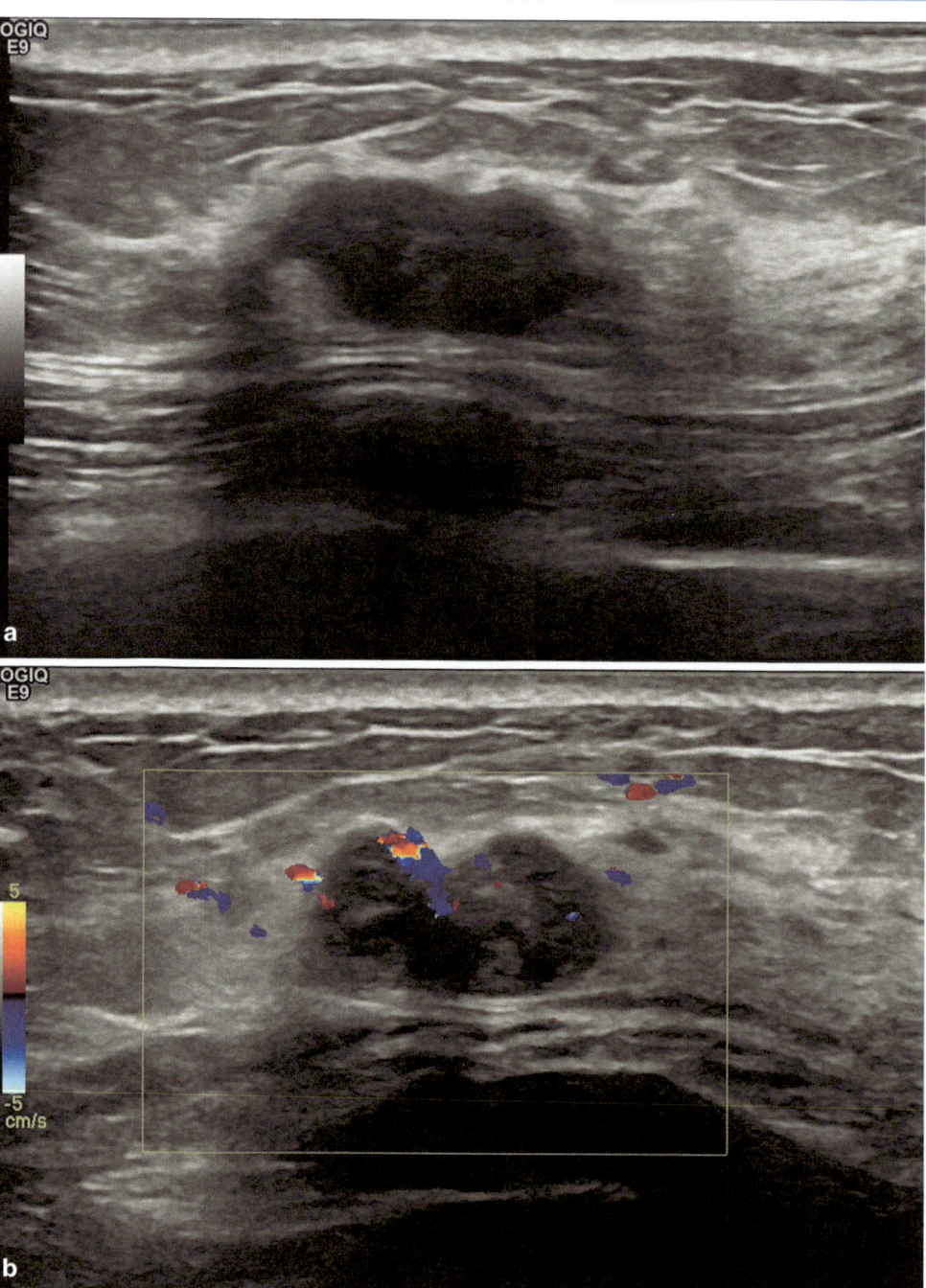

CASE 22
LACTATING ADENOMA

PATIENT HISTORY

A 30-year-old pregnant female with a palpable mass in the right breast.

RADIOLOGY FINDINGS

Fig. 1.1 Grayscale (**a**) transverse and (**b**) sagittal ultrasound images show a gently lobulated circumscribed hypoechoic mass.

Fig. 1.2 Color Doppler ultrasound image shows no vascular flow within the mass.

BI-RADS ASSESSMENT

BI-RADS 2. Benign finding (following diagnostic workup and biopsy).

DIAGNOSIS

Lactating adenoma

DISCUSSION

- Lactating adenoma is a benign breast mass thought to occur in response to the physiologic changes seen in pregnancy and lactation.

- There is often spontaneous regression of a lactating adenoma following pregnancy and lactation.
- Lactating adenoma is a fibroepithelial lesion that is similar in imaging and histologic appearance to a fibroadenoma.
- On mammogram, a circumscribed mass with a benign appearance is seen.
- On ultrasound, a circumscribed hypoechoic mass is commonly seen.
- Less frequently, a lactating adenoma with spiculated margins and posterior acoustic shadowing is seen by ultrasound, suggesting malignancy.
- Radiolucent or hyperechoic areas can be seen on mammogram and ultrasound, respectively, representing the fat content of milk secondary to lactational hyperplasia.

REFERENCES

Chung EM, Cube R, Hall GJ, Gonzalez C, Stocker JT, Glassman LM. Breast masses in children and adolescents: radiologic-pathologic correlation. Radiographics. 2009;29:907–31.

Harvey JA, March DE. Making the diagnosis: a practical guide to breast imaging. Philadelphia: Elsevier; 2013. p. 303.

Sabate JM, Clotet M, Torrubia S. Radiologic evaluation of breast disorders related to lactation and pregnancy. Radiographics. 2007;27:S101–124.

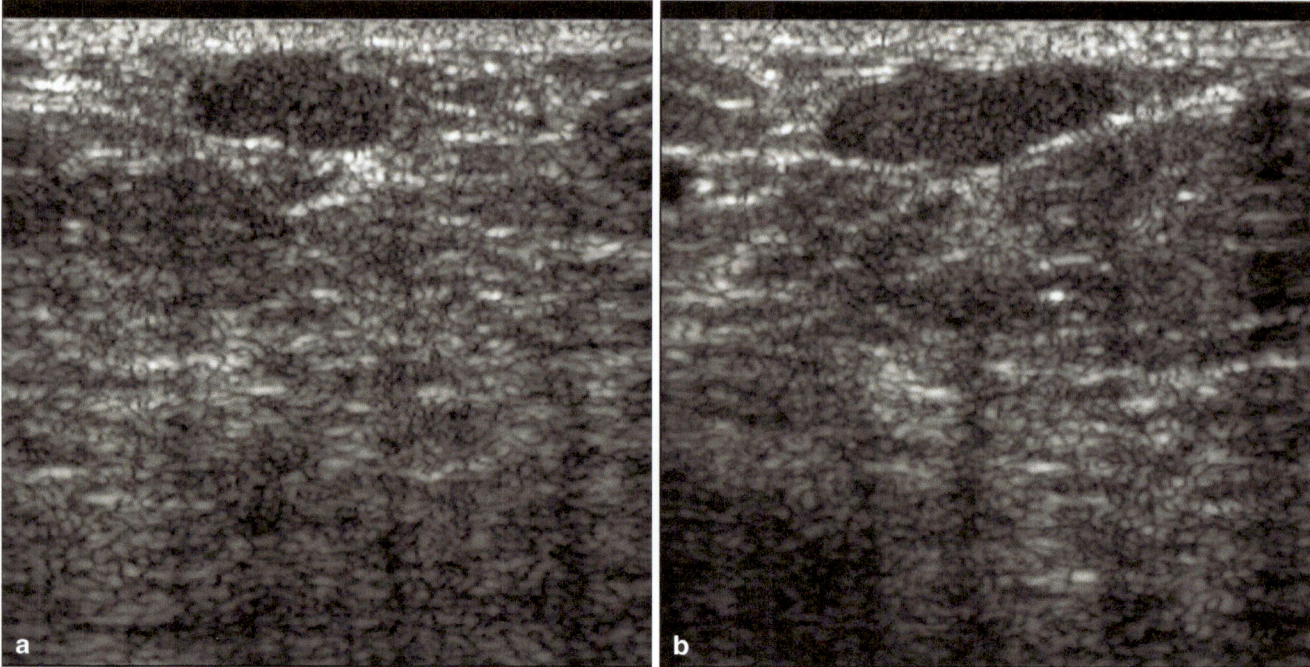

Fig. 1.1

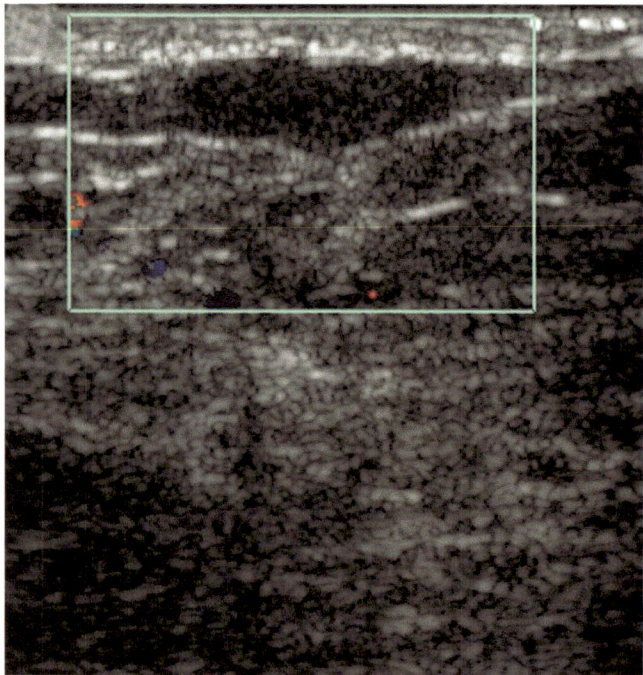

Fig. 1.2

CASE 23
SILICONE GRANULOMA

PATIENT HISTORY

A 50-year-old female with a history of removal of ruptured silicone implants.

RADIOLOGY FINDINGS

Fig. 1.1 (**a**) CC and (**b**) MLO views demonstrate a dense irregular mass in the lower inner right breast at posterior depth.

Fig. 1.2 Grayscale ultrasound image demonstrates a "snowstorm" appearance.

BI-RADS ASSESSMENT

BI-RADS 2. Benign finding (following diagnostic workup).

DIAGNOSIS

Silicone granuloma

DISCUSSION

- Silicone granuloma is a mass caused by foreign body reaction to free silicone in tissues.

- Most common locations are at the edge of implants and axilla.
- They are usually easy to recognize due to their high density. Their margins may be circumscribed or indistinct.
- Patients may be asymptomatic or present with a palpable mass.
- Silicone in an axillary node is an indication of extracapsular implant rupture.
- Presence of silicone granulomas indicates extracapsular rupture of a current or prior implant.
- If asymptomatic, no treatment is necessary. If symptomatic, supportive therapy and/or excision is recommended.
- Silicone in the axilla can involve the brachial plexus causing neuropathy.

REFERENCES

Berg WA, Birdwell RL, Gombos EC, et al. Diagnostic imaging breast. 1st ed. Salt Lake City: Amirsys; 2006. Section: IV-4, p. 36–7.

Caskey C, Berg WA, Hamper UM, Sheth S, Chang BW, Anderson ND. Imaging spectrum of extracapsular silicone: correlation of ultrasound, MR. imaging, mammographic and histopathologic findings. Radiographics. 1999;19:F39–51.

Harvey JA, March DE. Making the diagnosis: a practical guide to breast imaging. Philadelphia: Elsevier; 2013. p. 511–2.

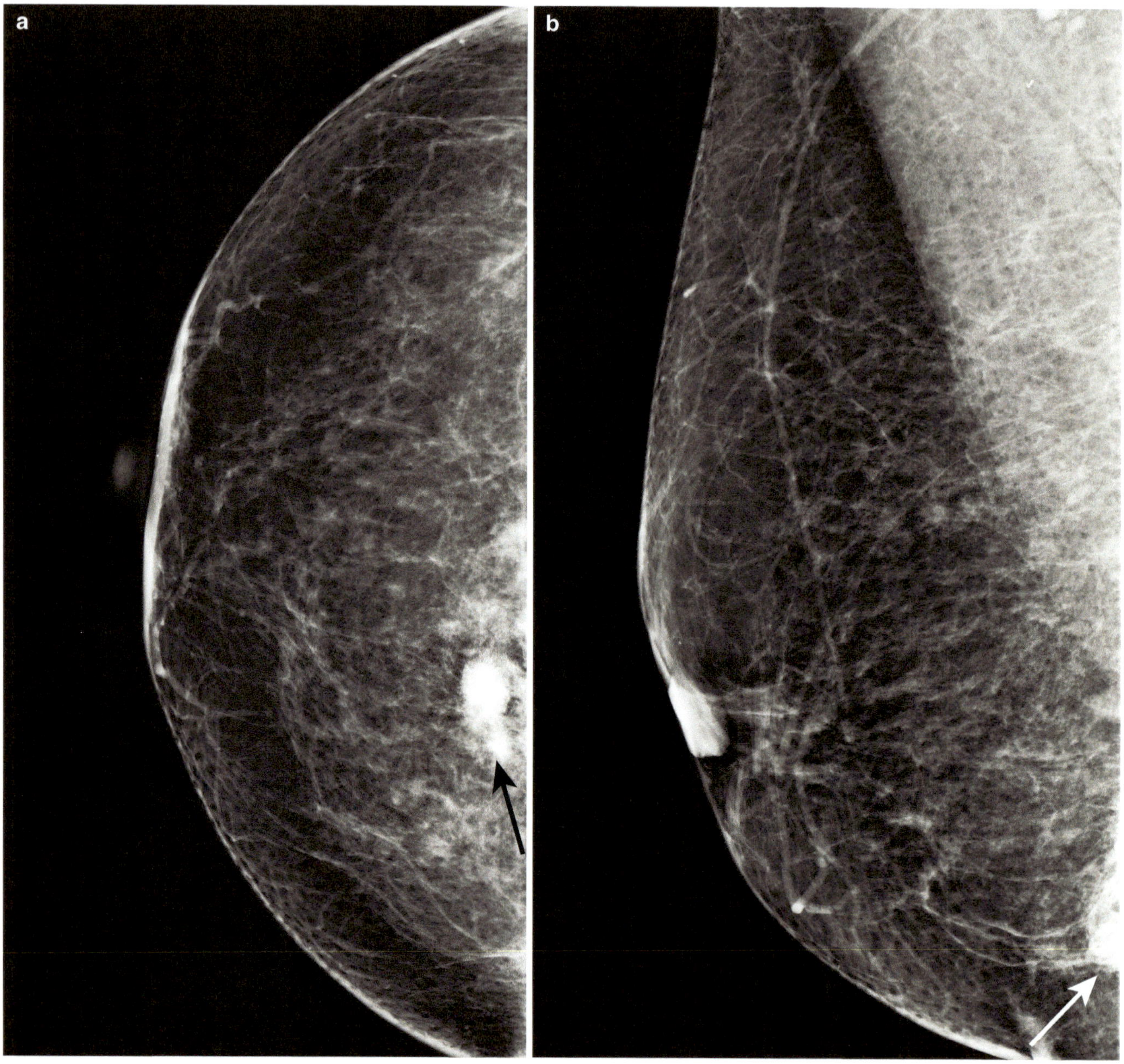

a

b

Fig. 1.1

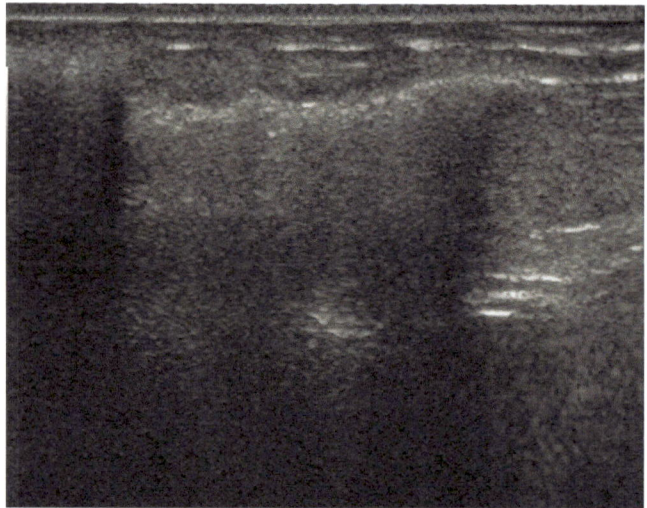

Fig. 1.2

CASE 24
LIPOMA

PATIENT HISTORY

A 58-year-old male with a palpable left breast mass for 1 month.

RADIOLOGY FINDINGS

Fig. 1.1 (**a**) CC, (**b**) MLO, and (**c**) ML images show a radiolucent oval circumscribed mass, corresponding to a triangular marker indicating a palpable mass.
Fig. 1.2 Grayscale ultrasound image shows a nearly isoechoic oval circumscribed mass.

BI-RADS ASSESSMENT

BI-RADS 2. Benign finding.

DIAGNOSIS

Lipoma

DISCUSSION

- A lipoma is a benign fatty mass that presents as a radiolucent mass surrounded by a thin pseudocapsule on mammogram.
- Clinically, lipomas are soft and mobile.
- May distort the breast architecture on mammogram by displacing the adjacent normal breast tissue.
- On ultrasound, a lipoma is seen as a hypoechoic, isoechoic, or hyperechoic oval or round circumscribed mass parallel to the skin, with an echotexture similar to the subcutaneous fat.
- The diagnosis usually can be made on mammogram without the need for ultrasound.

REFERENCES

Applebaum AH, Evans GF, Levy KR, Amirkhan RH, Schumpert TD. Mammographic appearance of male breast disease. Radiographics. 1999;19:559–68.

Kopans DB. Breast imaging. 2nd ed. Philadelphia: Lippincott Williams and Wilkins; 1998. p. 551–4.

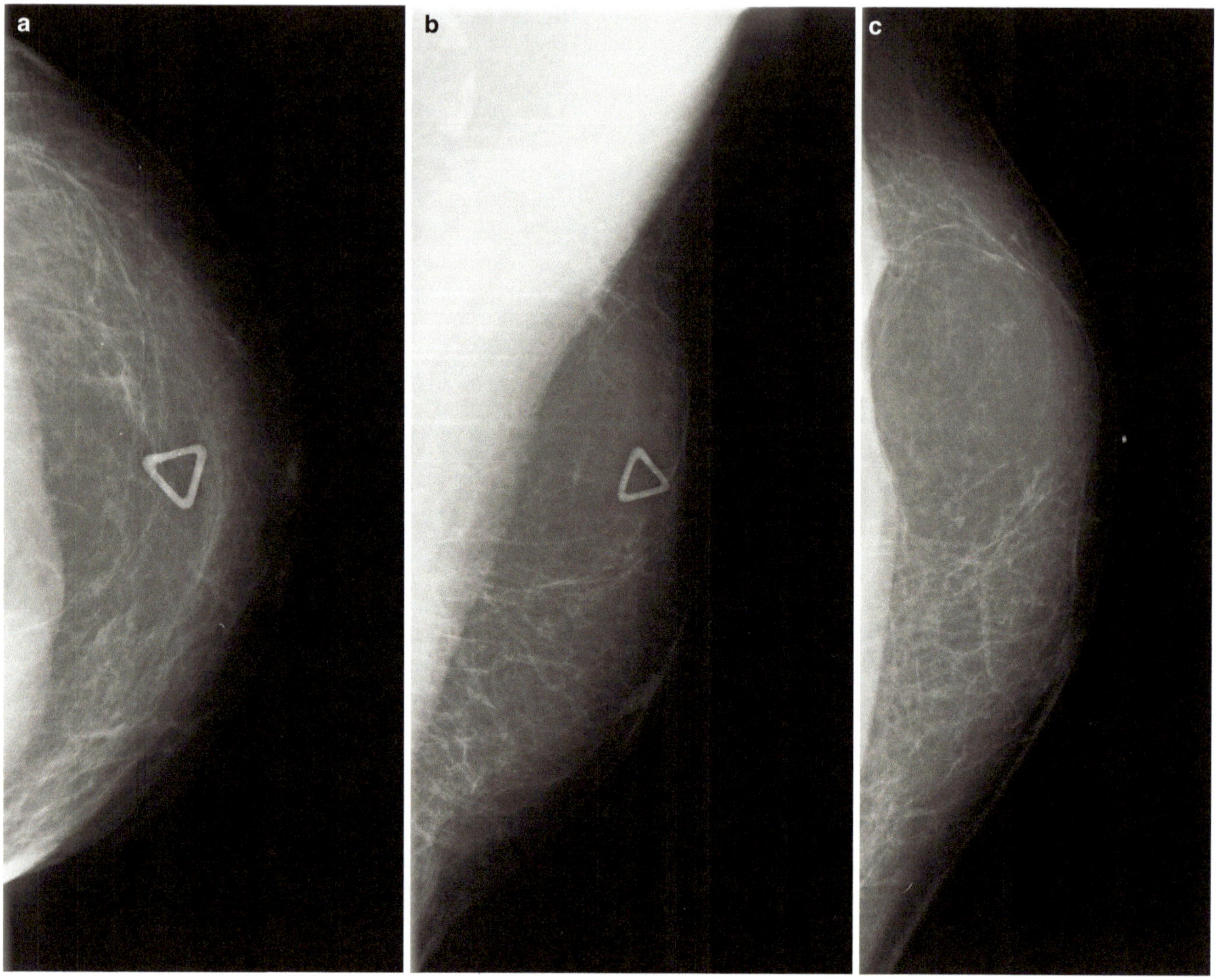

a   **b**   **c**

Fig. 1.1

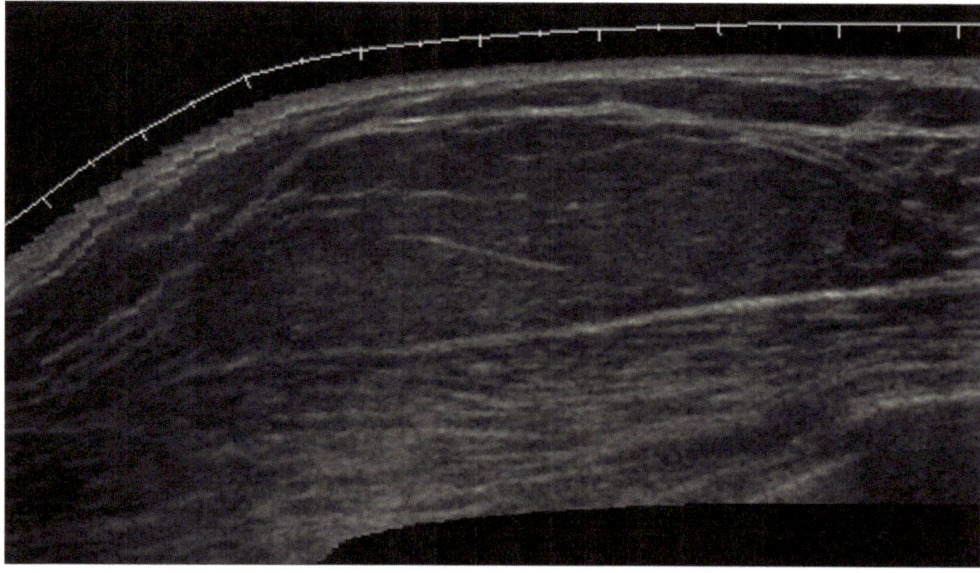

Fig. 1.2

CASE 25
ADENOID CYSTIC CARCINOMA

PATIENT HISTORY

A 47-year-old female with a history of focal left breast pain.

RADIOLOGY FINDINGS

Fig. 1.1 (a) CC, **(b)** MLO, and spot-compression **(c)** CC and **(d)** ML views show an oval mass with partially obscured margins in the subareolar region of the left breast.
Fig. 1.2 (a) Grayscale and **(b)** color Doppler images show an oval circumscribed avascular mass in the subareolar region of the left breast.

BI-RADS ASSESSMENT

BI-RADS 4. Suspicious abnormality (following diagnostic workup, prior to biopsy).

DIAGNOSIS

Adenoid cystic carcinoma

DISCUSSION

- Adenoid cystic carcinoma is a rare malignant breast tumor.
- Typically, a slow-growing lobular mass is seen clinically.
- Median size is 2 cm with a range between 0.2 and 12 cm.
- Commonly seen in the subareolar or central region but can occur anywhere in the breast.
- Excellent prognosis. Recurrence is possible if mass is not completely excised.
- Imaging characteristics vary and range from a circumscribed mass to ill-defined mass or focal asymmetries.

REFERENCES

Berg WA, Birdwell RL, Gombos EC, et al. Diagnostic imaging breast. 1st ed. Salt Lake City: Amirsys; 2006. Section IV-2, p. 102–3.
Ikeda DM. Breast imaging the requisites. 2nd ed. Philadelphia: Elsevier, Mosby; 2011. p. 131.
Santamarie G, Velasco M, Zanon G, et al. Adnoid cystic carcinoma of the breast: mammographic appearance and pathologic correlation. AJR. 1998;171:1679–83.

Fig. 1.1

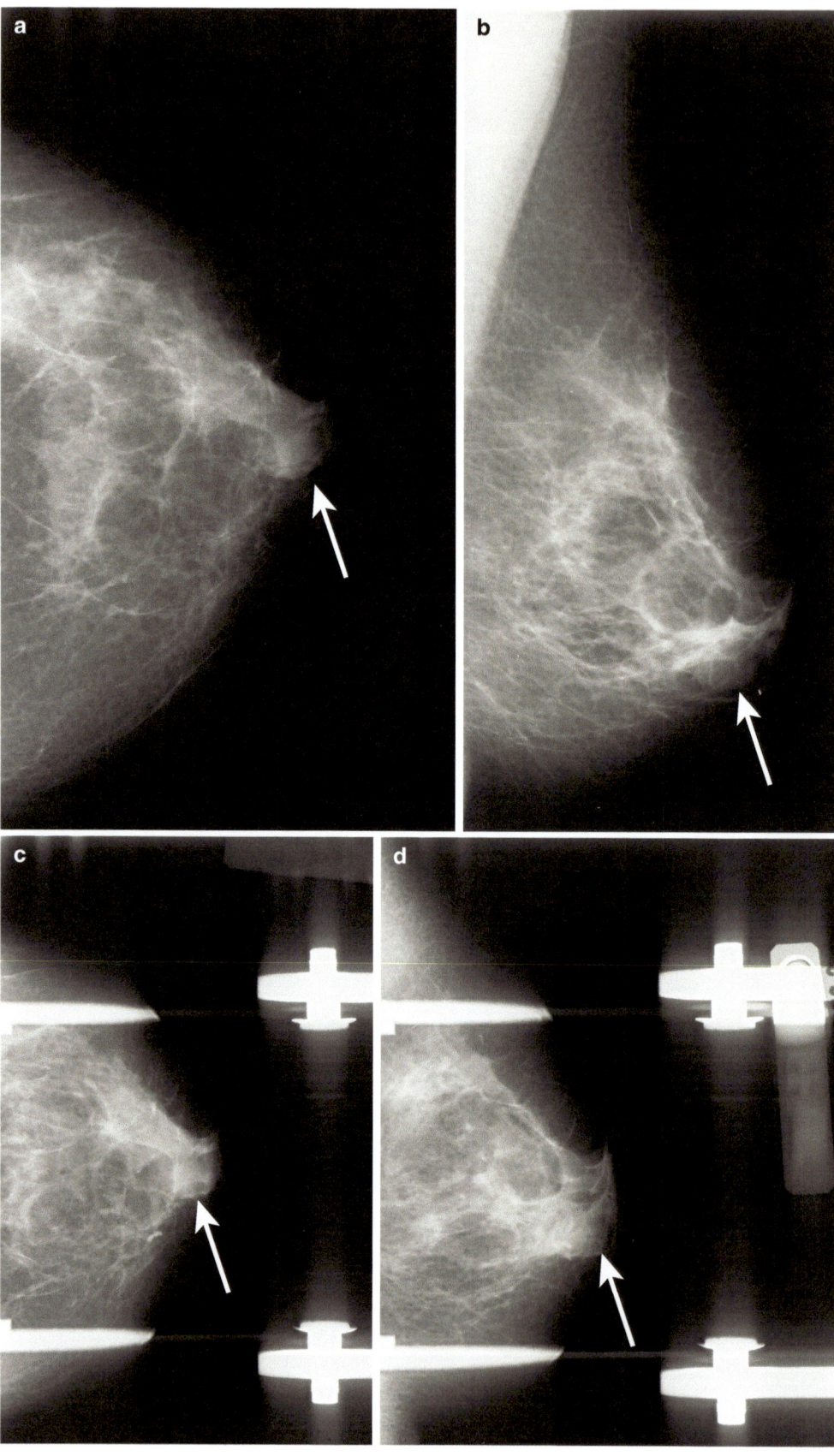

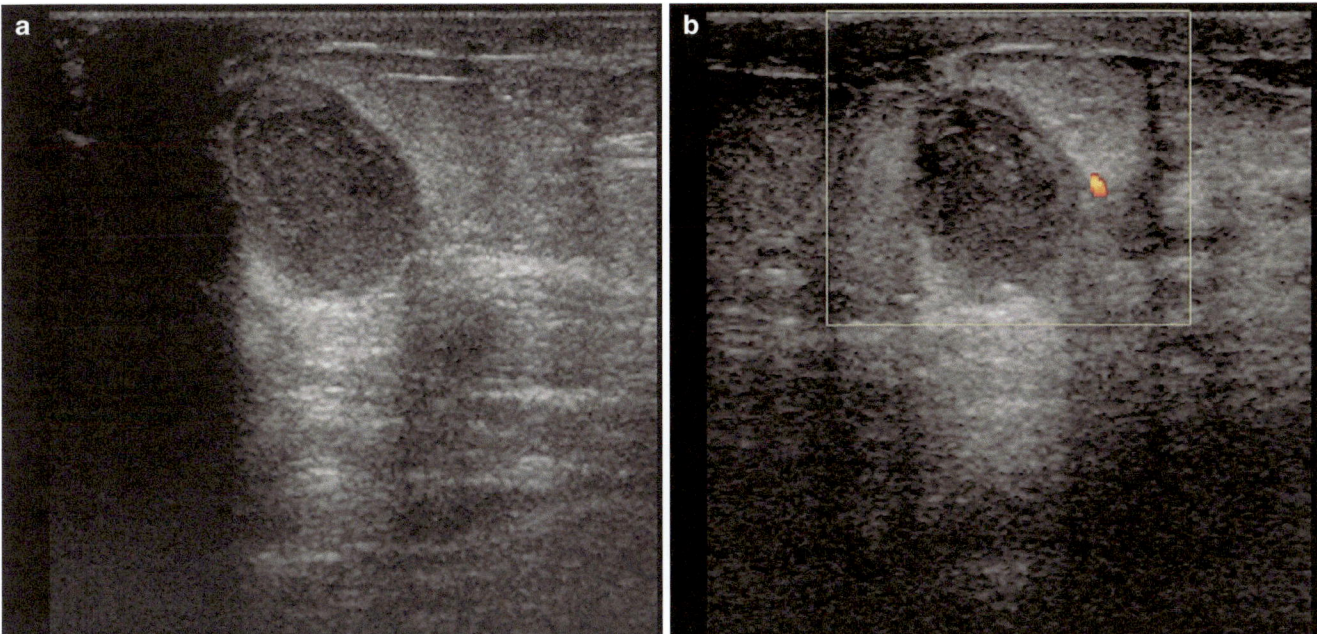

Fig. 1.2

Case 26
Diabetic Mastopathy

Patient History

A 31-year-old female with a palpable mass in the retroareolar right breast. The patient is on dialysis.

Radiology Findings

Fig. 1.1 Bilateral (**a**, **b**) CC and (**c**, **d**) MLO, and right spot-compression (**e**) CC and (**f**) MLO views show no discrete mass. There is a focal asymmetry in the retroareolar right breast when compared with that of the left. There is a perma-catheter incidentally seen in the upper right breast.

Fig. 1.2 (**a**, **b**) Grayscale and (**c**) color Doppler ultrasound images show a hypoechoic avascular mass with indistinct margins in the retroareolar region of the right breast, corresponding to the patient's palpable mass.

BI-RADS Assessment

BI-RADS 2. Benign finding (following diagnostic workup and biopsy).

Diagnosis

Diabetic mastopathy

Discussion

- Diabetic mastopathy is a variant of stromal fibrosis occurring in long-term insulin-dependent diabetics, in premenopausal women with long-standing insulin-dependent diabetes, or in rare patients with thyroid disease.
- Diabetic mastopathy results from an autoimmune reaction to the accumulation of abnormal matrix proteins caused by hyperglycemia.
- Clinical symptoms include palpable and firm, nontender masses, thickening of the breasts, or hard breasts.
- On mammography, increased parenchymal density may be seen unilaterally or in both the breasts.
- On ultrasound, a hypoechoic mass with indistinct margins can be seen.
- A biopsy is needed to establish the diagnosis.
- Excellent prognosis, self-limited.

References

Berg WA, Birdwell RL, Gombos EC, et al. Diagnostic imaging breast. 1st ed. Salt Lake City: Amirsys; 2006. Section IV-5, p. 30–1.

Ikeda DM. Breast imaging the requisites. 2nd ed. Philadelphia: Elsevier, Mosby; 2011. p. 400–1.

Sabate JM, Clotet M, Gomez A, De las Heras P, Torrubia S, Salinas T. Radiologic evaluation of uncommon inflammatory and reactive breast disorders. Radiographics. 2005;25:411–24.

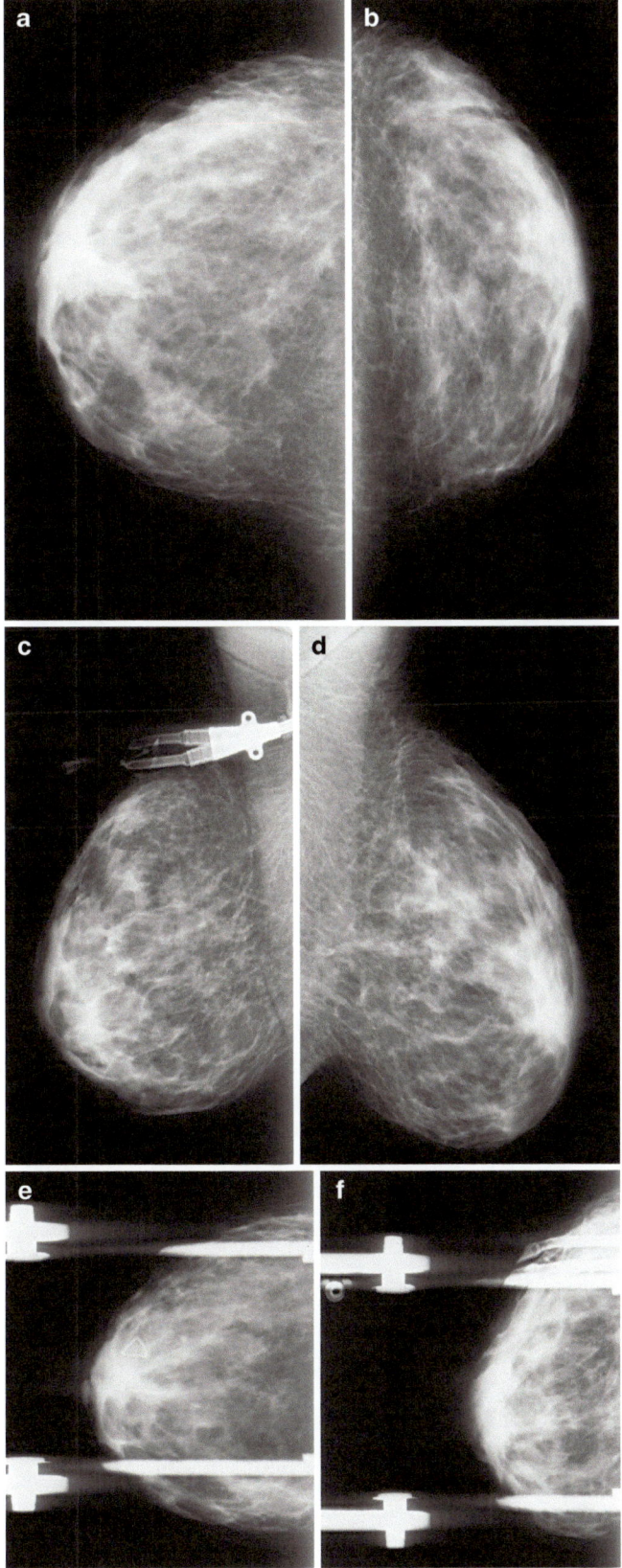

Fig. 1.1

Fig. 1.2

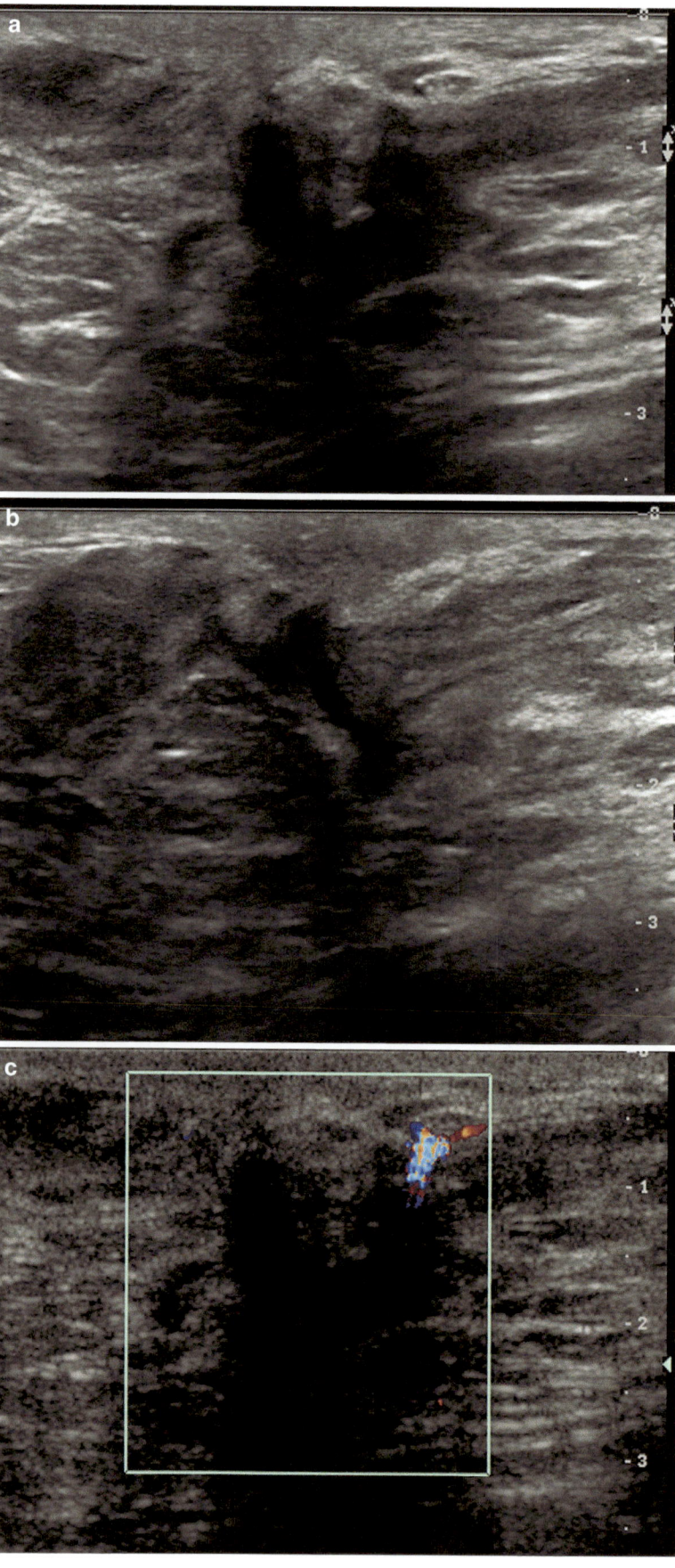

CASE 27
DIFFUSE BILATERAL BREAST CALCIFICATIONS

PATIENT HISTORY

A 79-year-old female for a bilateral screening mammogram.

RADIOLOGY FINDINGS

Fig. 1.1 (**a**, **b**) CC and (**c**, **d**) MLO views of both breasts show multiple diffuse secretory, vascular, round, and oval calcifications scattered diffusely bilaterally.

BI-RADS ASSESSMENT

BI-RADS 2. Benign findings.

DIAGNOSIS

Diffuse bilateral breast calcifications

DISCUSSION

- Multiple calcifications that are diffusely scattered throughout the breast are almost always benign.
- Diffuse calcifications must be randomly distributed to be considered benign.
- Round and punctuate calcifications are usually benign when they are scattered throughout both breasts.
- Round and punctuate calcifications usually develop within lobules.

REFERENCES

Harvey JA, March DE. Making the diagnosis: a practical guide to breast imaging. Philadelphia: Elsevier; 2013. p. 159.

Kopans D. Breast imaging. 3rd ed. Philadelphia: Lippincott Williams and Wilkins; 2006. p. 463.

Fig. 1.1

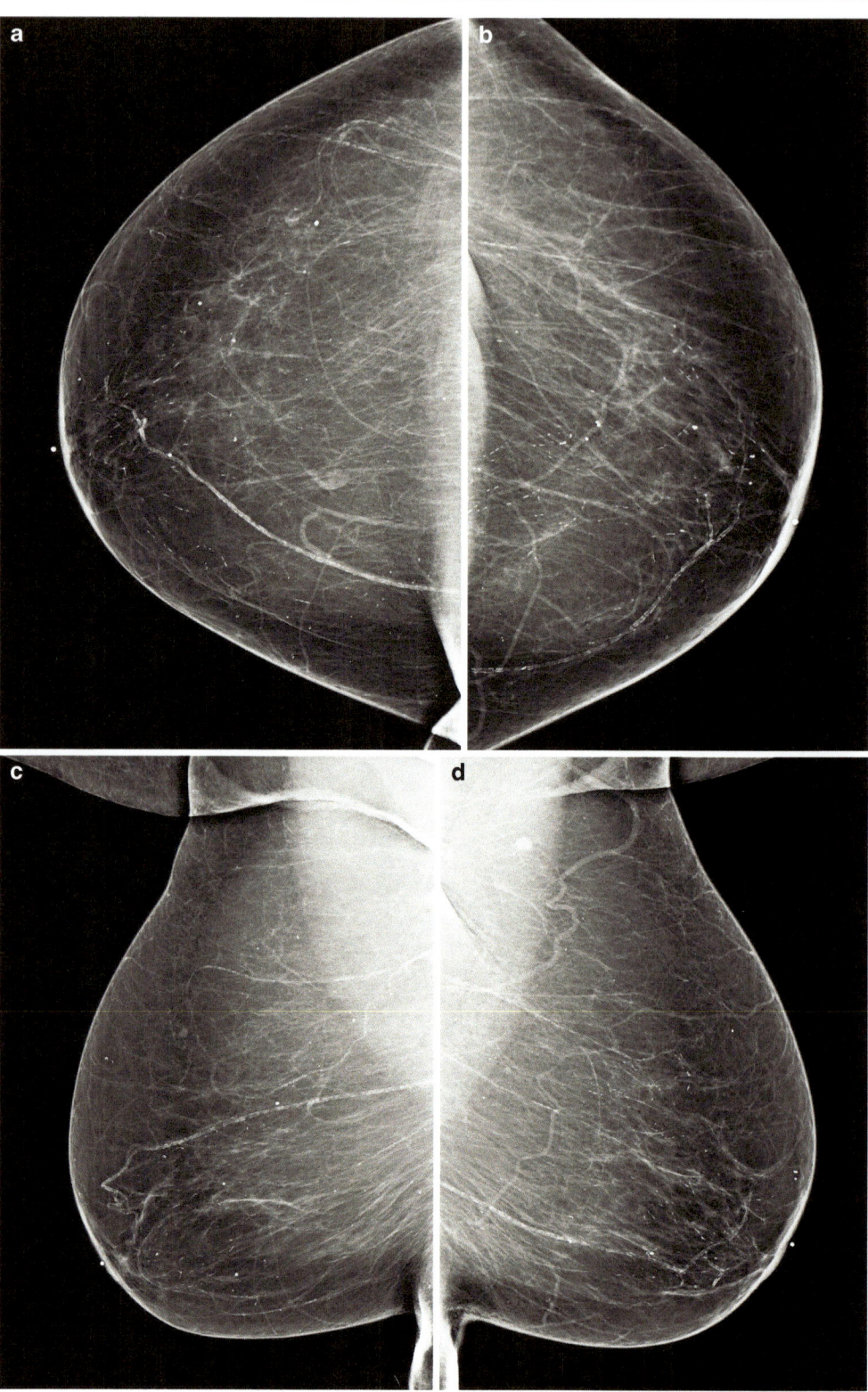

CASE 28
SUPERIOR VENA CAVA (SVC) SYNDROME

PATIENT HISTORY

Screening mammogram in a 62-year-old female recently diagnosed with lung cancer.

RADIOLOGY FINDINGS

Fig. 1.1 (**a**) CC and (**b**) MLO views demonstrate trabecular and skin thickening in the left breast. These findings were also seen in the contralateral breast (not shown).
Fig. 1.2 Axial contrast-enhanced CT of the thorax demonstrates an irregular heterogeneously enhancing mass in the anterior mediastinum causing displacement of the great vessels.
Fig. 1.3 PA view of the chest demonstrates a mass within the left anterior mediastinum causing deviation of the airway to the right.

DIAGNOSIS

Superior vena cava (SVC) syndrome

DISCUSSION

- SVC syndrome is caused by obstruction of flow in the SVC.
- Causes of obstruction include:
  - External compression
  - Intravascular mass
  - Thrombus
- Most common cause is bronchogenic carcinoma.
- Other malignancies causing SVC syndrome:
  - Metastases (commonly from breast)
  - Lymphoma
  - Thymoma
- Chest radiograph demonstrates widening of mediastinum with enlarged azygos vein.
- Right-sided mass is more common.
- Treatment depends on cause of obstruction.

REFERENCES

Berg WA, Birdwell RL, Gombos EC, et al. Diagnostic imaging breast. 1st ed. Salt Lake City: Amirsys; 2006. Section IV-5, p. 42–3.
Gurney J, Winer-Muram H, Stern E, et al. Diagnostic imaging chest. 1st ed. Salt Lake City: Amirsys; 2006. Section II-2, p. 48–51.

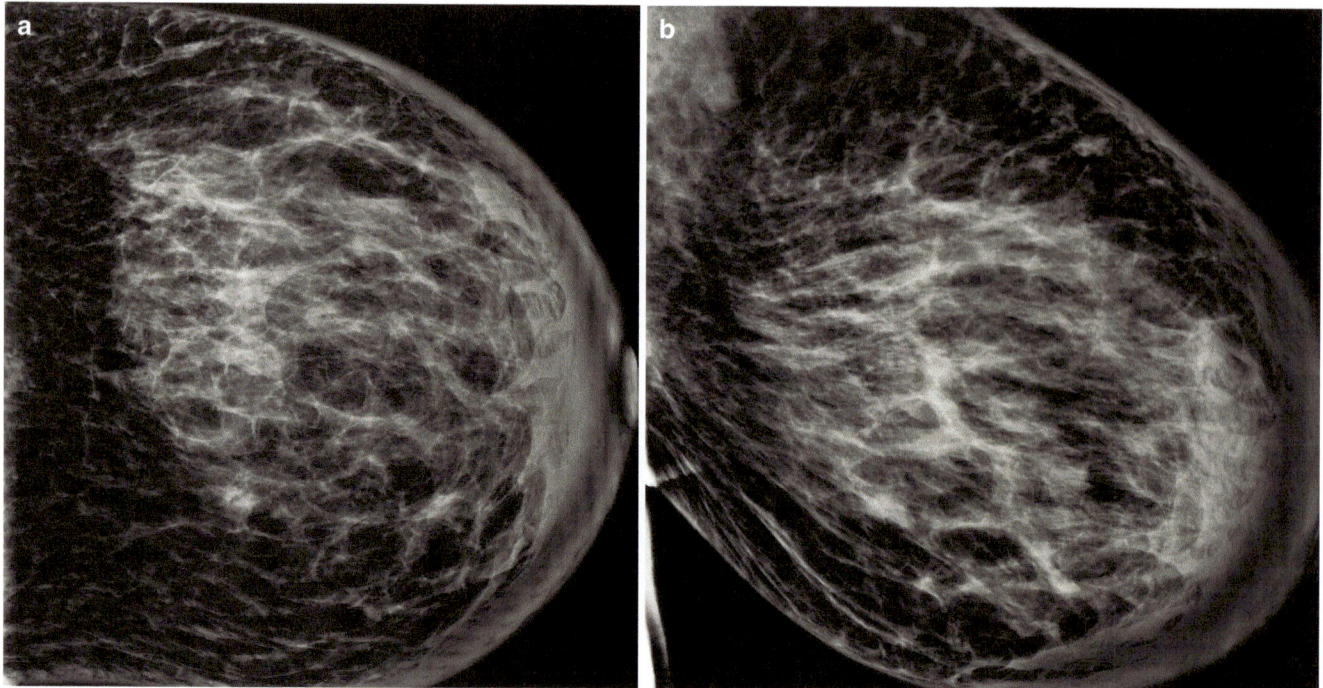

Fig. 1.1

Fig. 1.2

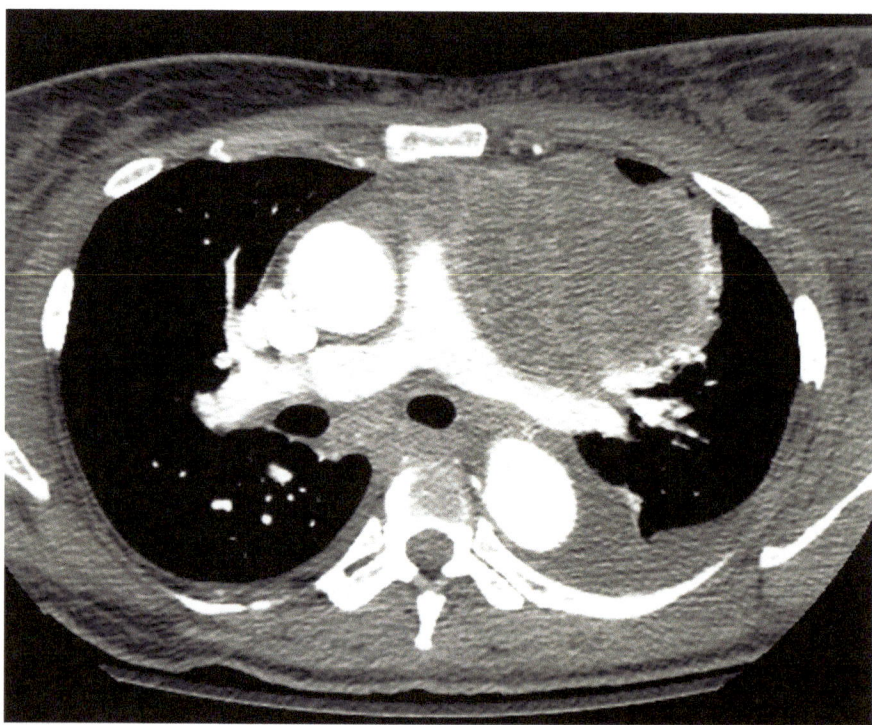

Fig. 1.3

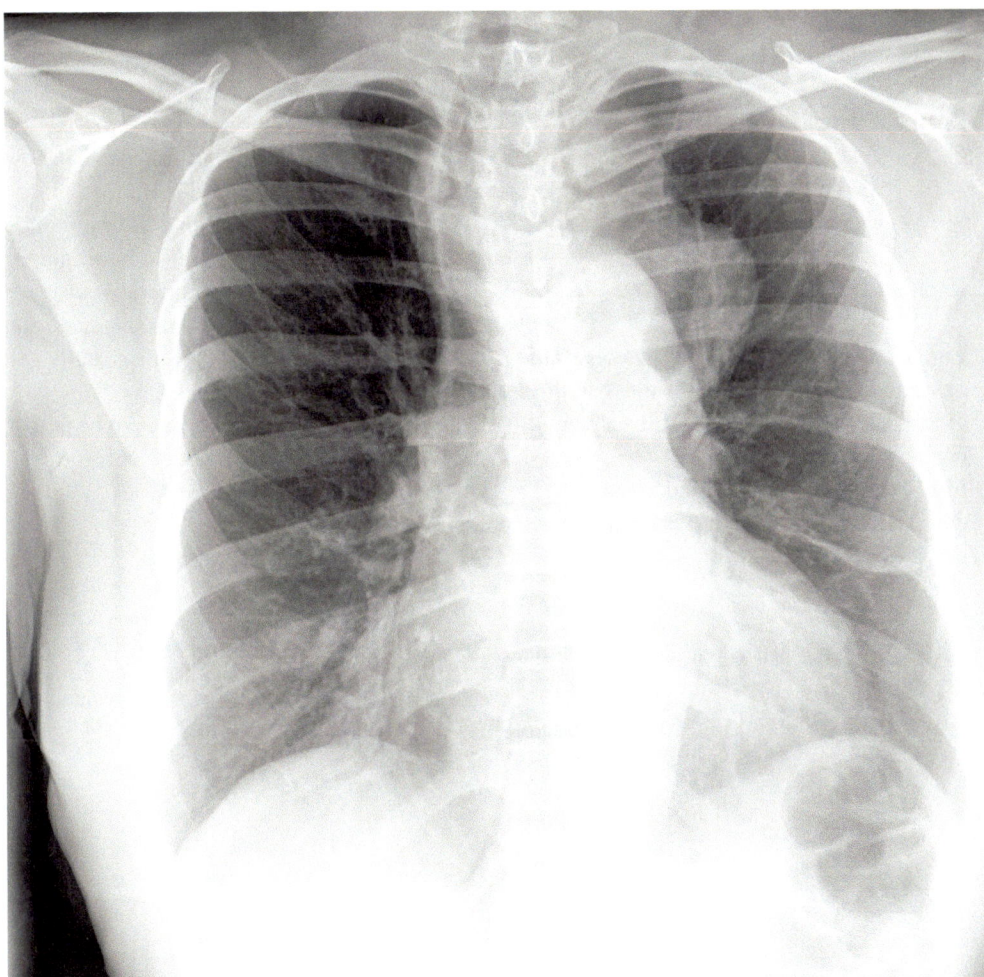

CASE 29
POSTOPERATIVE SEROMA

PATIENT HISTORY

A 64-year-old female who recently underwent lumpectomy.

RADIOLOGY FINDINGS

Fig. 1.1 (**a**) CC and (**b**) MLO views of the right breast demonstrate a high-density oval mass with circumscribed margins in the lower inner right breast extending from middle to posterior depth.

Fig. 1.2 (**a**) Grayscale and (**b**) color Doppler ultrasound demonstrate an anechoic avascular mass containing echogenic material.

BI-RADS ASSESSMENT

BI-RADS 2. Benign finding (following diagnostic workup).

DIAGNOSIS

Postoperative seroma

DISCUSSION

- Seromas are common complications of breast conservation surgery.
- Some studies have shown that risk factors for seroma formation include:
  - High body mass index
  - Increased drainage volume in the first 3 days postoperatively
  - Arterial hypertension
- Seromas are usually self-limited and can resolve on their own.
- Aspiration can be performed if the seroma is large enough to cause discomfort.

REFERENCES

Bassett LW, Jackson VP, Fu KL, Fu YS. Diagnosis of diseases of the breast. 2nd ed. Philadelphia: Elsevier; 2005. p 570–71.

Kuroi K, Shimozuma K, Taquchi T, et al. Evidence based risk factors for seroma formation in breast surgery. Jpn J Clin Oncol. 2006;36(4):197–206.

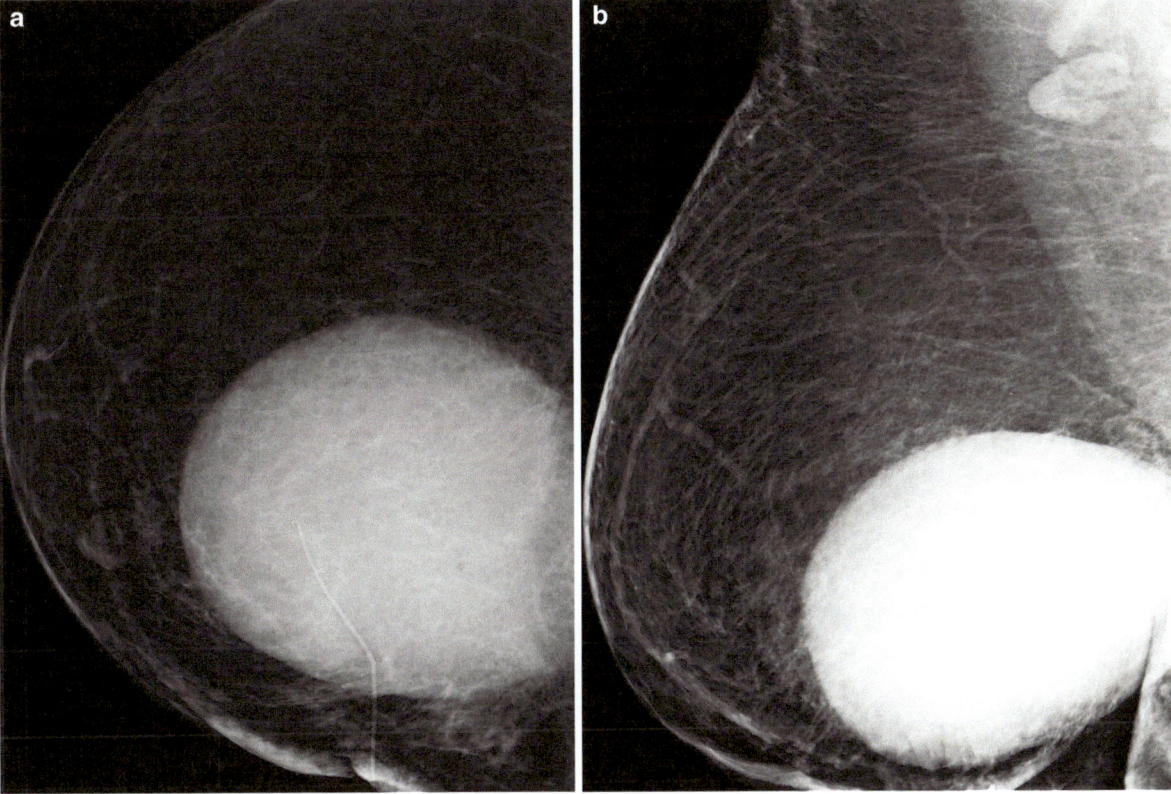

Fig. 1.1

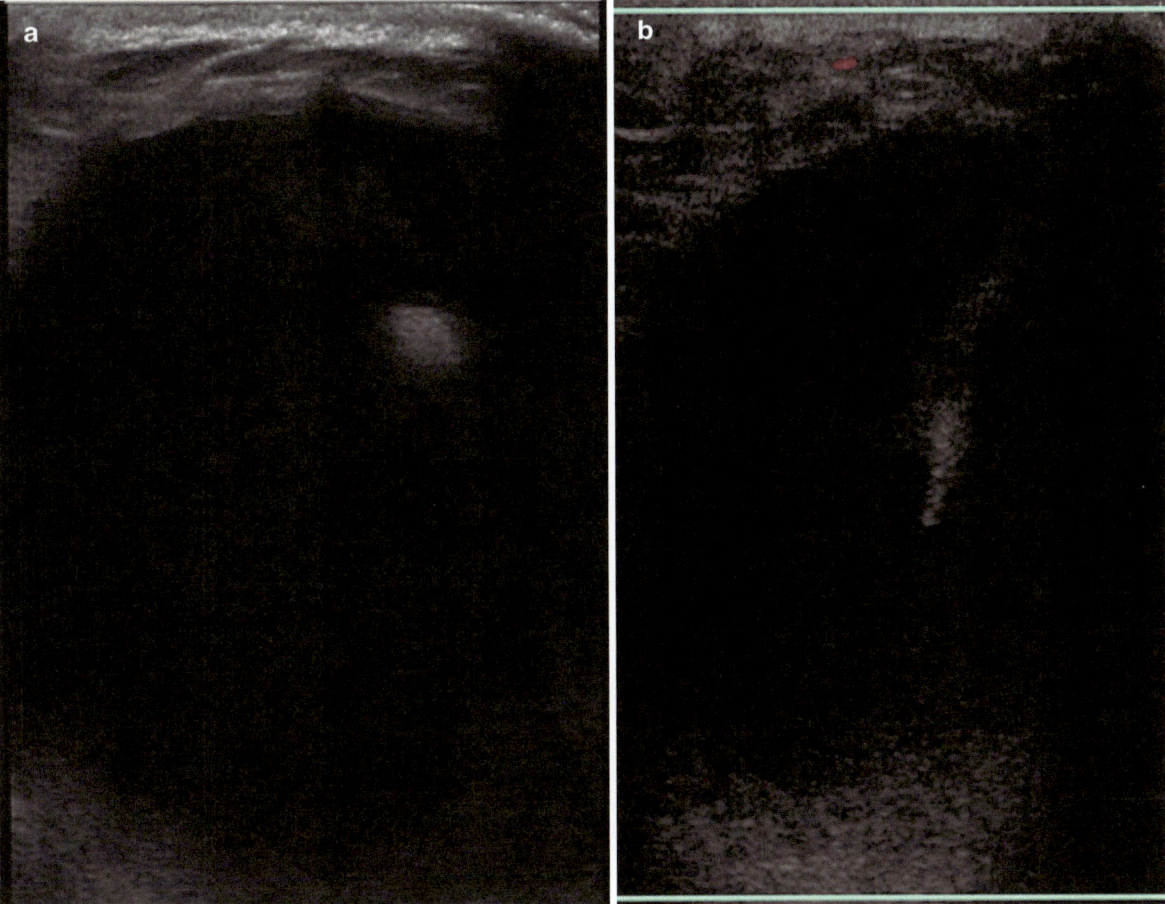

Fig. 1.2

Case 30
Medullary Carcinoma

Patient History

A 48-year-old female with a palpable left breast mass.

Radiology Findings

Fig. 1.1 (**a**) CC and (**b**) MLO images show a mass with partially obscured margins in the upper outer left breast at middle depth.

Fig. 1.2 Color Doppler ultrasound image shows an oval hypoechoic mass with ill-defined margins and vascular flow.

Fig. 1.3 (**a**) Axial subtracted T1-weighted, (**b**) axial contrast-enhanced T1-weighted, and (**c**) sagittal contrast-enhanced delayed T1-weighted images show a rim-enhancing mass with spiculated margins in the upper outer left breast at middle depth.

BI-RADS Assessment

BI-RADS 5. Highly suggestive of malignancy (following diagnostic workup, prior to biopsy).

Diagnosis

Medullary carcinoma

Discussion

- Medullary carcinoma accounts for 5–7 % of all breast cancers.
- More common in younger women.
- Fast growth rate, locally aggressive.
- On mammogram, medullary carcinoma is a uniformly dense, round, or oval noncalcified mass with indistinct or circumscribed margins.
- On ultrasound, a solid homogeneously hypoechoic mass is seen.
- As medullary cancer can have smooth margins and firm consistency, a fibroadenoma is often considered in the clinical and imaging differential diagnosis.
- A moderately enhancing mass is seen on MRI.

References

Cardenosa G. Breast imaging companion. 2nd ed. Philadelphia: Lippincott Williams and Wilkins; 2001. p. 258.

Meyer JE, Amin E, Lindfors KK, Lipman JC, Stomper PC, Genest D. Medullary carcinoma of the breast: mammographic and ultrasound appearance. Radiology. 1989;170:79–82.

Morris EA, Liberman L, editors. Breast MRI diagnosis and intervention. New York: Springer; 2005. p. 179.

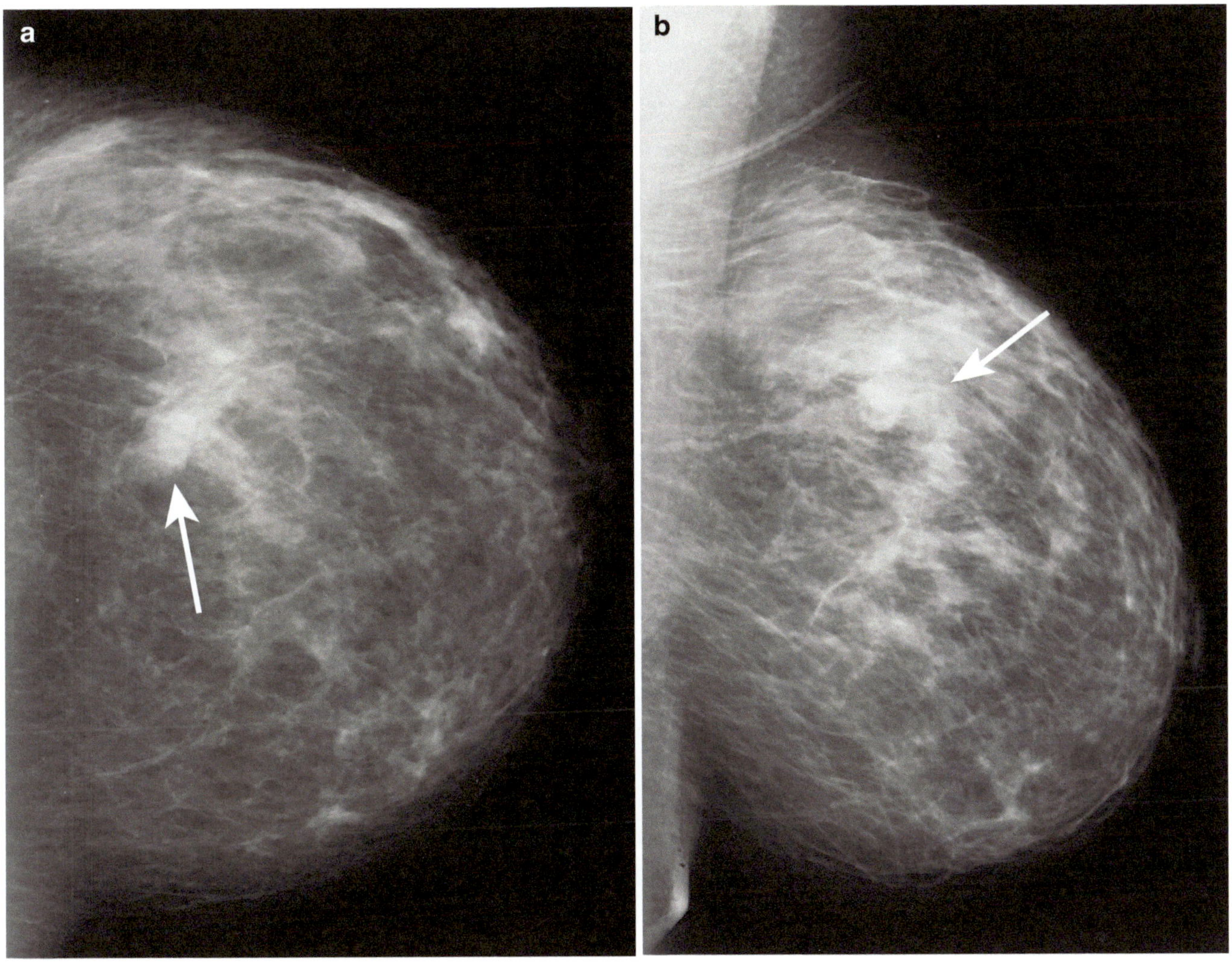

a

b

Fig. 1.1

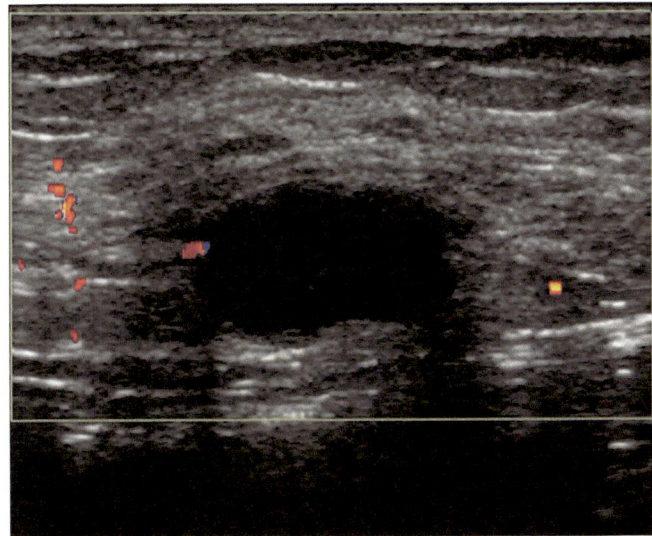

Fig. 1.2

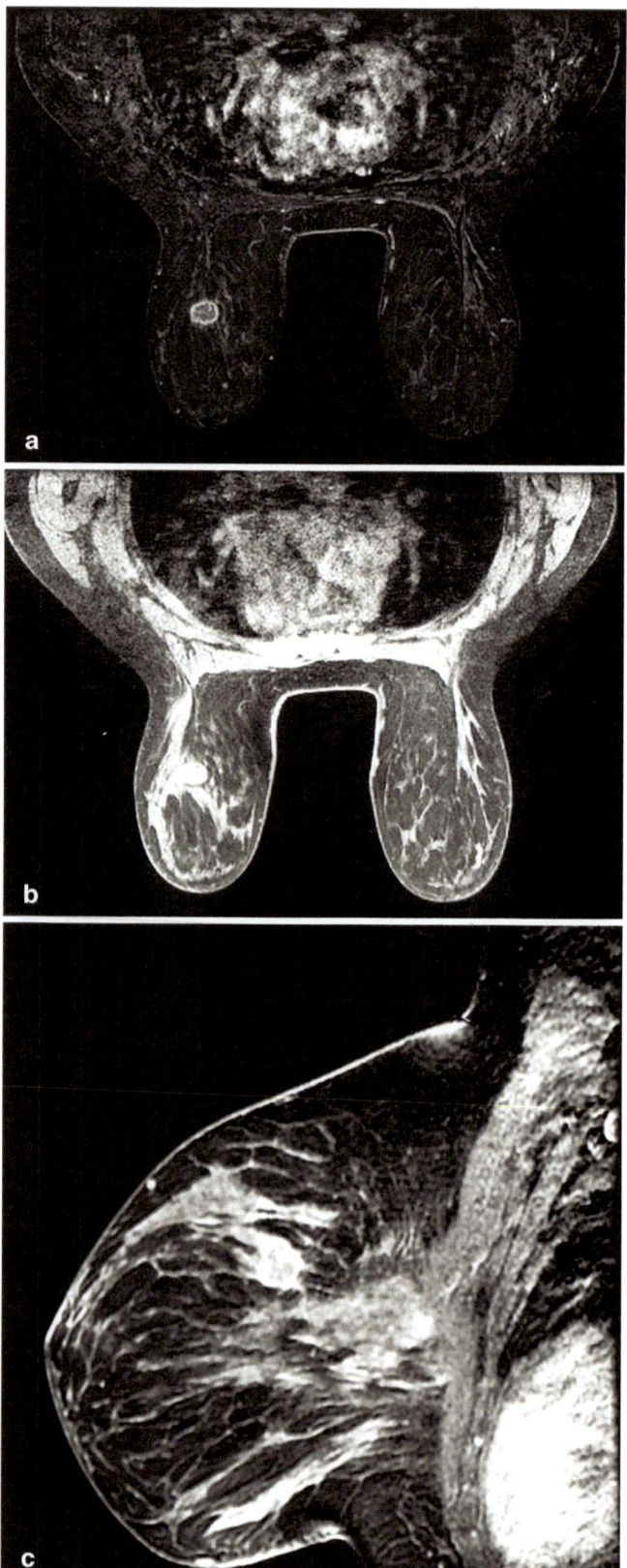

Fig. 1.3

CASE 31
LOBULAR CARCINOMA IN SITU (LCIS)

PATIENT HISTORY

A 46-year-old female for a screening mammogram.

RADIOLOGY FINDINGS

Fig. 1.1 (**a**) Spot magnification CC and (**b**) spot-magnification ML images show clustered pleomorphic calcifications at 12 o'clock middle depth in the left breast.

ASSESSMENT

High-risk lesion.

DIAGNOSIS

Lobular carcinoma in situ (LCIS)

DISCUSSION

- LCIS is a high-risk lesion associated with an increased risk of malignancy in either breast.

- There is an 11 times increased risk of breast cancer with the diagnosis of LCIS.
- LCIS is usually found as an incidental finding at biopsy.
- There is no pathognomonic appearance of LCIS on mammogram or ultrasound.
- LCIS is characterized by a monomorphic population of cells expanding breast lobules.
- Management of LCIS on core needle biopsy is controversial, ranging from recommendation of surgical excision to a 6-month follow-up mammogram, depending on concordance of biopsy.

REFERENCES

Berg WA, Mrose HE, Ioffe OB. ALH or LCIS at core needle breast biopsy. Radiology. 2001;218:503–9.

Foster MC, Helvie MA, Gregory NE, Rebner M, Nees AV, Paramagul C. LCIS or ALH at core needle biopsy: is excisional biopsy necessary? Radiology. 2004;231:813–19.

Harvey JA, March DE. Making the diagnosis: a practical guide to breast imaging. Philadelphia: Elsevier; 2013. p. 295.

Fig. 1.1

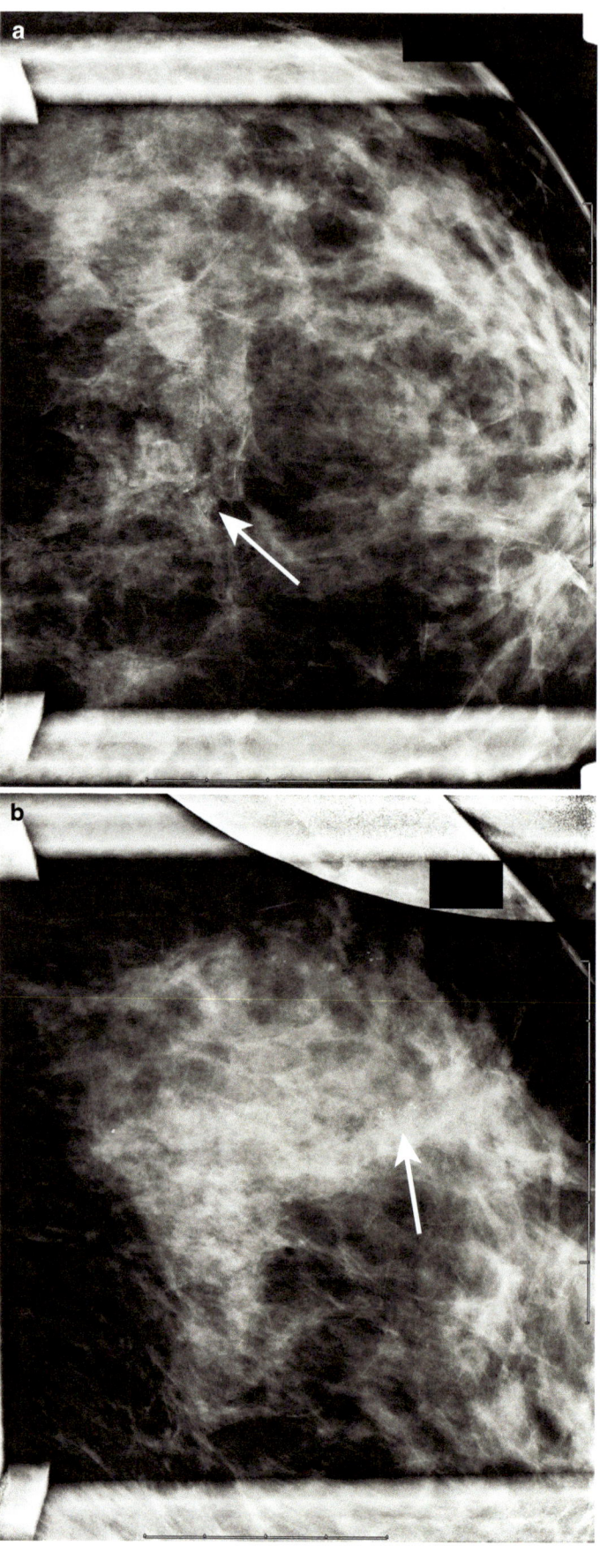

CASE 32
JUVENILE FIBROADENOMA

PATIENT HISTORY

An 18-year-old female with a palpable mass at 12 o'clock in the right breast.

RADIOLOGY FINDINGS

Fig. 1.1 (**a**, **b**) Grayscale and (**c**) color Doppler ultrasound images show an oval hypoechoic mass with circumscribed margins. There is vascular flow within the mass.

BI-RADS ASSESSMENT

BI-RADS 2. Benign findings (following diagnostic workup and biopsy).

DIAGNOSIS

Juvenile fibroadenoma

DISCUSSION

- The most common breast mass in girls younger than 20 years of age is a fibroadenoma.
- A juvenile fibroadenoma is an uncommon variant, accounting for 7–8 % of all fibroadenomas.
- Most common in African-American girls.
- Juvenile fibroadenomas grow quickly and can attain a very large size.
- Clinically, can be seen as a rapidly enlarging breast, skin ulceration, and/or distended superficial veins.
- On ultrasound, a hypoechoic circumscribed mass is seen.
- The differential diagnosis includes a fibroadenoma and phyllodes tumor.

REFERENCES

Cardenosa G. Breast imaging companion. 2nd ed. Philadelphia: Lippincott Williams and Wilkins; 2001. p. 291.
Chung EM, Cube R, Hall GJ, Gonzalez C, Stocker JT, Glassman LM. Breast masses in children and adolescents: radiologic-pathologic correlation. Radiographics 2009;29:907–31.

Fig. 1.1

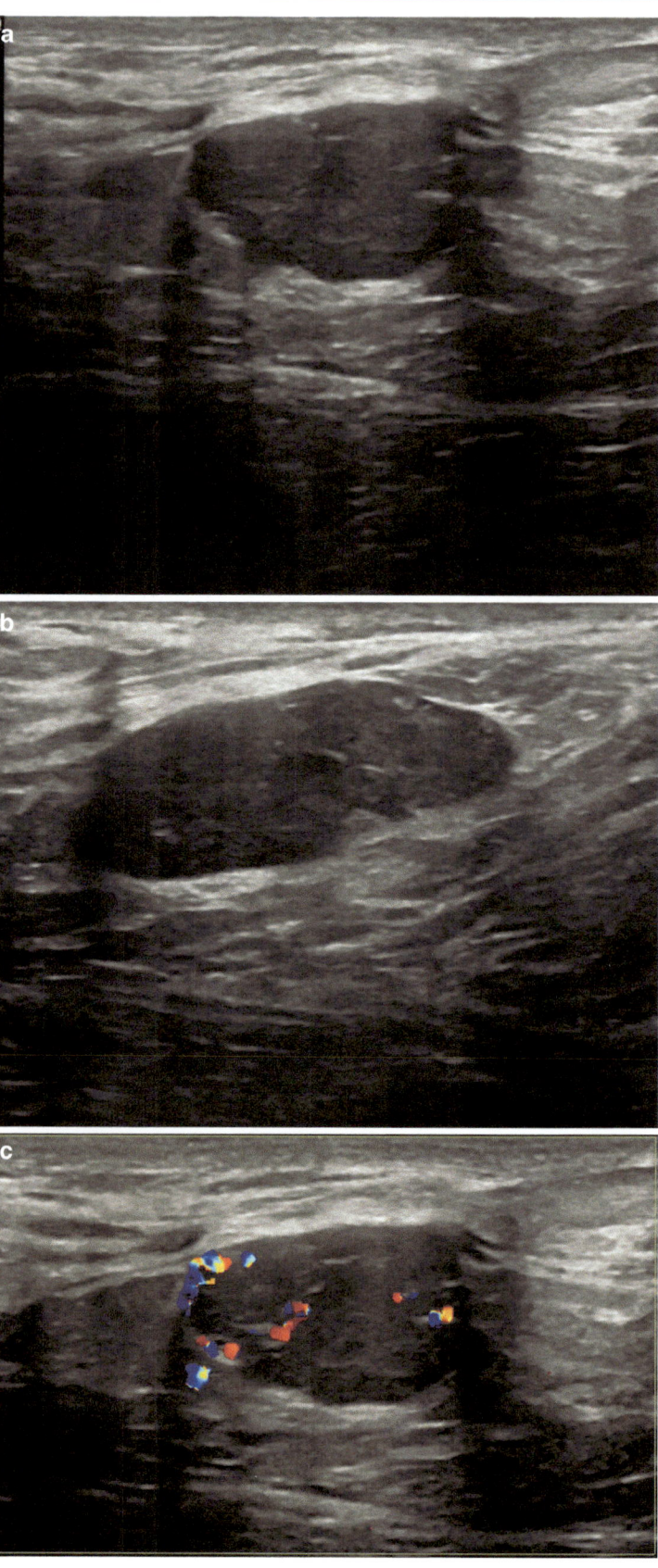

CASE 33
SIMPLE CYST

PATIENT HISTORY

A 41-year-old female with a palpable mass at 1 o'clock of the left breast.

RADIOLOGY FINDINGS

Fig. 1.1 (**a**) Spot-compression CC and (**b**) spot-compression MLO views demonstrate an oval mass with circumscribed and partially obscured margins in the upper outer left breast at middle depth.
Fig. 1.2 (**a**, **b**) Grayscale ultrasound images demonstrate an anechoic mass with imperceptible walls and posterior acoustic enhancement.

BI-RADS ASSESSMENT

BI-RADS 2. Benign finding. (Following diagnostic workup).

DIAGNOSIS

Simple cyst

DISCUSSION

- Cysts are collections of fluid with an epithelial lining.
- Most common breast mass in women.
- More common between 40 and 50 years.
- Rare in postmenopausal females.
- Cannot distinguish cysts from circumscribed solid masses on mammography.
- Simple cysts have no malignant potential.
- May fluctuate in size due to menstrual cycle.
- Asymptomatic, nonpalpable simple cysts do not require intervention.
- Painful or palpable cysts can be aspirated for patients' comfort.
- Benign cyst fluid is typically cloudy yellow or greenish black.

REFERENCES

Bassett L, Jackson V, Fu KL, Fu YS. Diagnosis of diseases of the breast. 2nd ed. Philadelphia: Elsevier; 2005. p. 432–7.
Berg W, Campassi C, Ioffe O. Cystic lesions of the breast: sonographic – pathologic correlation. Radiology. 2003;227:183–91.
Berg WA, Birdwell RL, Gombos EC, et al. Diagnostic imaging breast. 1st ed. Salt Lake City: Amirsys; 2006. Section IV-1, p. 48–51.

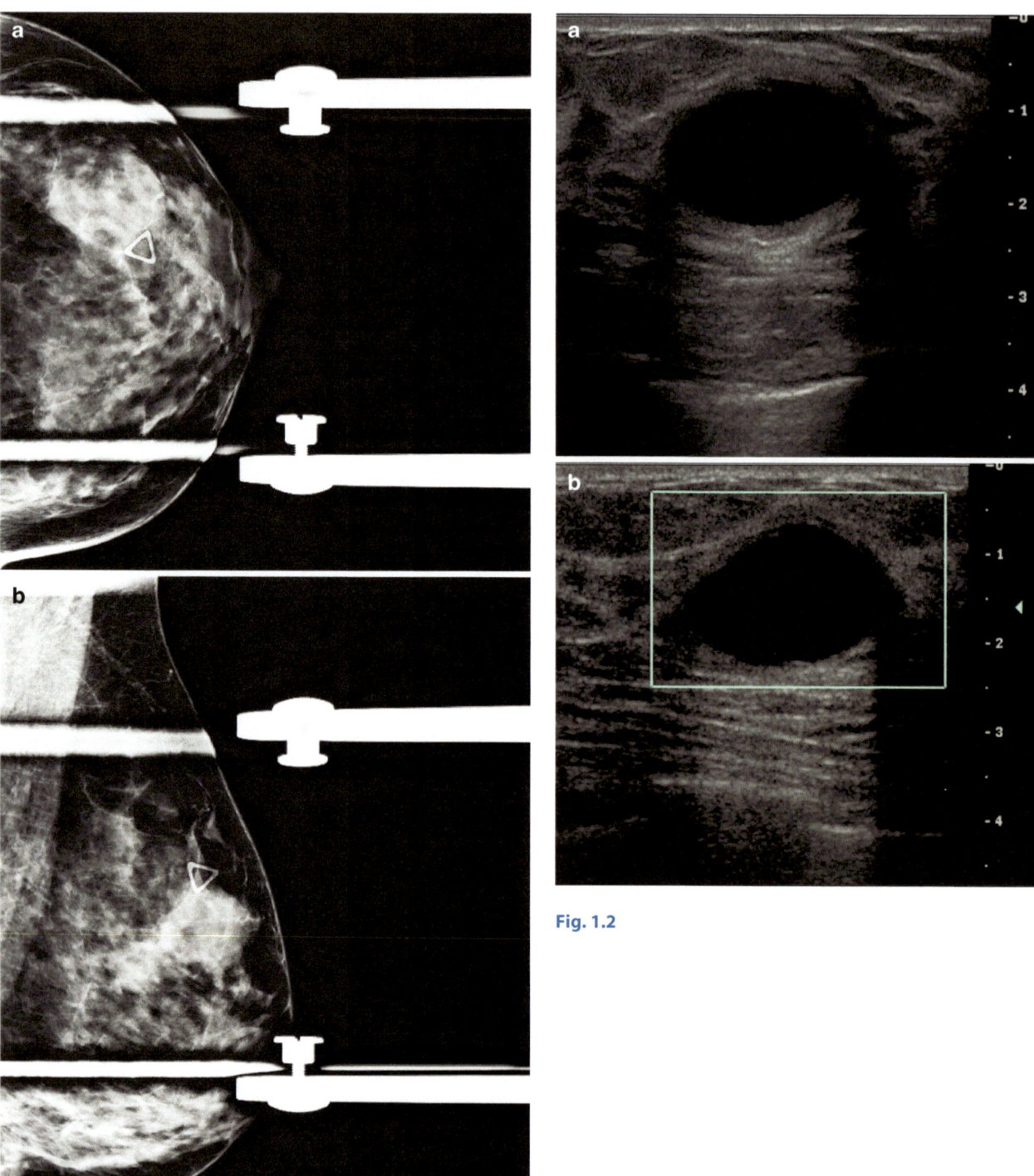

Fig. 1.1

Fig. 1.2

CASE 34
POLAND SYNDROME

PATIENT HISTORY

A 53-year-old female for a screening mammogram.

RADIOLOGY FINDINGS

Fig. 1.1 (**a**, **b**) Bilateral MLO views demonstrate absence of the (**b**) left pectoralis major muscle.

BI-RADS ASSESSMENT

BI-RADS 1. Negative.

DIAGNOSIS

Poland syndrome

DISCUSSION

- Poland syndrome is a congenital unilateral hypoplasia or absence of the pectoralis major muscle.
- More common in males.
- More common on the right side.
- Autosomal recessive.
- Associated with:
  - Ipsilateral syndactyly and brachydactyly
  - Absence of pectoralis minor
  - Hypoplasia of ipsilateral breast
  - Atrophy of ipsilateral 2nd–4th ribs
  - Renal agenesis
- Associated with increased incidence of:
  - Breast cancer
  - Leukemia
  - Non-Hodgkin's lymphoma
  - Lung cancer
- Chest radiograph demonstrates unilateral hyperlucency.

REFERENCES

Berg WA, Birdwell RL, Gombos EC, et al. Diagnostic imaging breast. 1st ed. Salt Lake City: Amirsys; 2006. Section I, p. 11.
Gurney JW, Winer-Muram HT, Stern EJ, et al. Diagnostic imaging chest. 1st ed. Salt Lake City: Amirsys; 2006. Section III-2, p. 8–9.
Jeung MV, Gangi A, Gasser B, et al. Imaging of chest wall disorders. Radiographics 1999;19(3):617–37.

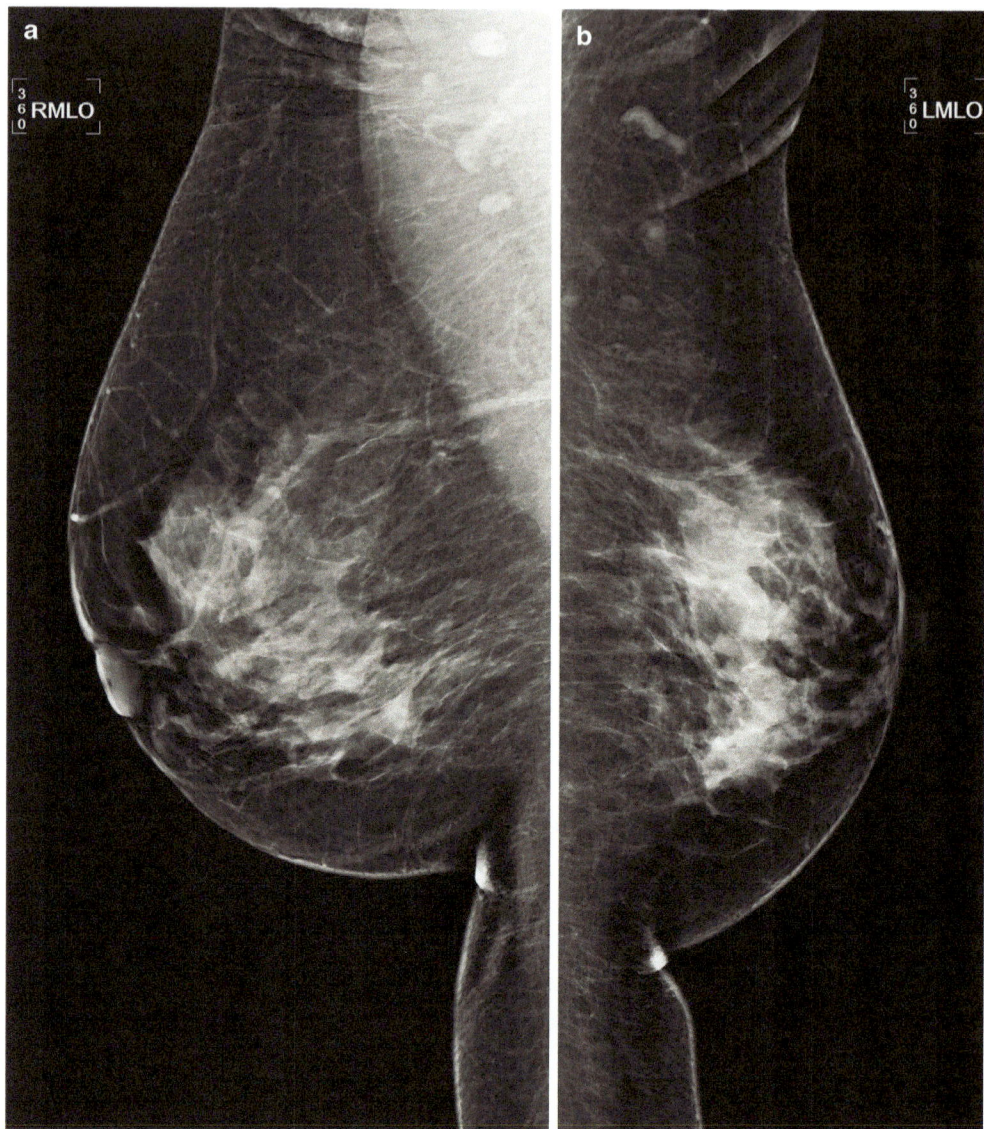

Fig. 1.1

Case 35
Intracystic Papillary Carcinoma

Patient History

A 76-year-old female for screening mammogram. Family history of mother with breast cancer.

Radiology Findings

Fig. 1.1 (**a**) CC, (**b**) ML, (**c**) spot-compression CC, and (**d**) spot-compression MLO images show an oval mass with predominantly circumscribed margins in the upper outer right breast at middle depth (*circle markers* correspond to skin moles).

Fig. 1.2 (**a**) Grayscale and (**b**) color Doppler ultrasound images show a hypoechoic mass with predominately circumscribed margins and an eccentric solid component with vascular flow.

BI-RADS Assessment

BI-RADS 4. Suspicious abnormality (following diagnostic workup, prior to biopsy).

Diagnosis

Intracystic papillary carcinoma

Discussion

- Intracystic papillary carcinoma is rare, representing 1–2 % of all breast cancers.
- Occurs most commonly in postmenopausal women.
- Slow growth rate; excellent prognosis.
- Can be asymptomatic or present as a palpable mass and/or bloody nipple discharge.
- Often a round or oval mass is seen in the retroareolar breast on mammogram.
- On ultrasound, an intracystic papillary carcinoma presents as a complex cystic mass which can contain:
  - Irregular septations
  - Hypoechoic mass within the cyst
  - Thickened cyst wall
  - Papillary projections
- MRI shows enhancement of cyst walls, septations, and mural nodules.

References

Dogan BE, Whitman GJ, Middleton LP, Phelps M. Intracystic papillary carcinoma of the breast. AJR. 2003;181:186.

Liberman L, Feng TL, Susnik B. Case 35: intracystic papillary carcinoma with invasion. Radiology. 2001;219:781–4.

Fig. 1.1

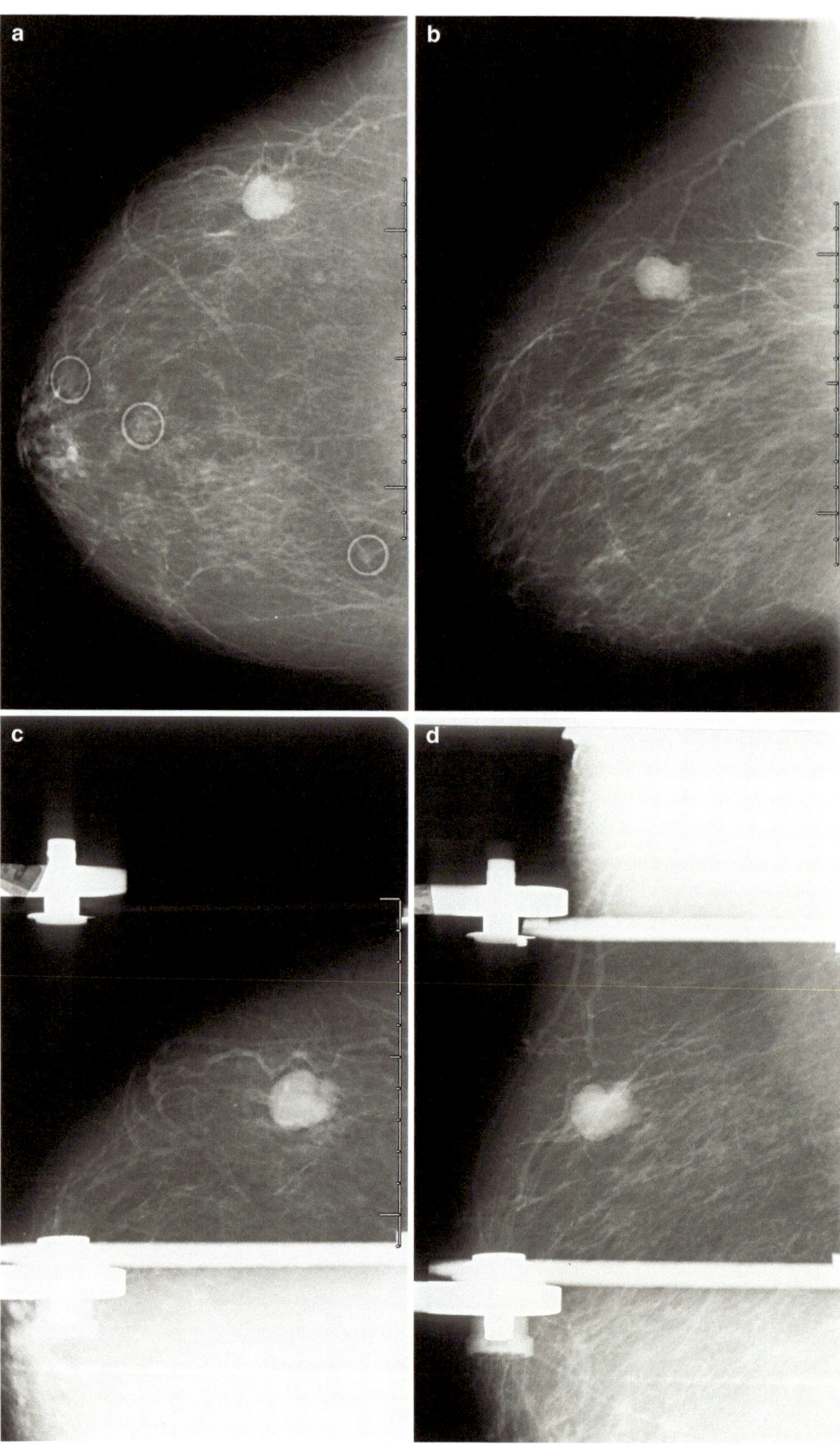

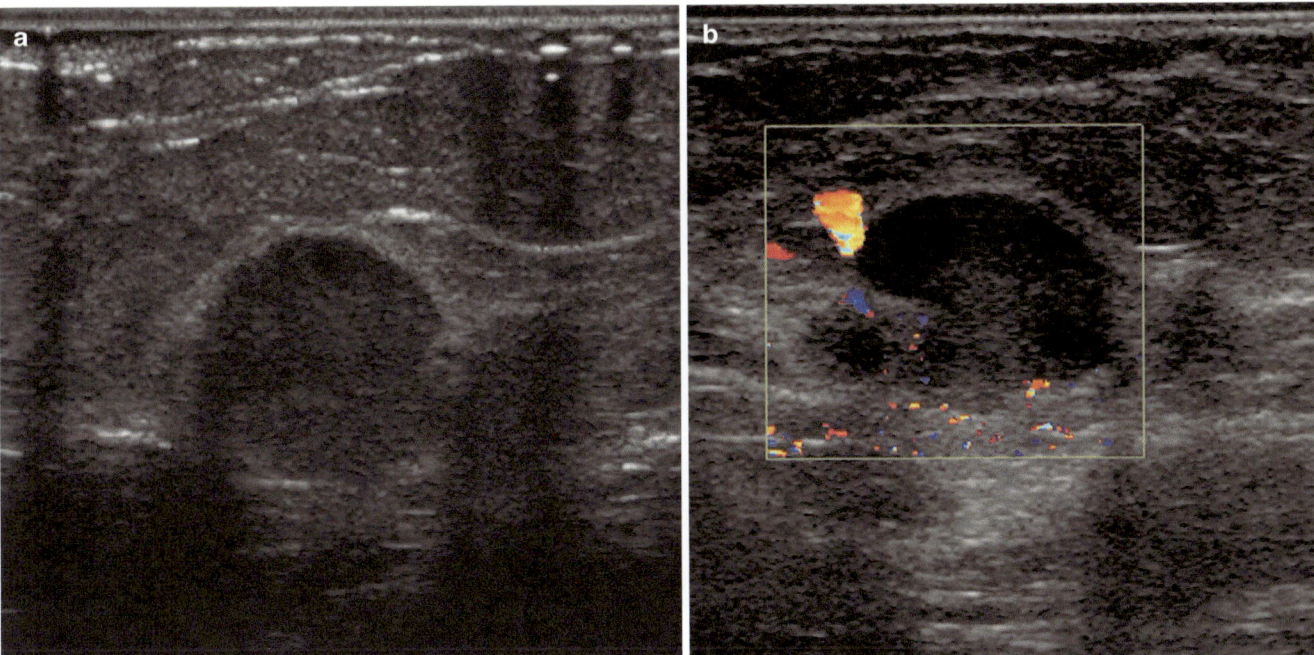

Fig. 1.2

CASE 36
INTRACAPSULAR RUPTURE OF SILICONE BREAST IMPLANT

PATIENT HISTORY

A 35-year-old female for evaluation of implant rupture.

RADIOLOGY FINDINGS

Fig. 1.1 (**a–c**) Grayscale ultrasound images show hyperechoic lines within the implant, often referred to as a "stepladder" appearance.

BI-RADS ASSESSMENT

BI-RADS 2. Benign finding (following diagnostic workup).

DIAGNOSIS

Intracapsular rupture of silicone breast implant

DISCUSSION

- Intracapsular rupture of a breast implant is defined as a disruption or tear of the implant shell, in which silicone gel moves outside of the implant shell but stays within the fibrous capsule.
- Intracapsular rupture occurs more commonly than extracapsular rupture.
- On ultrasound, an intracapsular rupture of a silicone implant is seen as pairs of hyperechoic lines, often referred to as a "stepladder" appearance.
- A rupture or tear of a saline implant is identified clinically, and imaging is not necessary to make the diagnosis.

REFERENCES

Berg WA, Caskey CI, Hamper UM, et al. Diagnosing breast implant rupture with MR imaging, ultrasound and mammography. Radiographics. 1993;13:1323–36.

Deangelis GA, Lange EE, Miller LR, Morgan RF. MR imaging of breast implants. Radiographics. 1994;14:783–94.

Everson LI, Parantainen H, Detlie T, et al. Diagnosis of breast implant rupture: imaging findings and relative efficacies of imaging techniques. AJR. 1994;163:57–60.

Fig. 1.1

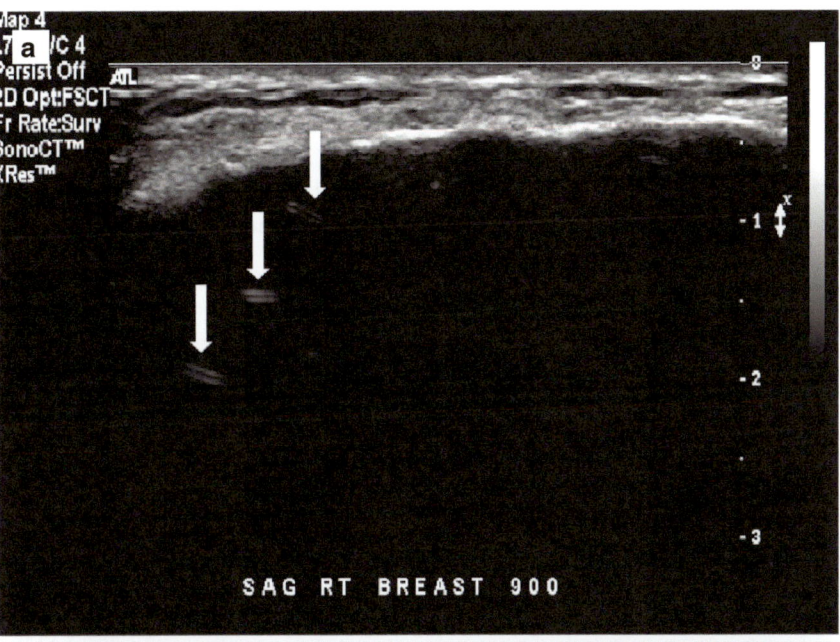

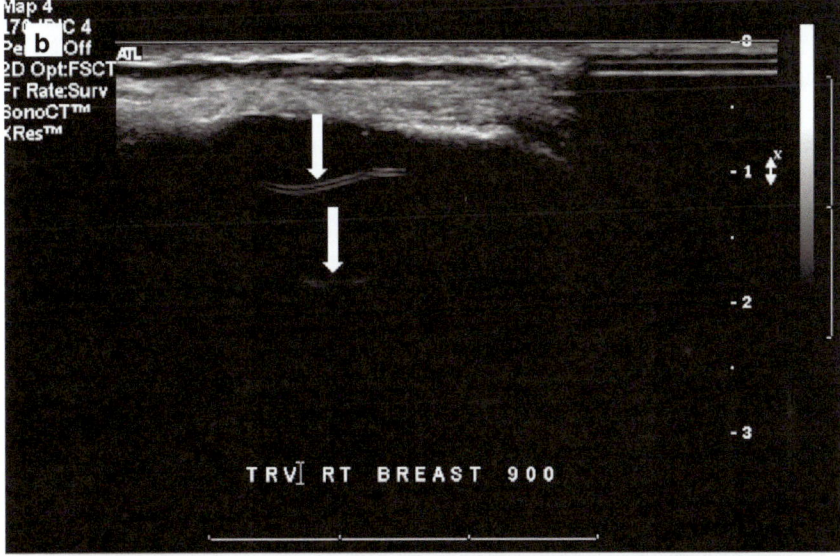

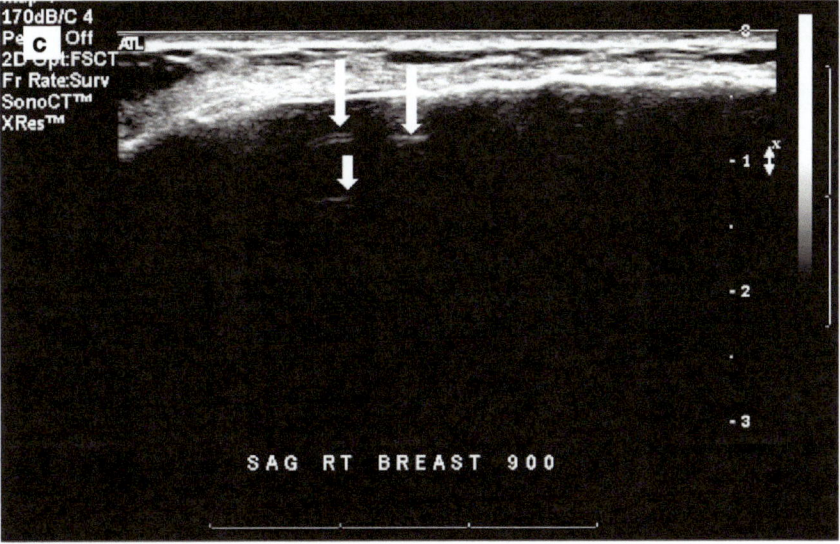

CASE 37
EXTRACAPSULAR RUPTURE OF SILICONE BREAST IMPLANT

PATIENT HISTORY

A 47-year-old female with a history of bilateral breast augmentation. The patient complains of deformity of the right breast.

RADIOLOGY FINDINGS

Fig. 1.1 Grayscale ultrasound of the right breast shows a hyperechoic area or "snowstorm" appearance.

BI-RADS ASSESSMENT

BI-RADS 2. Benign finding (following diagnostic workup).

DIAGNOSIS

Extracapsular rupture of silicone breast implant on ultrasound

DISCUSSION

• Classic appearance of extracapsular rupture on ultrasound is an intense echogenic area that obscures all findings posteriorly. This finding is referred to as a "snowstorm" appearance.
• Extracapsular rupture can appear as a hypoechoic mass that can be confirmed mammographically as an area of free silicone.
• Extracapsular rupture on MRI shows free silicone that is outside of the implant shell and fibrous capsule, best seen on MRI sequences that clearly demonstrate silicone, such as water-suppressed images.
• Extracapsular rupture is often caused by a strong external force such as trauma from a motor vehicle accident or closed capsulotomy (manual compression to break up a capsule causing pain).

REFERENCES

Ikeda DM. Breast imaging the requisites. 2nd ed. Philadelphia: Elsevier, Mosby; 2011. p. 348–50.
Mandell J. Core radiology: a visual approach to diagnostic imaging. 1st ed. Cambridge: Cambridge University Press; 2013. p. 647–9.
Molleran VM, Mahoney M. Breast MRI. 1st ed. Philadelphia; Saunders; 2014. p. 148–50.
Morris EA, Liberman L, editors. Breast MRI diagnosis and intervention. New York; Springer; 2005. p. 239–49.

Fig. 1.1

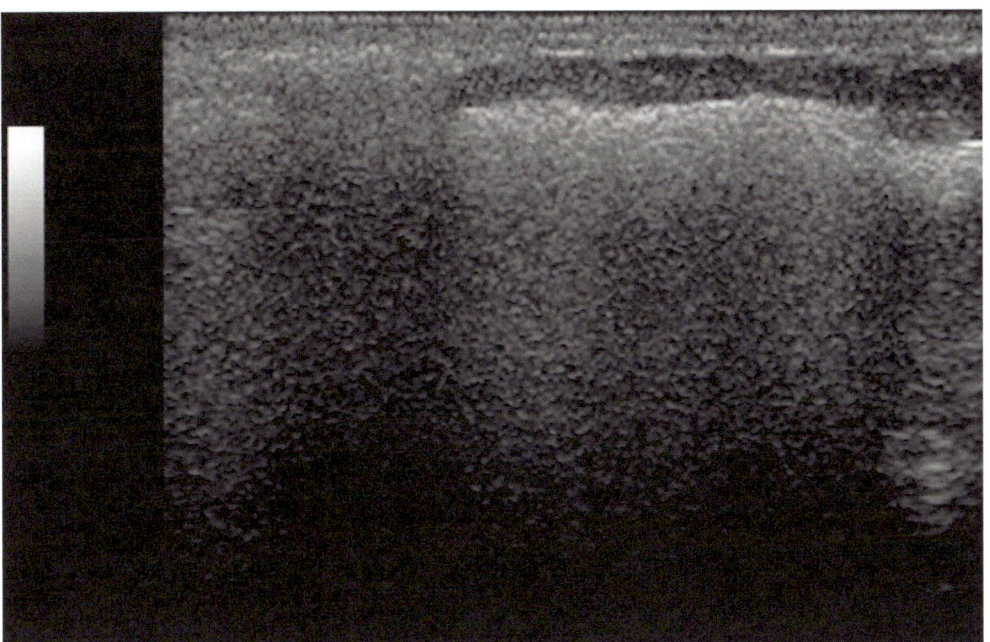

Case 38
Ductal Ectasia

Patient History

A 57-year-old female for a bilateral screening mammogram.

Radiology Findings

Fig. 1.1 Spot-compression (**a**) CC and (**b**) MLO views demonstrate an irregular mass in the retroareolar left breast.
Fig. 1.2 (**a**) Grayscale and (**b**) color Doppler images show a hypoechoic tubular mass in the retroareolar left breast.

BI-RADS Assessment

BI-RADS 2. Benign finding (following diagnostic workup).

Diagnosis

Ductal ectasia

Discussion

- Ductal ectasia is most commonly asymptomatic and less commonly can present with pain, tenderness, and possible palpable mass in the retroareolar breast.

- On mammography, prominence of the intramammary ducts in the retroareolar breast can be seen.
- On ultrasound, an anechoic tubular or branching structure in the retroareolar breast can be seen.
- On MRI, intraductal high signal tubular structure on T2-weighted images is seen. If the duct contains blood products and proteinaceous fluid, high signal may be seen on T1-weighted images.
- May be secondary to stasis, inflammation, obstruction, and glandular atrophy.
- Ductal ectasia can be seen in patients who have a smoking history, hyperprolactinoma, and prolonged phenothiazine exposure.

References

Berg WA, Birdwell RL, Gombos EC, et al. Diagnostic imaging breast. 1st ed. Salt Lake City: Amirsys; 2006. Section IV-1, p. 44–7.
Da Costa D, Taddese A, Luz Cure M, Gerson D, Poppiti R Jr, Esserman LE. Common and unusual diseases of the nipple-areolar complex. Radiographics. 2007;27:S65–77.

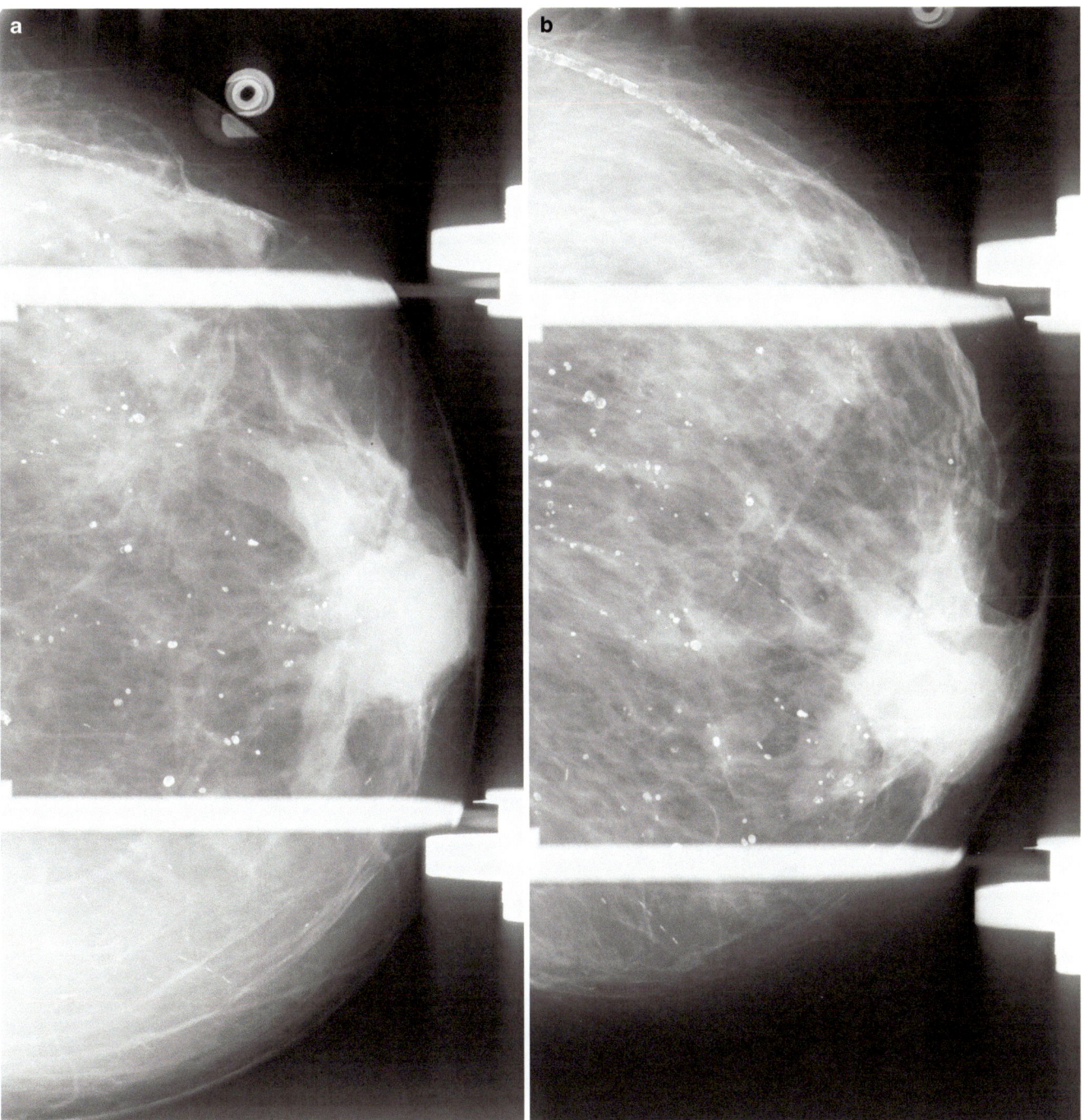

Fig. 1.1

Fig. 1.2

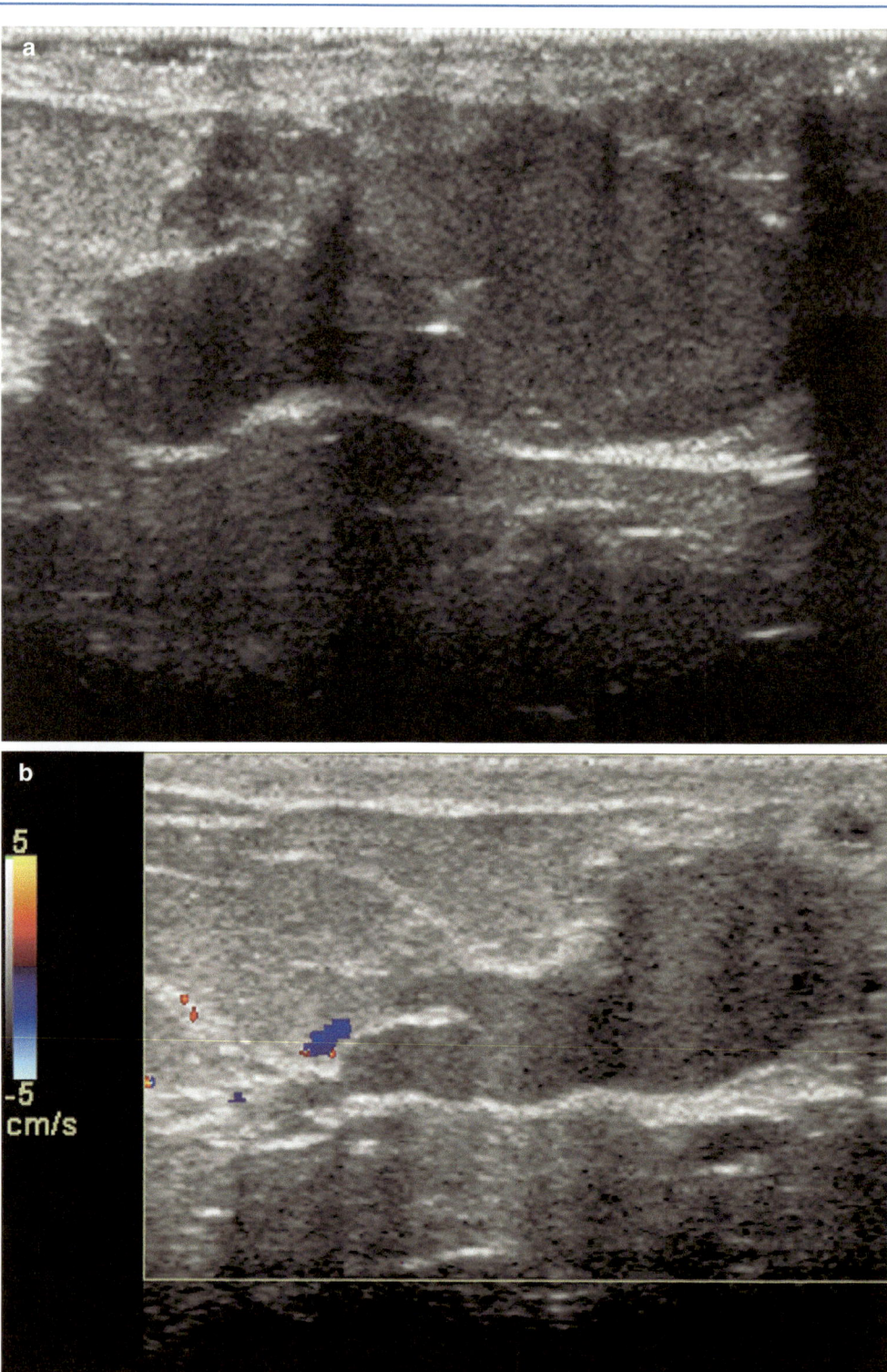

CASE 39
RADIAL SCAR

PATIENT HISTORY

A 59-year-old female for a screening mammogram

RADIOLOGY FINDINGS

Fig. 1.1 (**a**) CC, (**b**) MLO, (**c**) spot-compression CC, (**d**) spot-compression MLO, and (**e**) ML views demonstrate architectural distortion in the upper outer left breast at middle depth.

ASSESSMENT

High-risk lesion.

DIAGNOSIS

Radial scar

DISCUSSION

- Most commonly, radial scar presents as an incidental imaging finding on mammography.
- It appears as architectural distortion or a spiculated mass with central radiolucency on mammography.
- It is not a scar; it is not due to trauma or surgery.
- If sonographically visible, radial scar appears as an irregular, hypoechoic mass.

- If lesion is greater than 1–2 cm in size, it is called complex sclerosing lesion (CSL).
- Radial sclerosing lesion (RSL) is a generalized term that includes radial scar and CSL.
- Associated pathological findings include:
  - Tubular carcinoma
  - Invasive ductal carcinoma
  - DCIS
  - LCIS
  - ADH
- If radial scar has calcifications, there is a higher incidence of association with adenosis, ADH, or DCIS.
- If RSL is greater than 2 cm or palpable, there is an increased association with carcinoma.
- With a diagnosis of radial scar, there is a two times increased risk of developing invasive cancer in either breast.
- Radial scar can also mimic an invasive cancer. Myosin stain can be used to distinguish the two entities. Myoepithelial cells will be present in the basement membrane of radial scar but not in an invasive carcinoma.
- Excisional biopsy is recommended to exclude possible adjacent malignancy.

REFERENCES

Bassett LW, Jackson VP, Fu KL, Fu YS. Diagnosis of diseases of the breast. 2nd ed. Philadelphia: Elsevier; 2005. p. 449–51.

Berg WA, Birdwell RL, Gombos EC, et al. Diagnostic imaging breast. 1st ed. Salt Lake City; Amirsys; 2006. Section IV-2, p. 84–9.

Harvey JA, March DE. Making the diagnosis: a practical guide to breast imaging. Philadelphia: Elsevier; 2013. p. 295–6.

Kopans DB. Breast imaging. 2nd ed. Philadelphia: Lippincott Williams and Wilkins; 1998. p. 565–6.

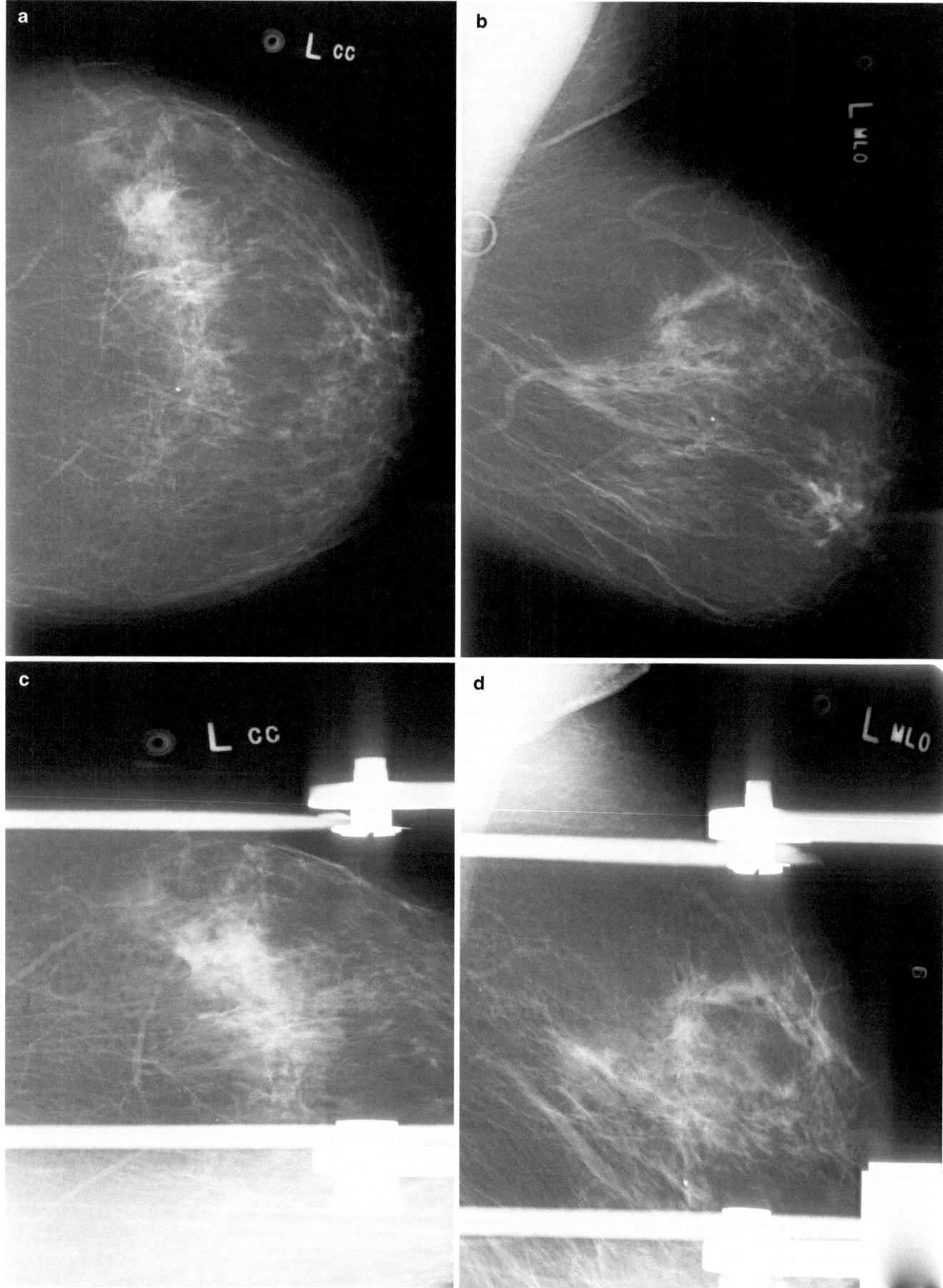

Fig. 1.1

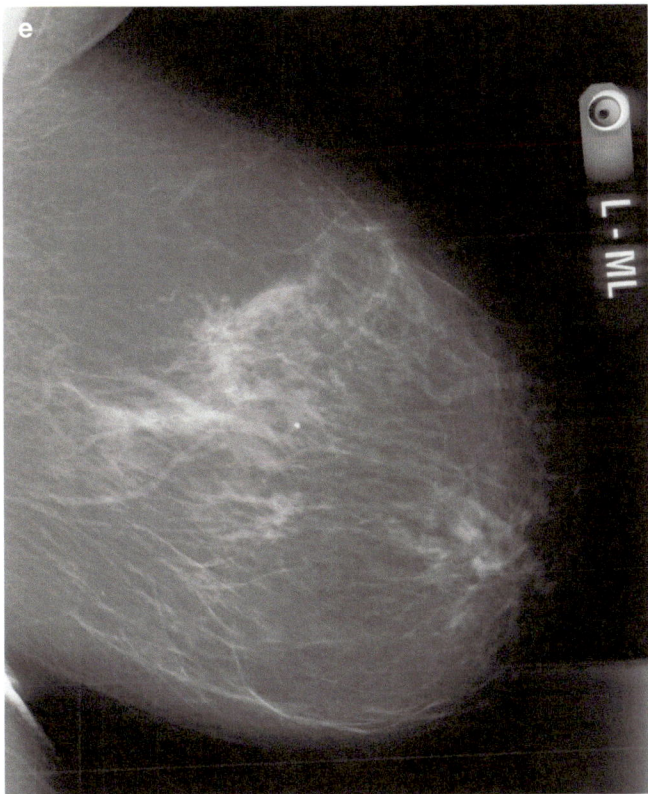

Fig. 1.1 (continued)

Case 40
Dermal Calcifications

Patient History

A 40-year-old female for a baseline screening mammogram.

Radiology Findings

Fig. 1.1 (**a**) CC and (**b**) MLO views demonstrate a cluster of calcifications at the 6 o'clock position, which have the same appearance on both the views.

Fig. 1.2 CC view with a fenestrated compression paddle demonstrates the cluster of calcifications with a superimposed BB marker.

Fig. 1.3 Tangential view demonstrates that the cluster of calcifications is within the skin directly under the BB.

BI-RADS Assessment

BI-RADS 2. Benign finding (following diagnostic workup).

Diagnosis

Dermal calcifications

Discussion

- Dermal calcifications may be single or clustered.
- Often have a calcified rim surrounding a lucent center.
- Suspected if calcifications are peripheral in location or close to the skin surface in any view.
- Occur most often in lower and inner breast.
- Dermal calcification workup:
  - Fenestrated compression paddle is placed on the skin surface closest to the calcifications.
  - BB is superimposed over the calcifications.
  - Tangential view is obtained demonstrating calcifications in the skin.

References

American College of Radiology (ACR) BI-RADS® Atlas. ACR BI-RADS® atlas-mammography. 5th ed. Reston: American College of Radiology; 2013. p. 38–9.

Bassett LW, Jackson VP, Fu KL, Fu YS, et al. Diagnosis of diseases of the breast. 2nd ed. Philadelphia: Elsevier; 2005. p. 402–4.

Ikeda DM. Breast imaging the requisites. 2nd ed. Philadelphia: Elsevier, Mosby; 2011. p. 76–9.

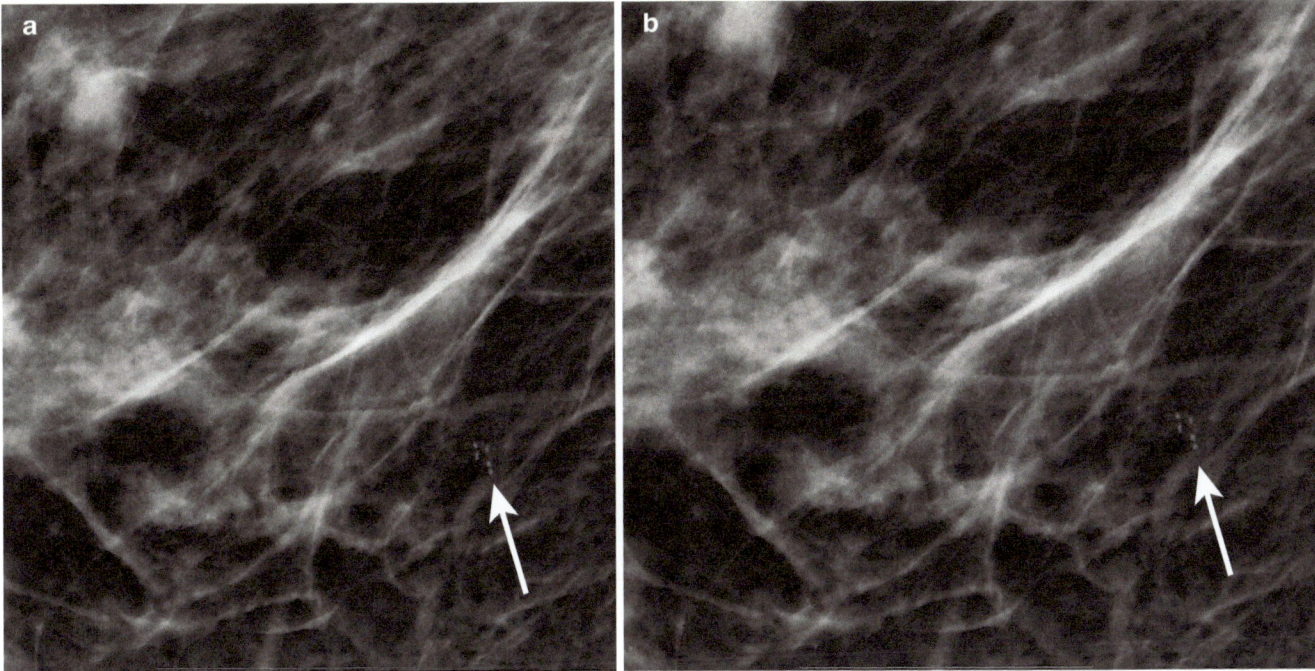

Fig. 1.1

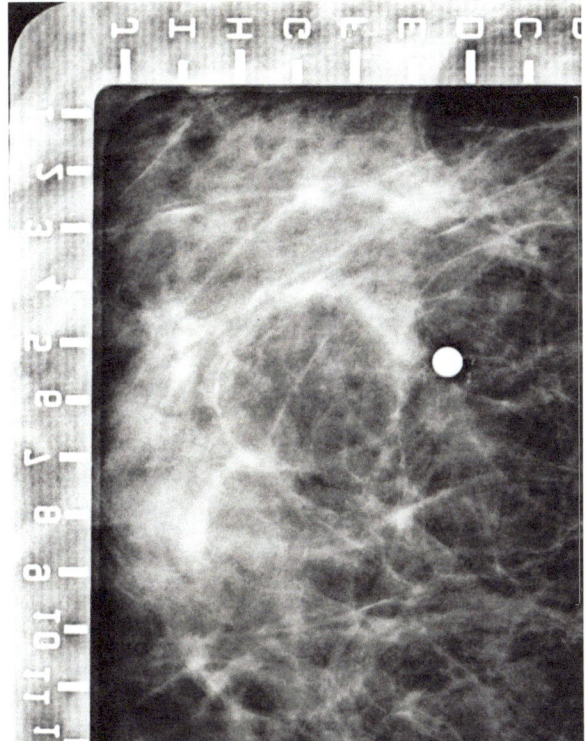

Fig. 1.2

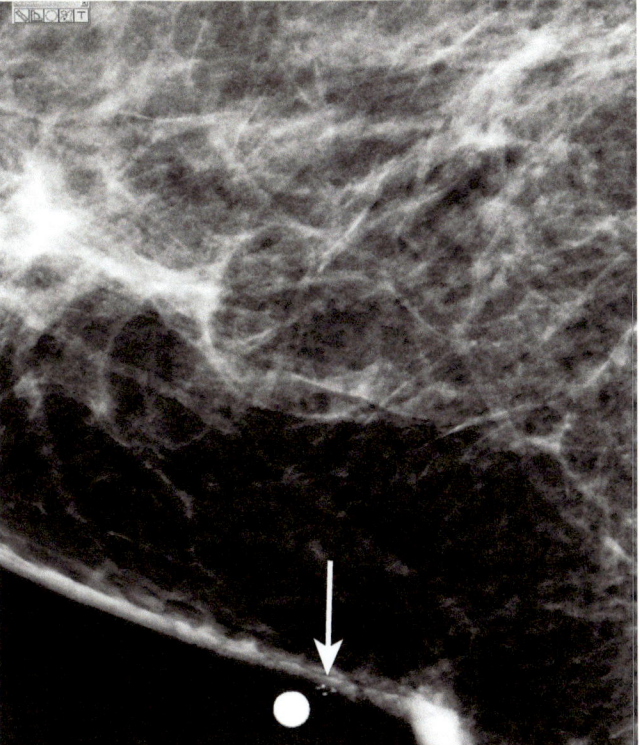

Fig. 1.3

CASE 41
TURNER'S SYNDROME

PATIENT HISTORY

A 42-year-old female for a baseline screening mammogram.

RADIOLOGY FINDINGS

Fig. 1.1 Bilateral (**a**, **b**) CC and (**c**, **d**) MLO views demonstrate mostly fatty breast tissue with minimal fibroglandular development. Circular markers represent skin moles.

BI-RADS ASSESSMENT

BI-RADS 2. Benign finding.

DIAGNOSIS

Turner's syndrome

DISCUSSION

- XO karyotype.
- Incidence is 1:3,000–5,000 live births.
- Associated with:
  - Horseshoe kidney
  - Coarctation of aorta
  - Aortic stenosis
  - Cystic hygroma
- Primary amenorrhea and absence of secondary sex characteristics.
- Widely spaced nipples.
- Annual mammography screening is recommended.

REFERENCES

Brant WE, Helms CA, editors. Fundamentals of diagnostic radiology. 2nd ed. Philadelphia: Lippincott Williams and Wilkins; 1999. p. 319, 576.
Saenger P. Clinical review 48: the current status of diagnosis and therapeutic intervention in Turner's syndrome. J Clin Endocrinol Metable. 1993;77:297–301.

Case 41   Turner's Syndrome

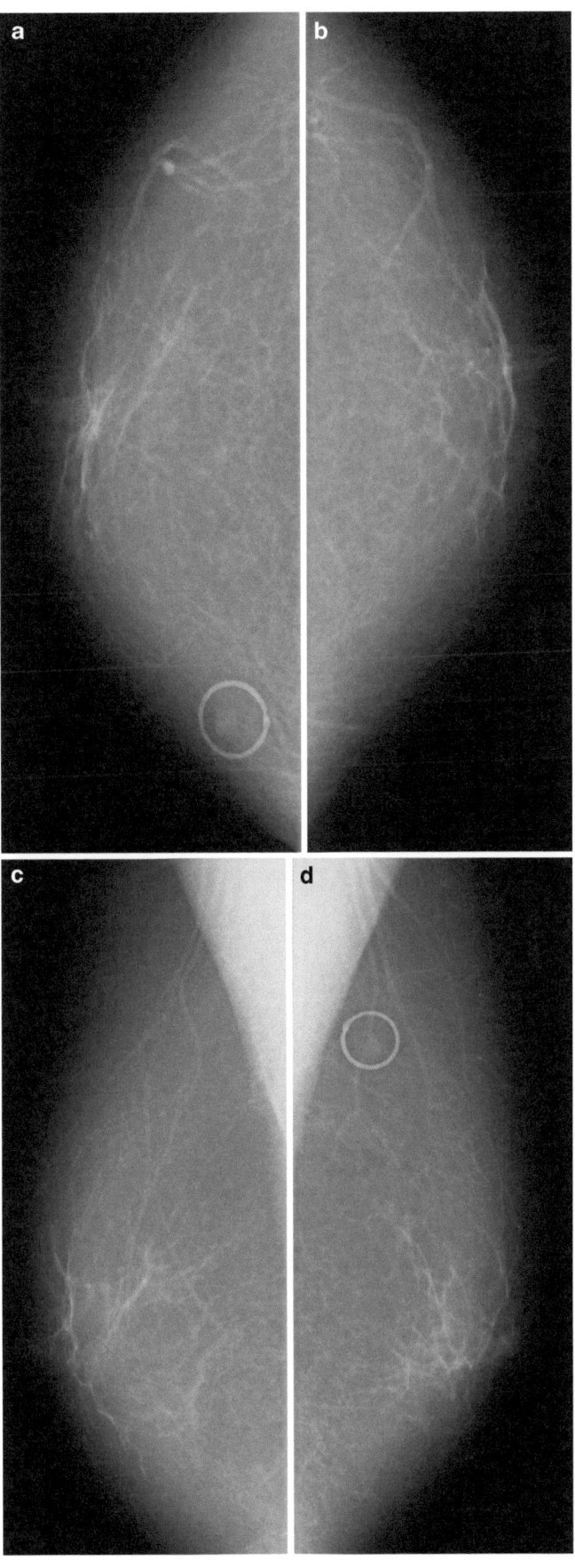

Fig. 1.1

Case 42
Invasive Ductal Carcinoma (IDC) in a Male Patient

Patient History

An 81-year-old-male with palpable left breast mass and nipple inversion.

Radiology Findings

Fig. 1.1 (**a**) CC and (**b**) ML images show an oval mass with spiculated margins and associated microcalcifications in the left breast at 6 o'clock middle depth, which corresponds to the triangular marker indicating a palpable mass.

Fig. 1.2 (**a**) Grayscale and (**b**) color Doppler ultrasound images show a hypoechoic oval mass with microlobulated margins and posterior acoustic shadowing. There is vascular flow within the mass.

Fig. 1.3 PET/CT fused images show a hypermetabolic mass in the left breast.

BI-RADS Assessment

BI-RADS 5. Highly suggestive of malignancy (following diagnostic workup, prior to biopsy).

Diagnosis

IDC in a male patient

Discussion

- Male breast cancer accounts for 0.7 % of all breast cancers, with 85 % of primary male breast cancers being IDC, not otherwise specified.

- Risk factors for male breast cancer include:
  - Advanced age
  - Prior irradiation of the chest
  - Exogenous estrogen for prostate cancer treatment or gender reassignment procedures
  - Diseases associated with hyperestrogenism, such as liver disease
  - Androgen deficiency owing to testicular dysfunction
  - BRCA-2 mutation
  - Klinefelter's disease
  - Family history of breast cancer
- Male breast cancer frequently presents as a palpable mass.
- On mammography, IDC is usually seen as an irregular mass with spiculated or microlobulated margins.
- On ultrasound, IDC is seen as a hypoechoic mass with angulated, microlobulated, or spiculated margins with or without posterior acoustic shadowing.
- Most common location is retroareolar, because male breast cancers arise from central ducts.
- Secondary signs of malignancy include skin thickening, nipple retraction, or axillary lymphadenopathy.
- Diagnostic workup includes mammogram and ultrasound, followed by image-guided biopsy.

References

Chen L, Chantra PK, Larsen LH, et al. Imaging characteristics of malignant lesions of the male breast. Radiographics. 2006;26:993–1006.

Kopans DB. Breast imaging. 2nd ed. Philadelphia: Lippincott Williams and Wilkins; 1998. p. 498–508.

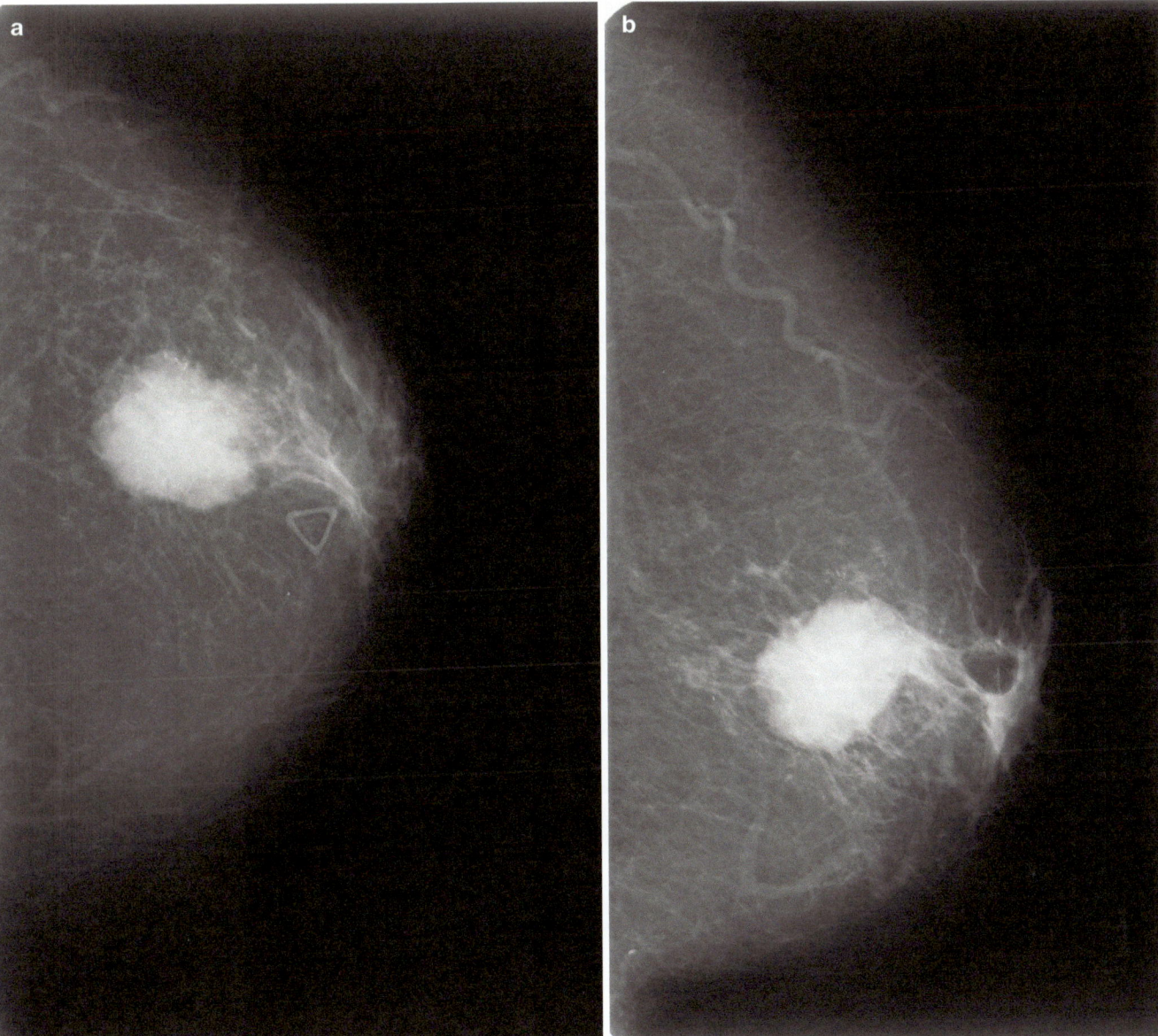

Fig. 1.1

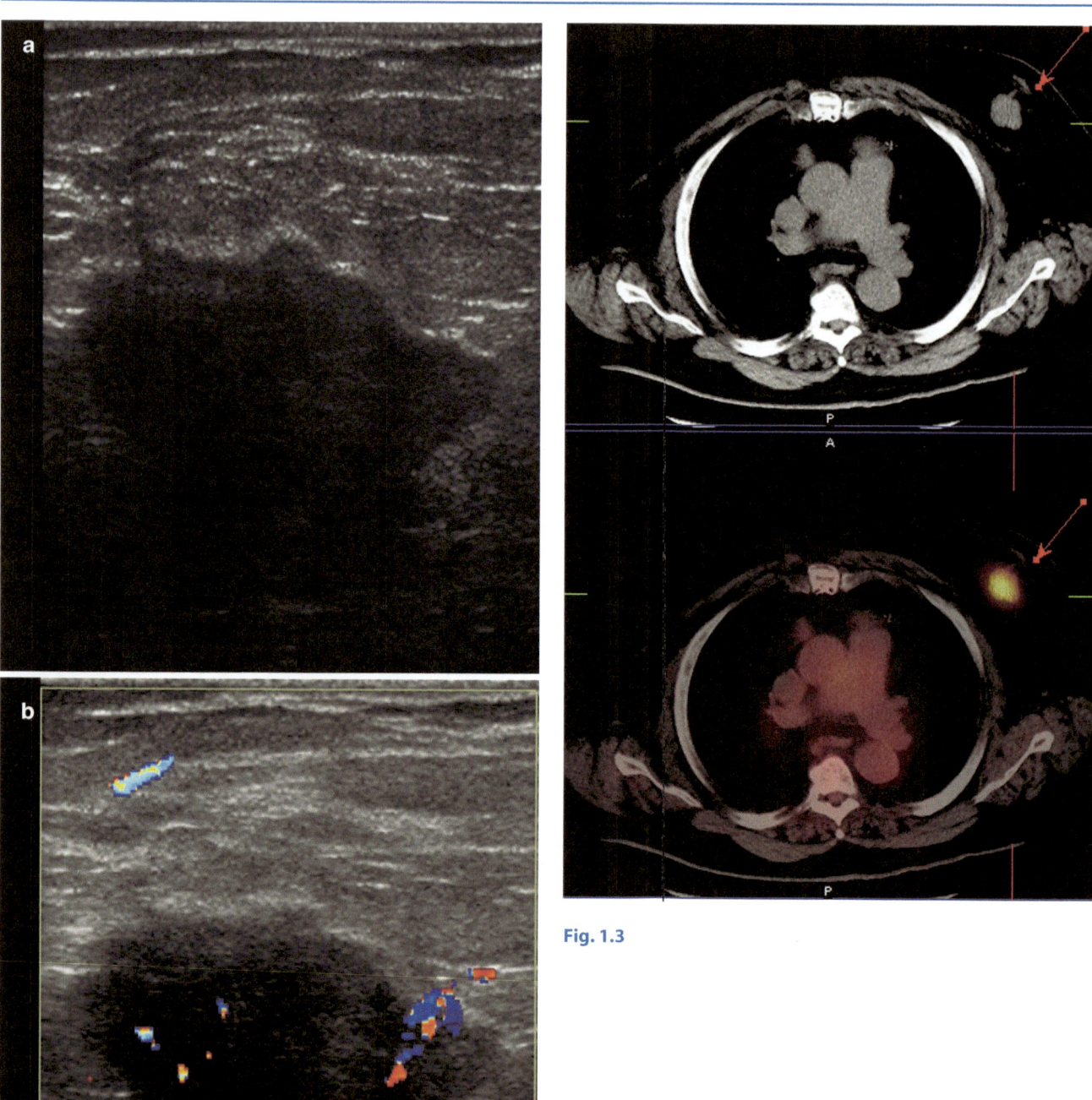

Fig. 1.2

Fig. 1.3

CASE 43
MONDOR'S DISEASE (SUPERFICIAL THROMBOPHLEBITIS)

PATIENT HISTORY

A 36-year-old female with a palpable cord-like structure and associated pain and tenderness.

RADIOLOGY FINDINGS

Fig. 1.1 (**a**) CC, (**b**) MLO, and (**c**) spot-compression CC images show a tubular structure in the upper inner left breast, corresponding to a triangular marker indicating a palpable cord-like structure.

Fig. 1.2 (**a**) Grayscale and (**b**) color Doppler ultrasound images show a superficial beaded tubular structure with no vascular flow.

BI-RADS ASSESSMENT

BI-RADS 2. Benign findings (following diagnostic workup).

DIAGNOSIS

Mondor's disease (superficial thrombophlebitis)

DISCUSSION

- Mondor's disease refers to thrombophlebitis of a superficial vein in the breast.

- May be the result of direct trauma, breast surgery, or extreme physical activity.
- Associated with breast carcinoma in up to 12 % of the cases.
- Clinically presents as a palpable cord-like mass, which may have associated pain, tenderness, or erythema.
- Mammographically, a thickened cord-like structure is seen, representing the thrombosed portion of the vein.
- On ultrasound, a superficial tubular structure filled with low-level internal echoes, representing thrombosis, is seen.
- Treatment is not needed, as Mondor's disease is self-limiting.
- Symptoms will last for a few weeks, with complete resolution expected within 6 weeks.
- Follow-up mammogram and ultrasound is recommended to assure complete resolution.

REFERENCES

American College of Radiology (ACR) BI-RADS® Atlas. ACR BI-RADS® Atlas-Ultrasound. 5th ed. Reston: American College of Radiology; 2013. p. 115.

Conant EF, Wilkes AN, Mendelson EB, Feig SA. Superficial thrombophlebitis of the breast (Mondor's disease): mammographic findings. AJR. 1993;160:1201–3.

Sabate JM, Clotet M, Gomez A, De las Heras P, Torrubia S, Salinas T. Radiologic evaluation of uncommon inflammatory and reactive breast disorders. Radiographics. 2005;25:411–24.

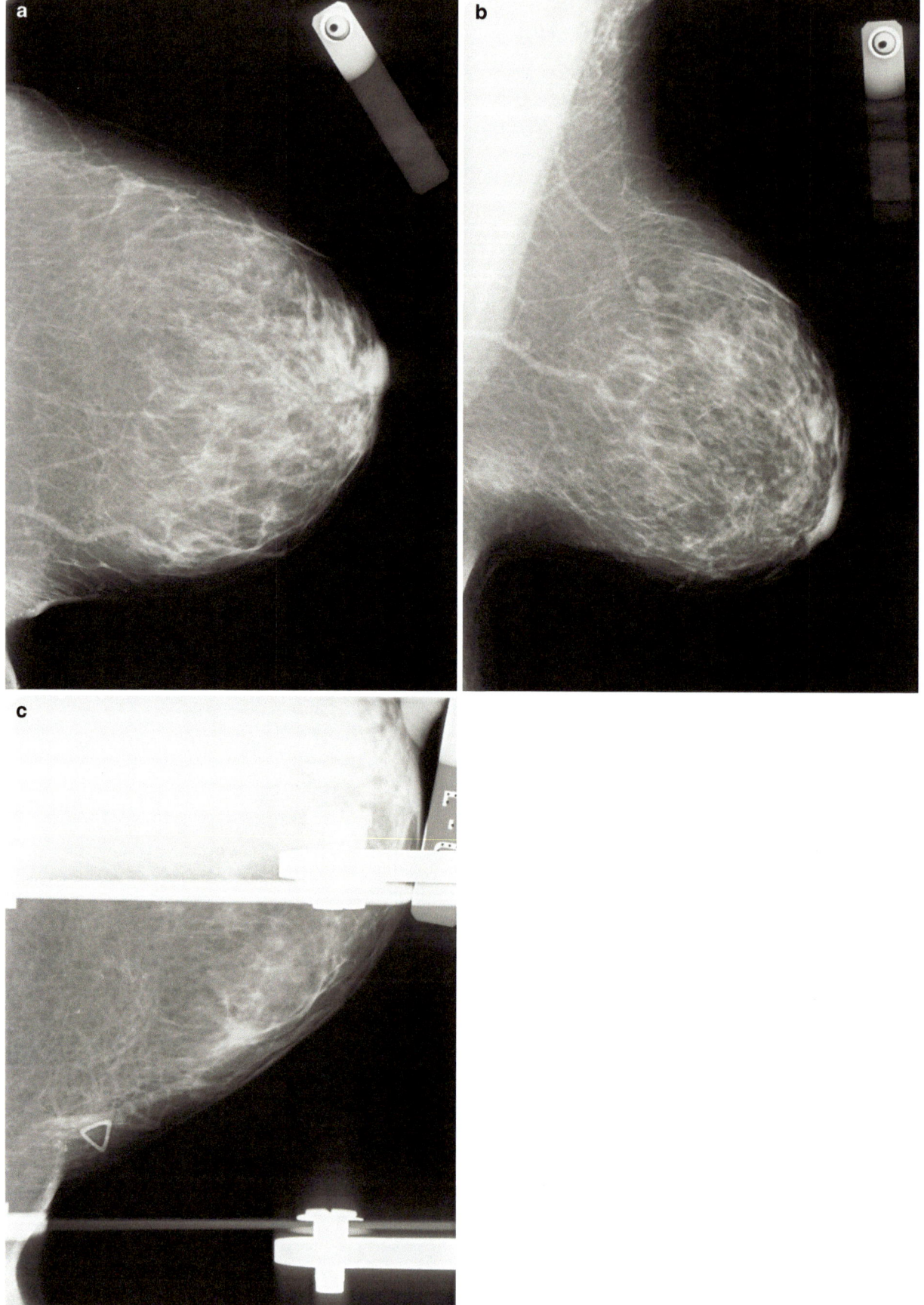

Fig. 1.1

Fig. 1.2

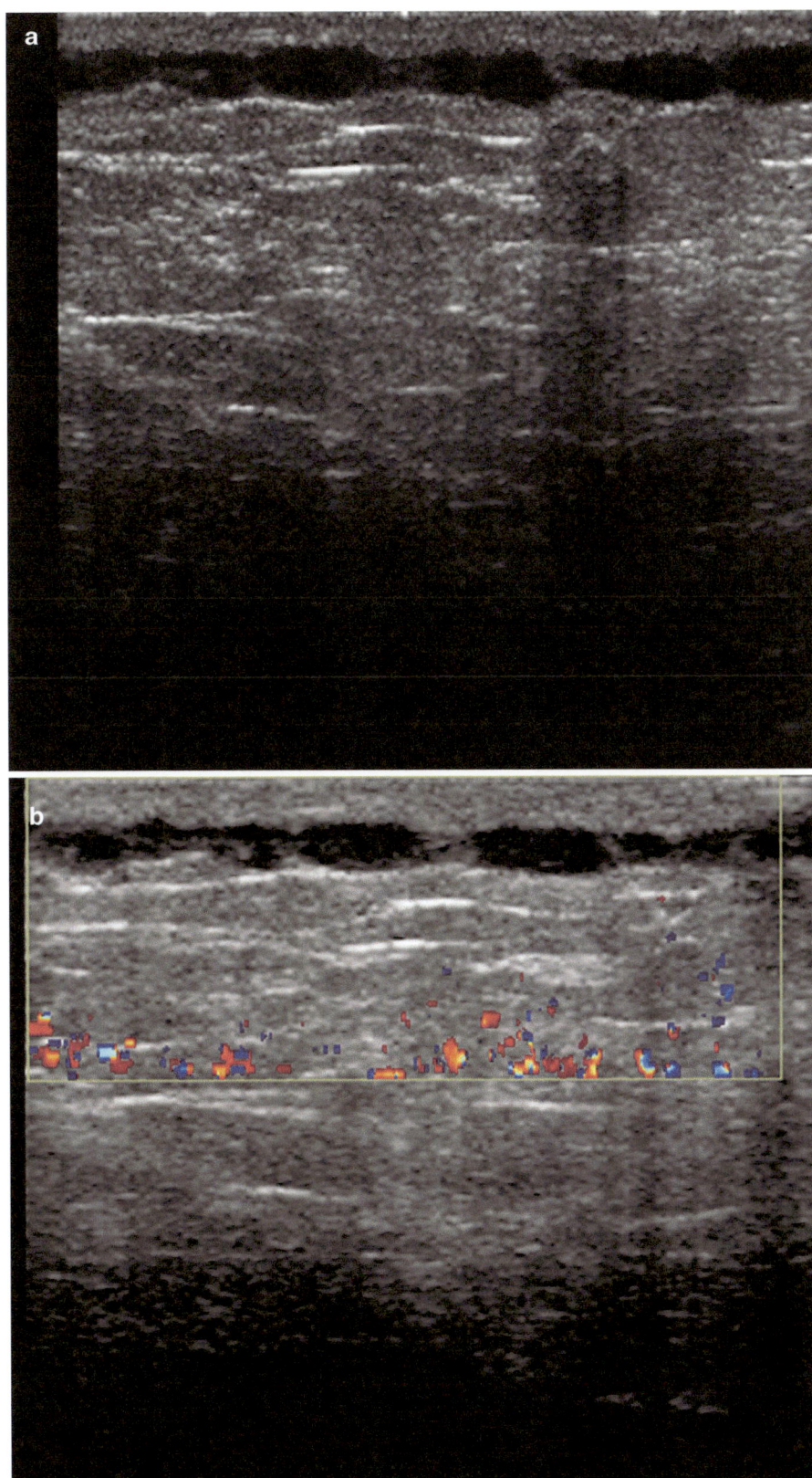

CASE 44
INTRADUCTAL PAPILLOMA

PATIENT HISTORY

A 47-year-old female with a palpable left breast mass for 6 months.

RADIOLOGY FINDINGS

Fig. 1.1 (**a**) Spot-compression CC and (**b**) spot-compression MLO images show an irregular mass in the retroareolar left breast corresponding to a triangular marker to indicate a palpable mass.
Fig. 1.2 (**a**) Grayscale and (**b**) color Doppler ultrasound images show an oval hypoechoic mass with irregular margins within a dilated duct. There is vascular flow within the hypoechoic mass.

ASSESSMENT

High-risk lesion.

DIAGNOSIS

Intraductal papilloma

DISCUSSION

- An intraductal papilloma is a benign papillary tumor, which arises in a duct as a single mass or multiple masses.
- Solitary masses are usually central in location, whereas multiple papillomas are usually more peripheral in location.
- May present clinically with bloody or clear nipple discharge or a palpable subareolar mass.
- Mammogram can be normal or can show a circumscribed mass, calcifications, or a single dilated duct in the subareolar breast.
- A dilated duct with a hypoechoic solid intraductal mass can be seen on ultrasound.
- Controversy over management exists.
- Surgical excision is often advocated following diagnosis of intraductal papilloma on core needle biopsy.
- Reasons to advocate for excision include:
  - Difficulty for pathologist to distinguish benign from malignant papillary lesion from a core needle biopsy sample
  - Sampling error
  - Premalignant potential in cases of multiple papillomas

REFERENCES

Cardenosa G. Breast imaging companion. 2nd ed. Philadelphia: Lippincott Williams and Wilkins; 2001. p. 224.
Harvey JA, March DE. Making the diagnosis: a practical guide to breast imaging. Philadelphia: Elsevier; 2013. p. 401–6.
Jacobs TW, Connolly JL, Schnitt SJ. Nonmalignant lesions in breast core needle biopsies. Am J Surg Path. 2002;26:1095–110.
Liberman L, Tornos C, Huzjan R, Bartella L, Morris EA, Dershaw DD. Is surgical excision warranted after benign concordant diagnosis of papilloma at percutaneous breast biopsy? AJR. 2006;186:1328–34.
Mercado Cl, Hamele-Bena D, Oken S, Singer CI, Cangiarella J. Papillary lesions of the breast at percutaneous core needle biopsy. Radiology. 2006;238:801–8.

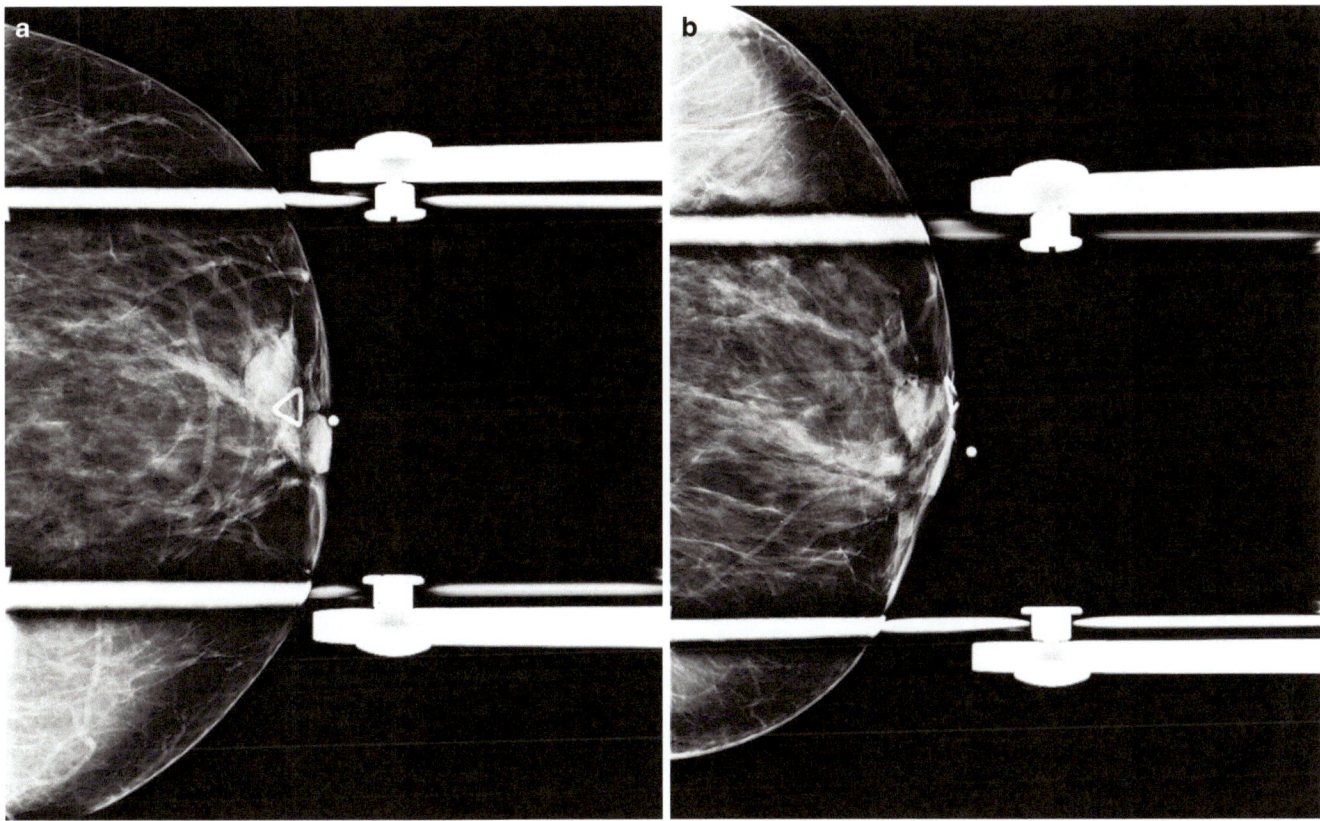

Fig. 1.1

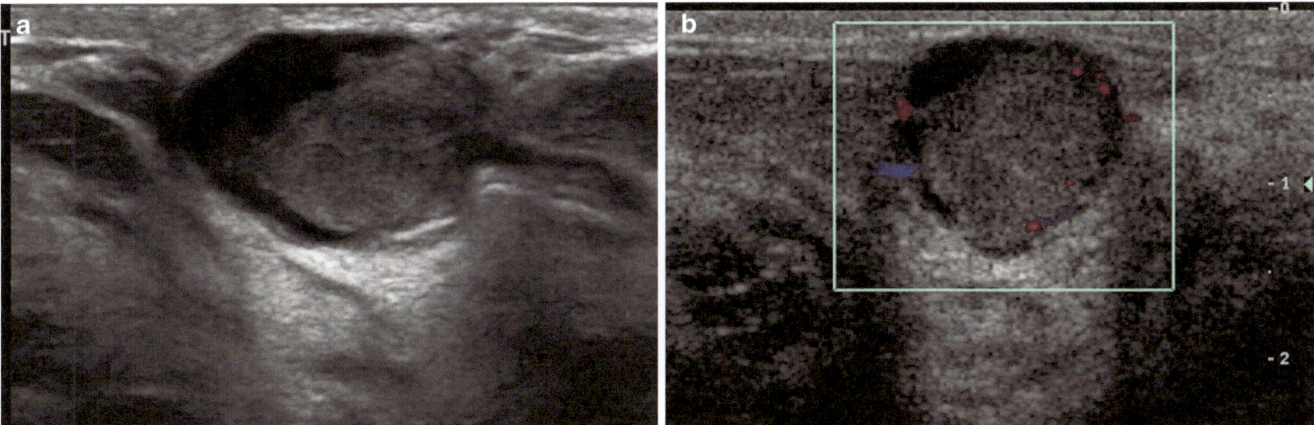

Fig. 1.2

CASE 45
FAT NECROSIS (MULTIPLE PRESENTATIONS)

PATIENT HISTORY

Screening mammograms in multiple different patients.

RADIOLOGY FINDINGS

Fig. 1.1 (**a**, **b**) Bilateral MLO views demonstrate multiple, bilateral, lucent-centered masses compatible with oil cysts.
Fig. 1.2 (**a**) Grayscale and (**b**) color Doppler ultrasound images demonstrate an irregular hypoechoic mass that is taller than wide. There is no internal vascular flow.
Fig. 1.3 CC view demonstrates two lucent-centered lesions with peripheral rim calcification in the retroareolar plane at anterior depth.

BI-RADS ASSESSMENT

BI-RADS 2. Benign finding (following possible diagnostic workup and biopsy).

DIAGNOSIS

Fat necrosis (multiple presentations)

DISCUSSION

- Fat necrosis is a benign, inflammatory process, which usually occurs after trauma or injury to the breast.
- Radiographic appearance may mimic malignancy and biopsy may be necessary.
- Can have multiple mammographic appearances:
  - Oil cysts
  - Calcifications
  - Spiculated opacities
  - Focal masses
- Fat necrosis may also present as a palpable mass with no mammographic findings.
- Oil cysts are a pathognomonic finding for fat necrosis.
- Calcifications may be pleomorphic or coarse.
- If fibrosis is a predominant component of fat necrosis, then it may appear as a spiculated mass.
- Steatocystoma multiplex:
  - Multiple sebaceous cysts on the trunk, back, external genitalia, and proximal extremities
  - Autosomal dominant
  - Predominantly in males
  - Multiple, bilateral oil cysts seen mammographically

REFERENCE

Hogge JP, Robinson RE, Magnant CM, Zuurbier RA. The mammographic spectrum of fat necrosis of the breast. Radiographics. 1995;15:1347–56.

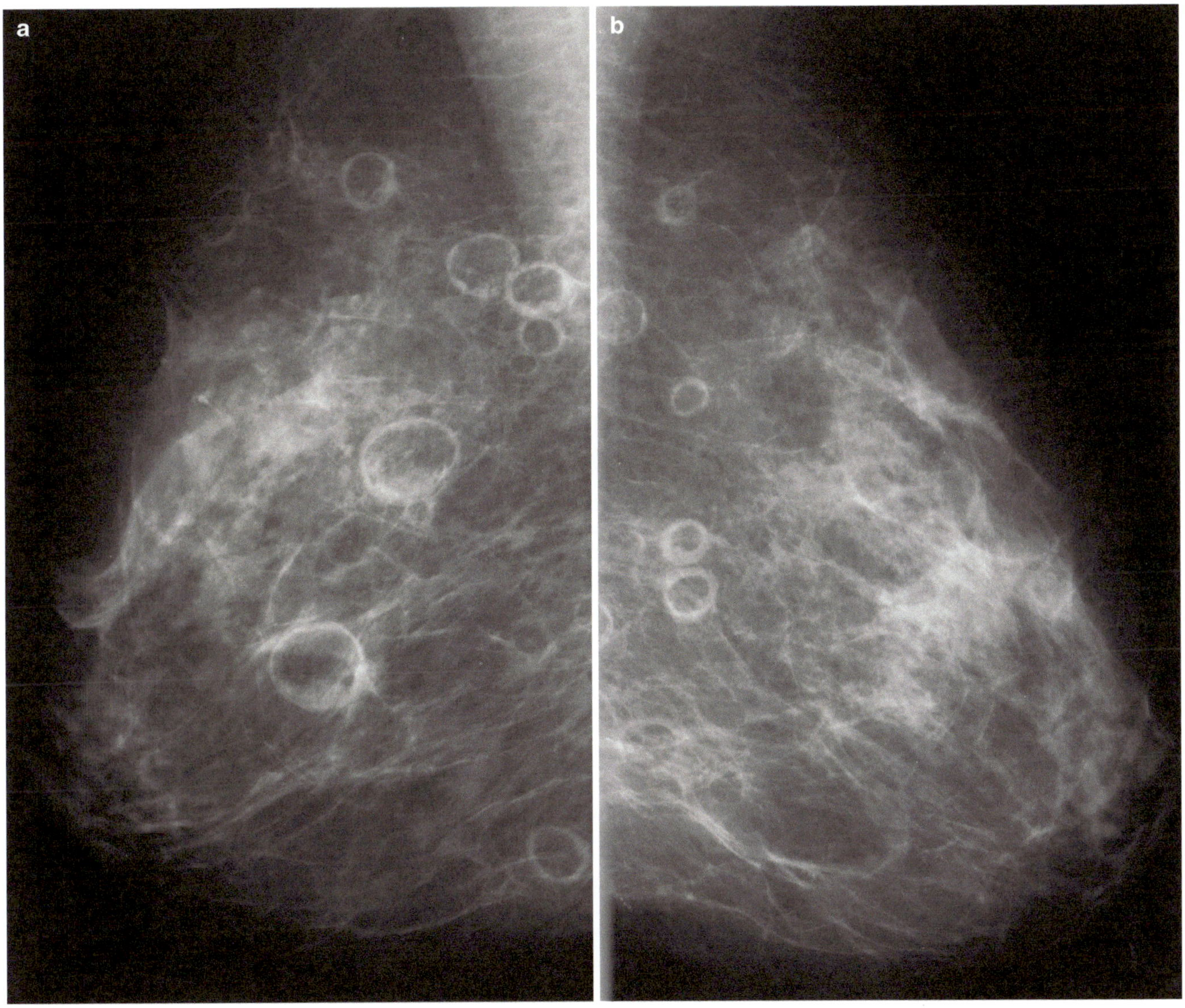

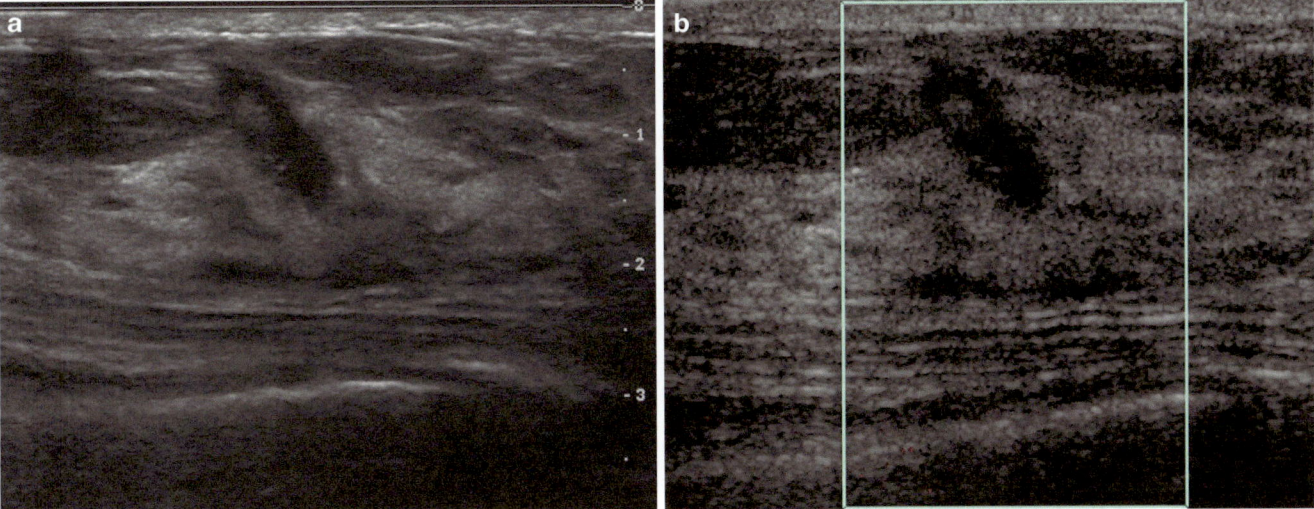

Fig. 1.1

Fig. 1.2

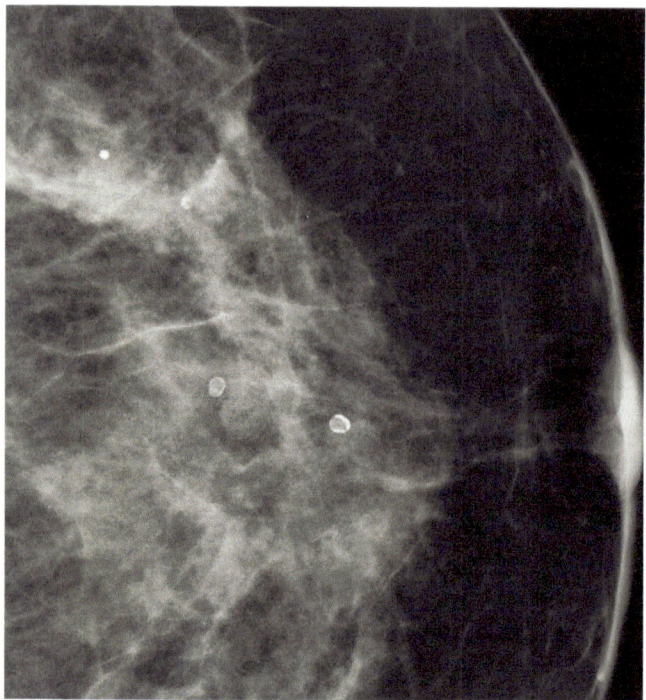

Fig. 1.3

CASE 46
RECURRENCE AT LUMPECTOMY SITE

PATIENT HISTORY

A 44-year-old female with a history of right breast cancer treated with breast-conserving therapy (BCT) and radiation therapy; screening mammogram.

RADIOLOGY FINDINGS

Fig. 1.1 (**a**) CC and (**b**) MLO views demonstrate architectural distortion with associated pleomorphic calcifications at the site of prior lumpectomy in the upper outer right breast at anterior depth.
Fig. 1.2 Grayscale ultrasound image demonstrates an irregular hypoechoic mass with posterior acoustic shadowing.
Fig. 1.3 PET and PET/CT fused images demonstrate an area of hypermetabolism in the right breast.

BI-RADS ASSESSMENT

BI-RADS 4. Suspicious abnormality (following diagnostic workup, prior to biopsy).

DIAGNOSIS

Recurrence at lumpectomy site

DISCUSSION

- Recurrent breast carcinoma is defined as invasive or non-invasive cancer in a breast that has been treated for a prior cancer.
- Can be divided into:
  - True recurrence – cancer at the original tumor site, typically <5 years after BCT
  - Marginal miss – cancer near the original tumor site <5 years after BCT
  - Ipsilateral breast cancer – cancer, remote from original tumor site
    - Contralateral breast cancer – usually considered as a second primary
- Recurrences at the original tumor site generally represent true treatment failures.
- Approximately half of the recurrences are found by mammography and half present as palpable findings.
- On mammography, recurrences usually present as pleomorphic calcifications or masses.
- Recurrence is rare within 18 months of BCT.
- Most local recurrence occurs between 1 and 7 years post lumpectomy.
- After breast conservation therapy, local recurrence rates are 6–8 %. Without RT, rates of recurrence are higher, 30–40 %.
- Local recurrence usually occurs in the same ductal system as the original cancer.
- Prognosis is worse if:
  - Recurrence is <5 years, post BCT.
  - Tumor size at recurrence is >2 cm.
  - There is associated metastatic disease.
- Recurrence after mastectomy is usually always detected clinically.
- Women who are BRCA gene carriers have a similar rate of recurrence when compared with the normal-risk women.
- FDG PET has a sensitivity of 89 % and specificity of 84 % for local recurrence.
- FDG PET and PET/CT are most useful for staging recurrent or metastatic breast cancer.
- Treatment for recurrence:
  - Salvage mastectomy.
  - If there has been no prior radiation therapy, BCT can be considered.
  - Postmastectomy recurrence is treated with radiation therapy.

REFERENCES

Berg WA, Birdwell RL, Gombos EC, et al. Diagnostic imaging breast. 1st ed. Salt Lake City: Amirsys; 2006. Section IV-4, p. 54–7.
Harvey JA, March DE. Making the diagnosis: a practical guide to breast imaging. Philadelphia: Elsevier; 2013. p. 478.
Ikeda DM. Breast imaging the requisites. 2nd ed. Philadelphia: Elsevier, Mosby; 2011. p. 314, 324–8.
Rosen EL, Eubank WB, Mankoff DA. FDG PET, PET/CT, and breast cancer imaging. Radiographics. 2007;27:S215–29.

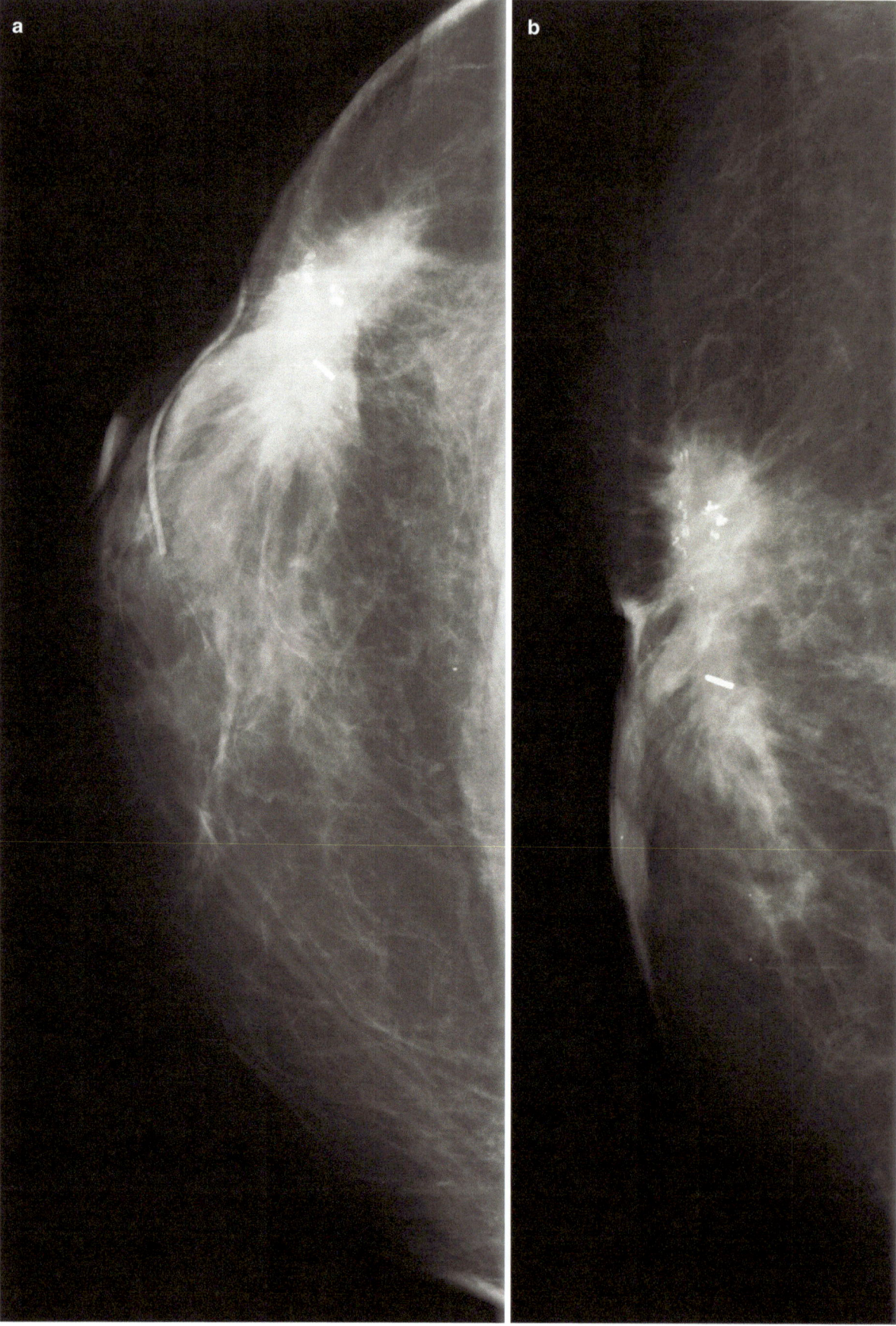

Fig. 1.1

Fig. 1.2

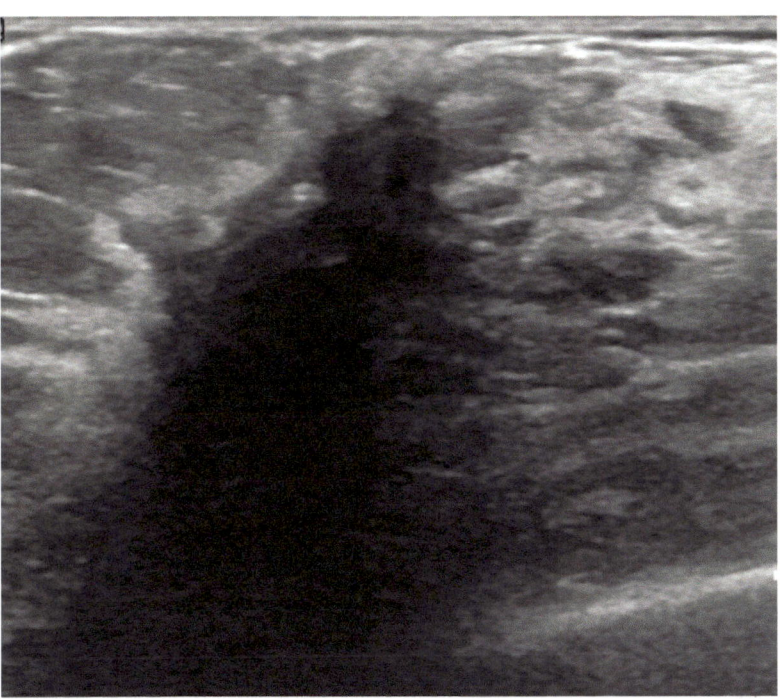

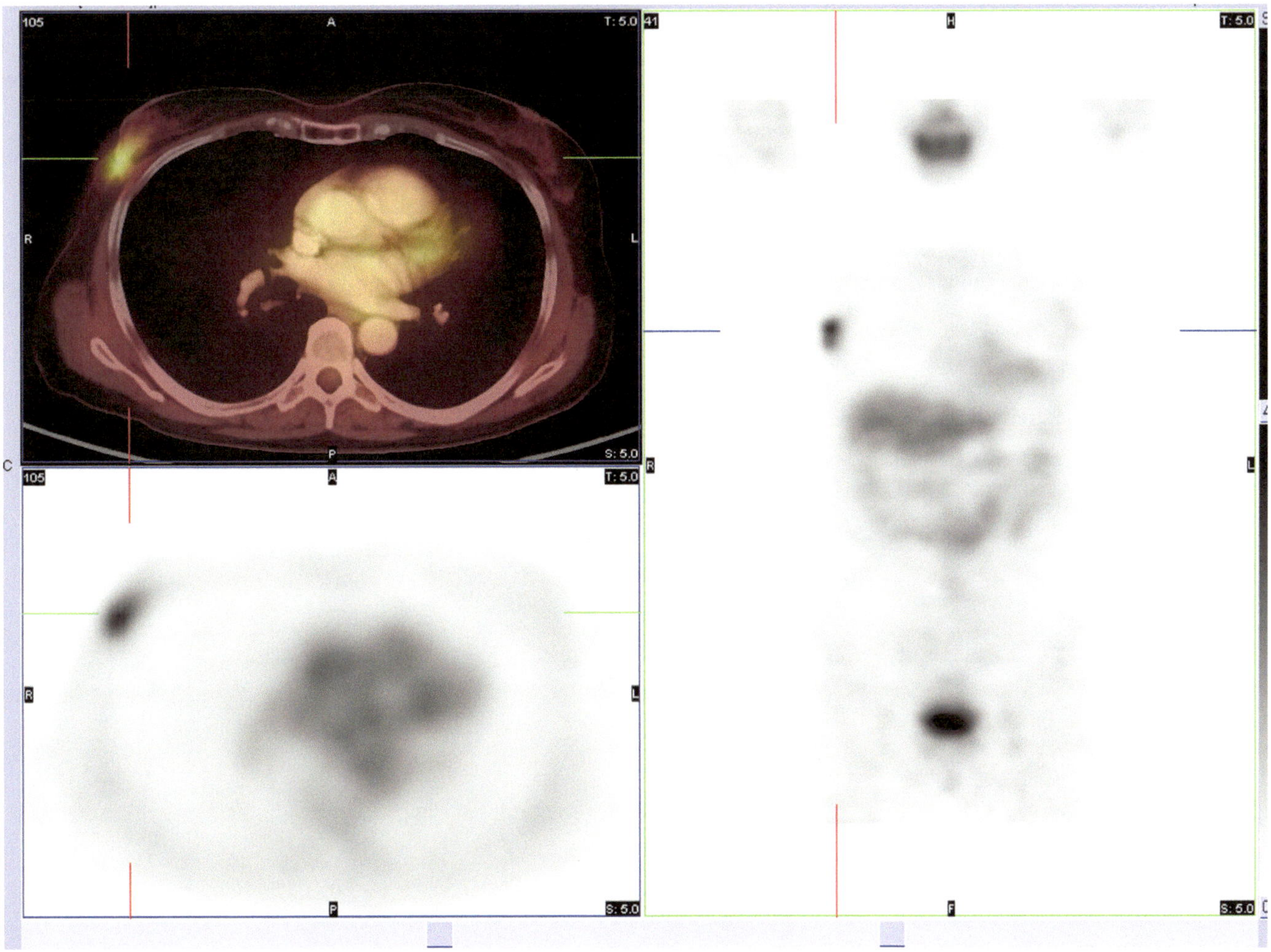

Fig. 1.3

CASE 47
ENLARGED AXILLARY LYMPH NODES

PATIENT HISTORY

A 70-year-old female for a screening mammogram.

RADIOLOGY FINDINGS

Fig. 1.1 (**a**) MLO and (**b**) axillary tail views demonstrate a round, high-density lobular mass in the axillary tail. Circle marker indicates an adjacent skin lesion.

Fig. 1.2 (**a**) Grayscale and (**b**) color Doppler ultrasound images demonstrate a hypoechoic oval mass with slight vascular flow. A discrete fatty hilum is not seen.

BI-RADS ASSESSMENT

BI-RADS 4. Suspicious abnormality (following diagnostic workup, prior to biopsy).

DIAGNOSIS

Enlarged axillary lymph nodes

DISCUSSION

- Axillary lymphadenopathy is defined as an axillary lymph node of >2 cm.

- If normal, lymph nodes maintain reniform shape and radiolucent fatty hilum.
- If abnormal, lymph nodes show increased density, and their shape becomes round and irregular with possible loss of fatty hilum.
- On ultrasound, thickened cortex can be seen.
    - A uniformly thickened cortex favors inflammation.
    - An asymmetrically thickened cortex favors malignancy.
- Loss or compression of hilum is highly indicative of malignancy.
- Differential diagnosis includes:
    - Metastases (breast, melanoma, lung)
    - Primary breast cancer in axilla (can appear as adenopathy)
    - Mastitis
    - Inflammation/infection
    - Ruptured silicone implant
- In case of metastatic nodes with unknown primary, MRI is useful.

REFERENCES

American College of Radiology (ACR) BI-RADS® Atlas. ACR BI-RADS® atlas-ultrasound. 5th ed. Reston: American College of Radiology; 2013. p. 108–13.

Bassett LW, Jackson VP, Fu KL, Fu YS. Diagnosis of diseases of the breast. 2nd ed. Philadelphia: Elsevier; 2005. p. 407–9.

Berg WA, Birdwell RL, Gombos EC, et al. Diagnostic imaging breast. 1st ed. Salt Lake City: Amirsys; 2006. Section IV-3, p. 30–3.

Lim ET, O'Doherty A, Hill AD, Quinn CM. Pathological axillary lymph nodes detected at mammographic screening. Clin Radiol. 2004;59(1):86–91.

Patel T, Given-Wilson R, Thomas V. The clinical importance of axillary lymphadenopathy detected on screening mammography: revisited. Clin Radiol. 2005;60(1):64–71.

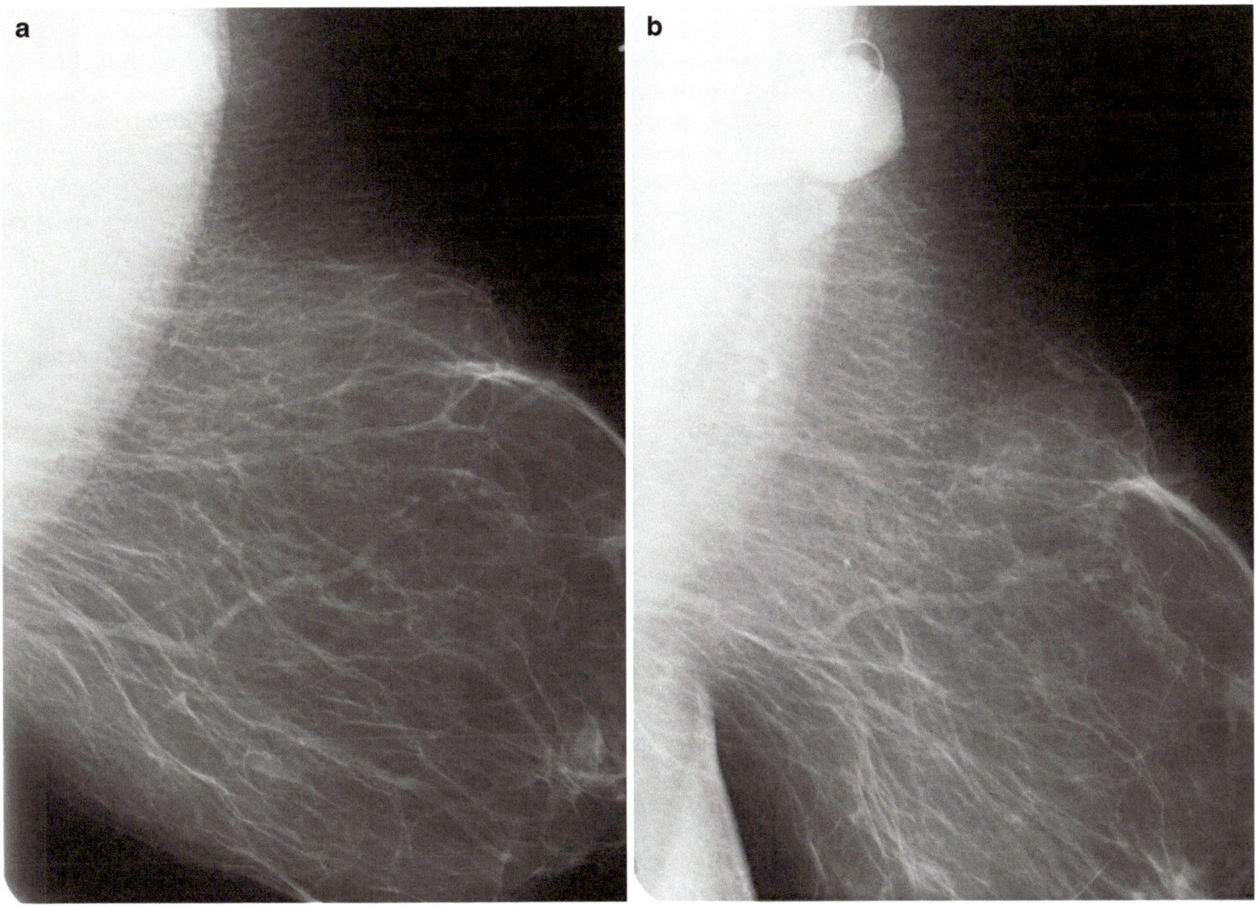

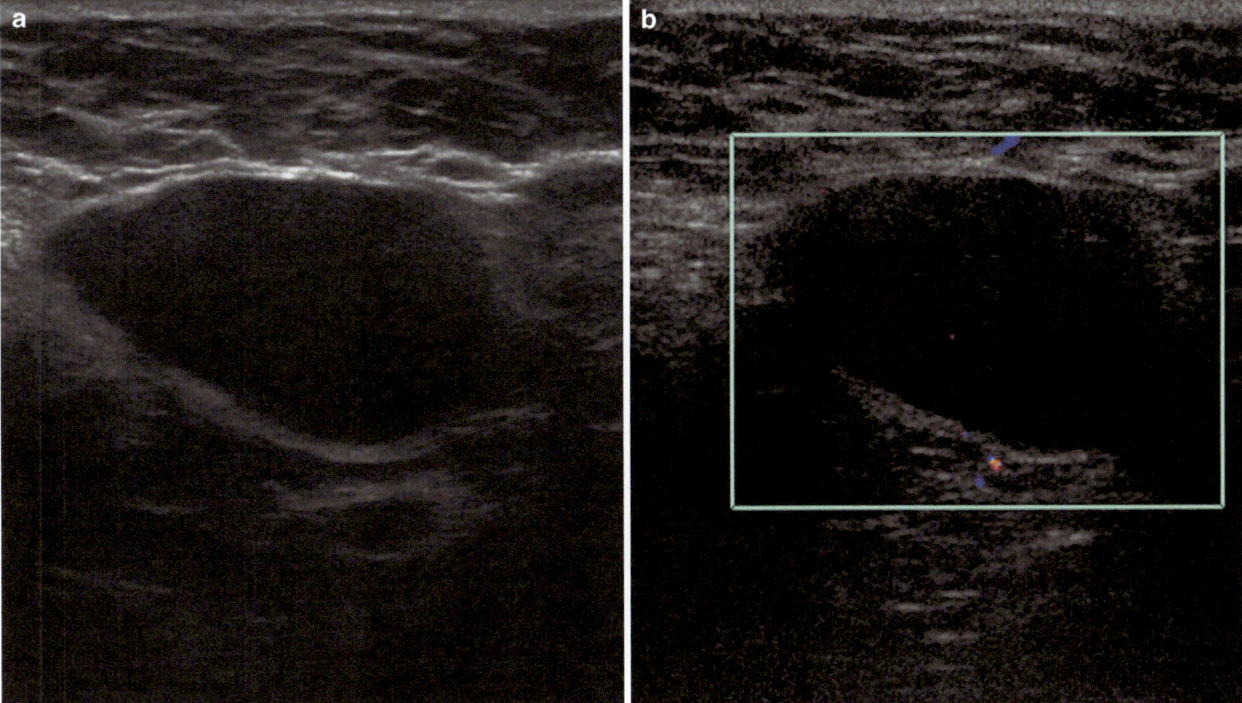

Fig. 1.1

Fig. 1.2

CASE 48
INFLAMMATORY BREAST CARCINOMA (IBC)

PATIENT HISTORY

An 83-year-old female with right breast erythema.

RADIOLOGY FINDINGS

Fig. 1.1 Bilateral (**a**, **b**) CC and (**c**, **d**) MLO images show skin thickening and trabecular thickening of the right breast. The left breast is negative.

BI-RADS ASSESSMENT

BI-RADS 4. Suspicious abnormality (following diagnostic workup, prior to biopsy).

DIAGNOSIS

Inflammatory breast carcinoma (IBC)

DISCUSSION

- IBC accounts for 1–4 % of breast cancers, with the average age of onset between 45 and 54 years of age.

- The pathologic feature that defines IBC is dermal lymphatic invasion, which is a diagnosis made by performing a skin-punch biopsy.
- IBC is an aggressive malignancy, which tends to metastasize at an early stage.
- Clinically, one can observe skin edema (peau d'orange), skin erythema, palpable mass, breast enlargement, nipple retraction, and breast pain.
- Skin thickening, trabecular thickening, and diffuse increase in breast density can be seen mammographically. Less frequently, a mass with or without associated calcifications can be present.
- Skin thickening and diffuse edema is commonly seen on ultrasound.
- The main differential diagnosis is mastitis, and differentiation from IBC is done by performing a skin-punch biopsy.

REFERENCES

Bassett LW, Feig SA, Hendrick RE, Jackson VP, Sickles EA. Breast disease (third series) test and syllabus. Reston: American College of Radiology; 2000. p. 76.
Bilgren-Gunhan I, Ustun EE, Memis A. Inflammatory breast carcinoma: mammographic, sonographic, clinical and pathologic findings in 142 cases. Radiology. 2002;223:829–38.

Fig. 1.1

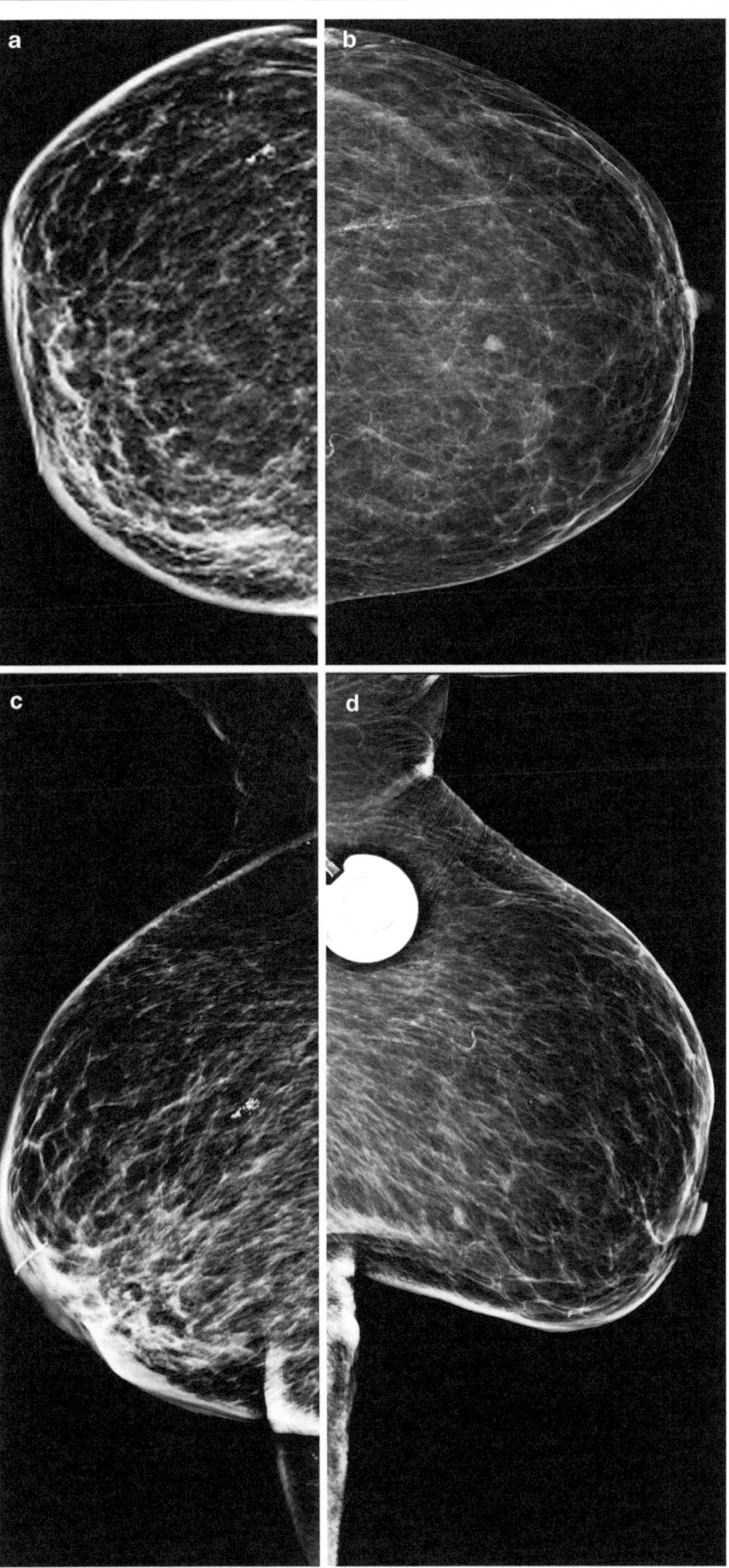

Case 49
Intramammary Lymph Node

Patient History

A 56-year-old female for a screening mammogram.

Radiology Findings

Fig. 1.1 (**a**) CC, (**b**) MLO, (**c**) spot-compression CC, and (**d**) spot-compression MLO images show a circumscribed mass in the upper outer right breast at middle depth.

Fig. 1.2 (**a**) Grayscale and (**b**) color Doppler ultrasound images show a circumscribed mass with a hypoechoic outer cortex and a hyperechoic central fatty hilum. There is vascular flow seen within the hilum.

BI-RADS Assessment

BI-RADS 2. Benign finding (following possible diagnostic workup).

Diagnosis

Intramammary lymph node

Discussion

- Intramammary lymph nodes are seen in approximately 50 % of screening patient population.
- Most commonly located in the upper outer quadrant of the breast.
- On mammogram, a lobular circumscribed mass containing a radiolucent notch (representing the fat in the hilum of the lymph node) is seen.
- On ultrasound, pathognomonic findings include a circumscribed hypoechoic cortex with a round, oval, or lobular shape, and a hyperechoic central fatty hilum is seen. Usually, vascular flow to the fatty hilum is present.
- An intramammary lymph node can enlarge, with thickening of the cortex and loss of the fatty hilum as a response to hyperplasia, inflammation, or metastatic disease.

References

American College of Radiology (ACR) BI-RADS® Atlas. ACR BI-RADS® atlas-mammography. 5th ed. Reston: American College of Radiology; 2013. p. 97–8.

Meyer JE, Ferraro FA, Frenna TH, DePiro PJ, Denison CM. Mammographic appearance of normal intramammary lymph nodes in an atypical location. AJR. 1993;161:779–80.

Venta LA, Dudiak LM, Salomon CG, Flisak ME. Sonographic evaluation of the breast. Radiographics. 1994;14:29–50.

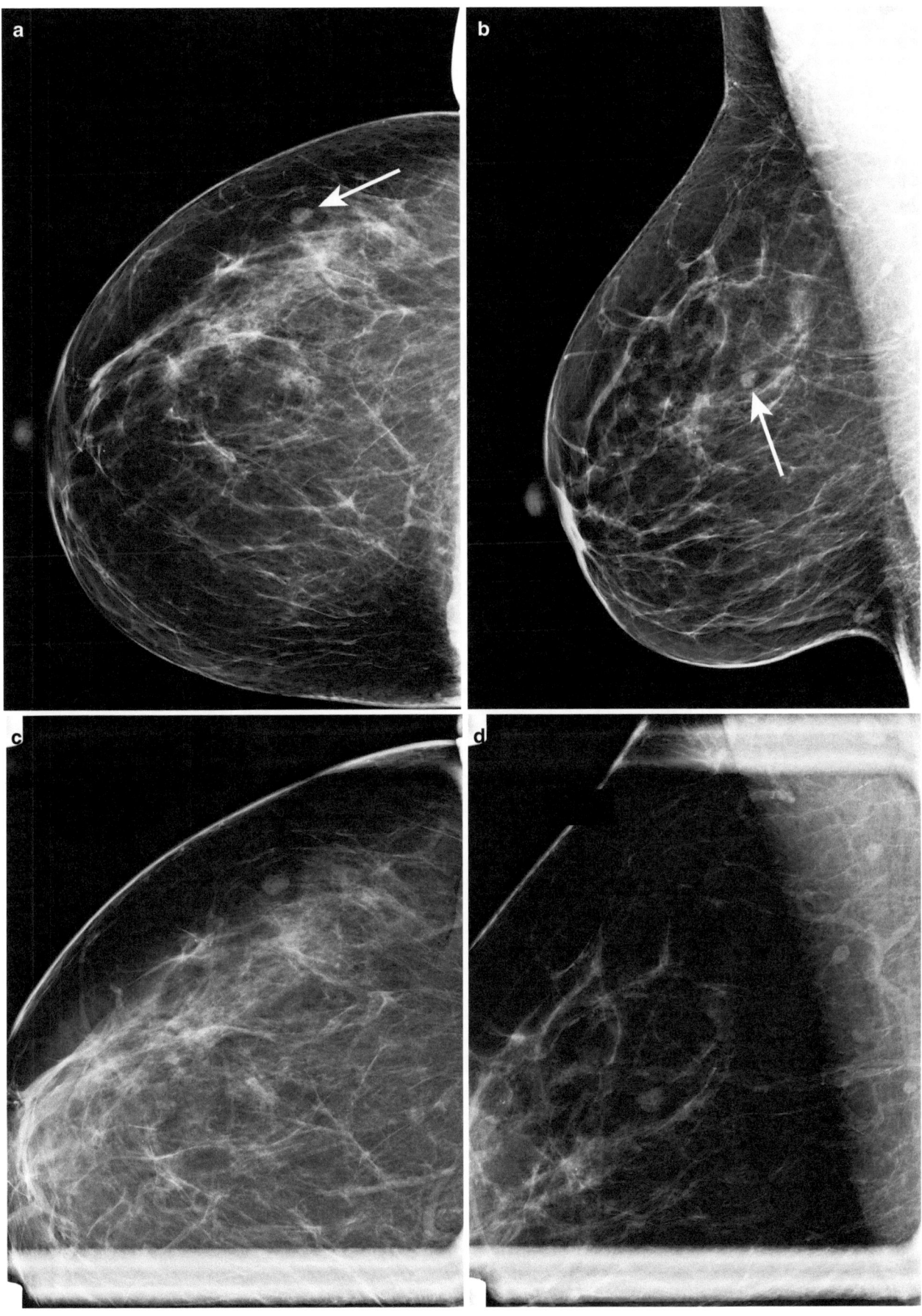

Fig. 1.1

Fig. 1.2

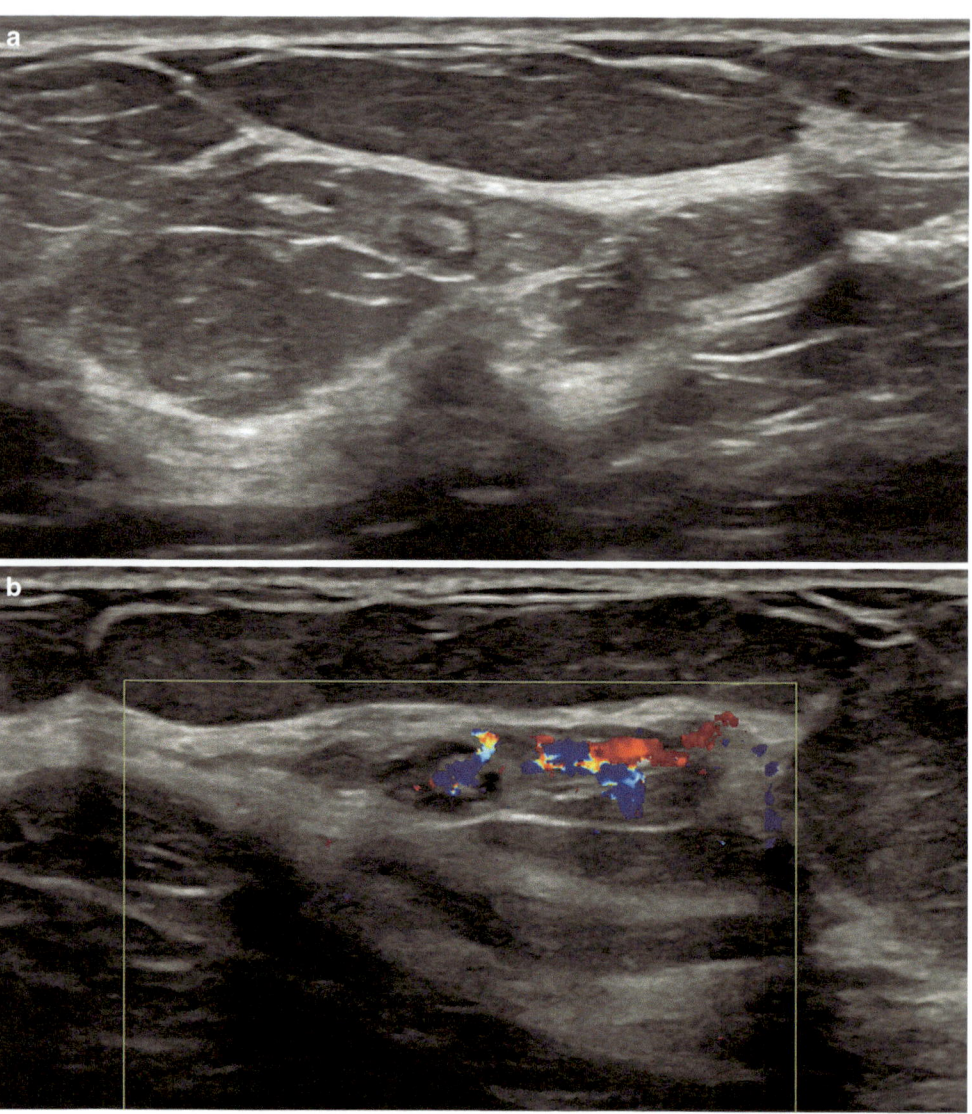

CASE 50
OIL CYST

PATIENT HISTORY

A 55-year-old female for a screening mammogram.

RADIOLOGY FINDINGS

Fig. 1.1 (**a**) CC and (**b**) MLO images demonstrate multiple circumscribed masses with rim calcification and lucent centers throughout the right breast.

BI-RADS ASSESSMENT

BI-RADS 2. Benign findings.

DIAGNOSIS

Oil cyst

DISCUSSION

- An oil cyst is a cavity containing oily fluid resulting from fat necrosis undergoing cystic degeneration.

- Surgery, accidental trauma, or radiation therapy can result in the formation of an oil cyst.
- Mammographically, an oil cyst is radiolucent. Curvilinear calcifications first develop around the periphery with central calcifications developing later.
- An oil cyst is a benign finding, not requiring any further workup.
- On ultrasound, the appearance of an oil cyst can be variable presenting as an anechoic mass or a mass of mixed echogenicity. The mass may be with or without shadowing (due to rim calcifications).
- Steatocystoma multiplex is a rare familial hamartomatous malformation that is characterized by the presence of multiple intradermal cysts, having the appearance of oil cysts on mammogram.

REFERENCES

American College of Radiology (ACR) BI-RADS® Atlas. ACR BI-RADS® atlas-mammography. 5th ed. Reston: American College of Radiology; 2013. p. 51–2.
Cardenosa G. Breast imaging companion. 2nd ed. Philadelphia: Lippincott Williams and Wilkins; 2001. p. 317–8.
Harvey JA, March DE. Making the diagnosis: a practical guide to breast imaging. Philadelphia: Elsevier; 2013. p. 181–2.
Taboada JL, Stephens TW, Krishnamurthy S, Brandt KR, Whitman GJ. The many faces of fat necrosis in the breast. AJR. 2009;192:815–25.

Fig. 1.1

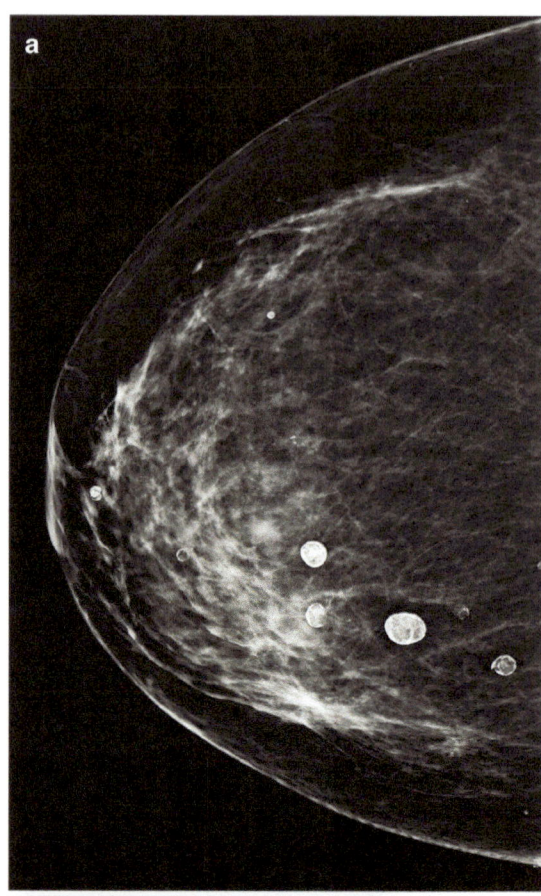

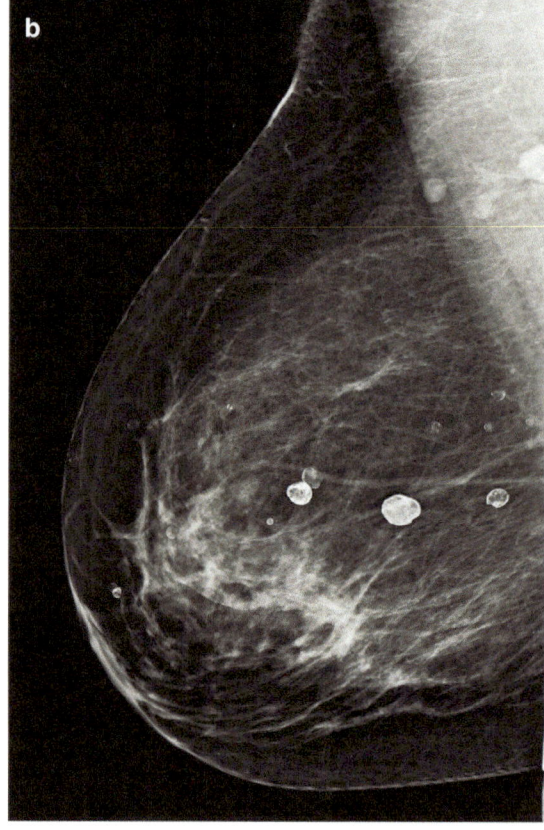

Case 51
Hormone Replacement Therapy (HRT)

Patient History

A 55-year-old female for a screening mammogram.

Radiology Findings

Fig. 1.1 (**a**) CC and (**b**) MLO images of the left breast with scattered fibroglandular densities prior to hormone replacement therapy (HRT).
Fig. 1.2 (**a**) CC and (**b**) MLO images of the left breast following HRT show an overall increase in breast density.

BI-RADS Assessment

BI-RADS 2. Benign findings.

Diagnosis

HRT

Discussion

- HRT is prescribed in menopausal patients to reduce vasomotor symptoms of menopause, prevent osteoporosis, and offer potential cardiovascular benefits.

- On mammogram, the use of HRT over time can result in diffuse increase in density and development of new asymmetries or cysts in about 25 % of patients.
- Cessation of HRT will usually result in breast parenchyma, returning to its prehormone replacement therapy density.
- If the development of a new asymmetry is attributed to the use of HRT, then discontinuing the HRT for 3 months may result in the regression of the asymmetry.
- Causes of bilateral increase in breast density include hormone therapy (estrogen with progesterone more commonly than estrogen alone), perimenopausal, follicular phase in premenopausal women, pregnancy and lactation, and elevated serum prolactin.

References

Berkowitz JE, Gatewood OM, Goldblum LE, Gayler BW. Hormonal replacement therapy: mammographic manifestations. Radiology. 1990;174:199–201.

Harvey JA, March DE. Making the diagnosis: a practical guide to breast imaging. Philadelphia: Elsevier; 2013. p. 139.

Kopans DB. Breast imaging. 2nd ed. Philadelphia: Lippincott Williams and Wilkins; 1998. p. 241–2.

Stomper PC, VanVoorhis BJ, Ravniker VA, Meyer JE. Mammographic changes associated with postmenopausal hormone replacement therapy: a longitudinal study. Radiology. 1990;174:487–90.

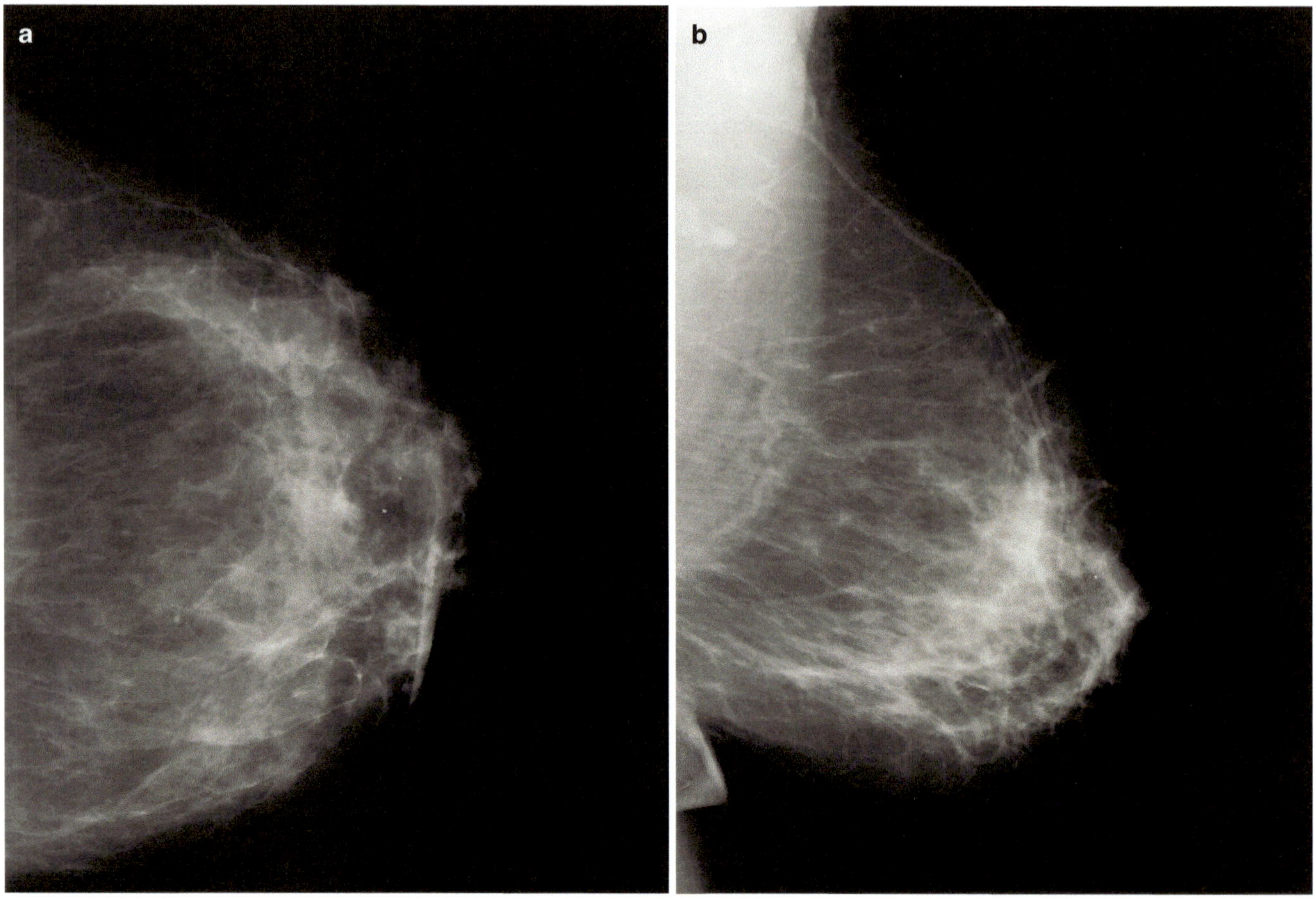

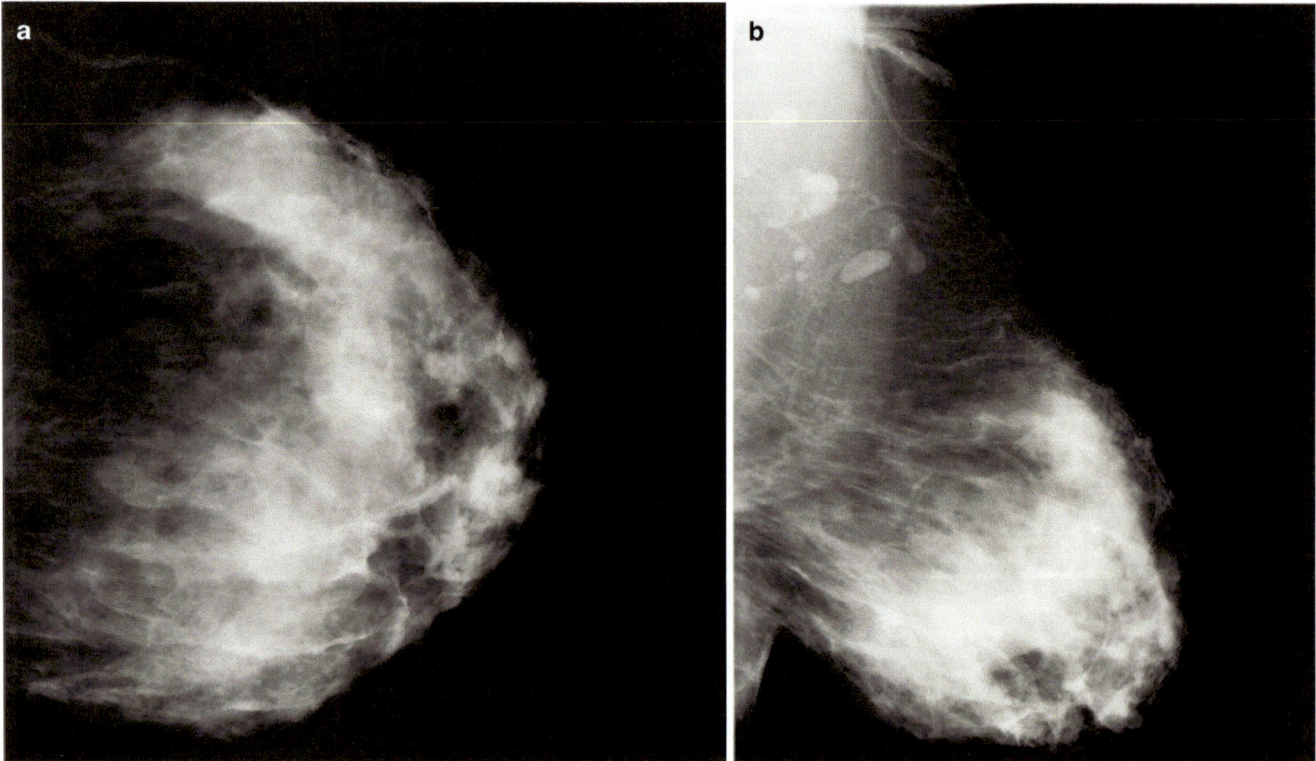

Fig. 1.1

Fig. 1.2

CASE 52
COMPLEX CYSTIC AND SOLID MASS

PATIENT HISTORY

A 48-year-old female with a mass in the upper outer right breast.

RADIOLOGY FINDINGS

Fig. 1.1 (**a**) Spot-compression CC, (**b**) spot-compression MLO, and (**c**) ML views show an oval mass in the upper outer right breast at middle to posterior depth.
Fig. 1.2 (**a**) Grayscale and (**b**) color Doppler images show an oval predominately anechoic mass with an intracystic hypoechoic mass with vascularity in the right breast.

BI-RADS ASSESSMENT

BI-RADS 4. Suspicious abnormality (following diagnostic workup, prior to biopsy)

DIAGNOSIS

Complex cystic and solid mass

DISCUSSION

- Complex cystic and solid mass can contain:
  - Both cystic and solid components
  - Thickened cystic wall
  - Irregular thickened septations
- Differential diagnosis of a complex cyst includes:
  - Benign intracystic papilloma
  - Invasive papillary carcinoma
  - Intracystic (papillary) DCIS
  - Tumefactive debris within a complicated cyst
  - Postsurgical seroma or hematoma
- Biopsy is recommended for definitive diagnosis by either ultrasound-guided wire localization or ultrasound-guided core needle biopsy of the solid component of the mass.

REFERENCES

American College of Radiology (ACR) BI-RADS® Atlas. ACR BI-RADS® atlas-breast ultrasound. 5th ed. Reston: American College of Radiology; 2013. p. 62–3.
Berg WA, Birdwell RL, Gombos EC, et al. Diagnostic imaging breast. 1st ed. Salt Lake City: Amirsys; 2006. Section IV-1, p. 56–65.
Doshi DJ, March DE, Crisi GM, Coughlin BF. Complex cystic breast masses: diagnostic approach and imaging-pathologic correlation. Radiographics. 2007;27:S53–64.

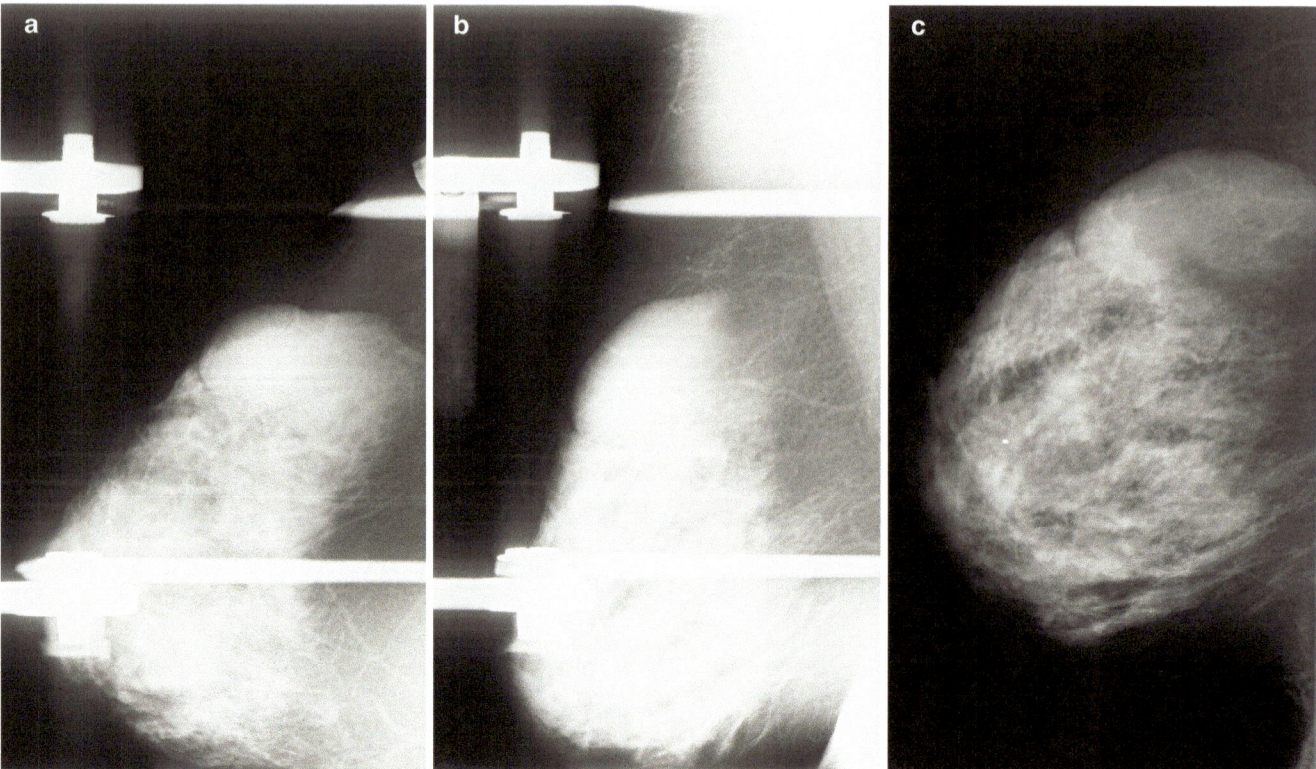

Fig. 1.1

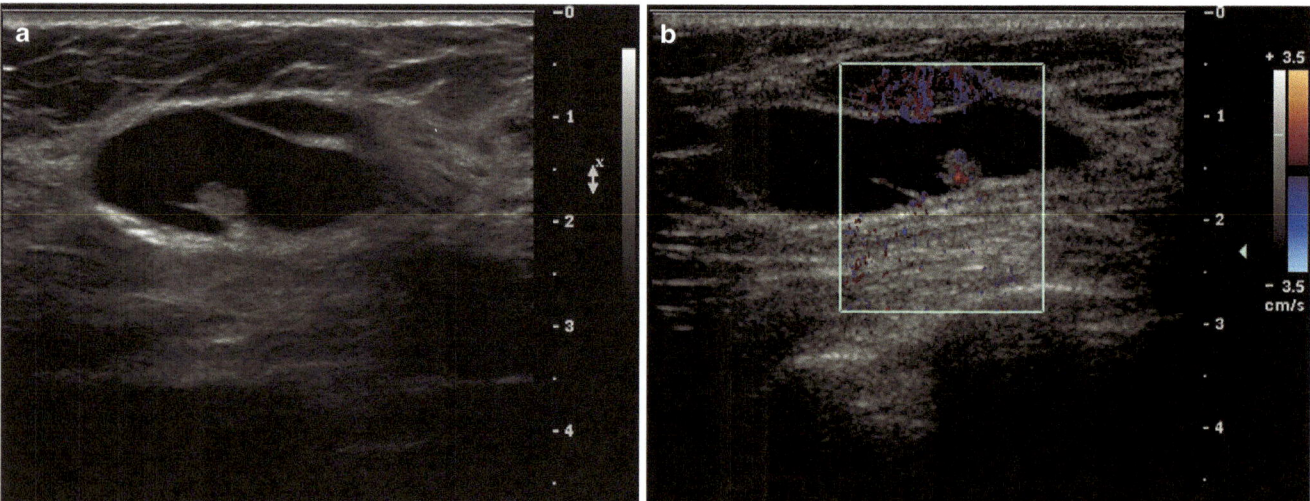

Fig. 1.2

CASE 53
FIBROADENOMA IN A TEENAGE PATIENT

PATIENT HISTORY

A 19-year-old female with a history of a palpable mass at 12 o'clock in the left breast.

RADIOLOGY FINDINGS

Fig. 1.1 (**a**) Grayscale and (**b**) color Doppler images show an oval hypoechoic avascular circumscribed mass at 12 o'clock corresponding to the patient's palpable mass. This mass is parallel to the chest wall.

BI-RADS ASSESSMENT

BI-RADS 2. Benign finding (following diagnostic workup and biopsy).

DIAGNOSIS

Fibroadenoma in a teenage patient

DISCUSSION

- Fibroadenoma is the most common benign breast mass.
- More common in younger women.
- Fibroadenomas contain epithelial and stromal elements. In younger patients, fibroadenomas contain more epithelial than stromal elements.
- Breast ultrasound is commonly used as the first modality in women under 30 years of age, lactating, pregnant, or presenting with a palpable lump. This is due to the dense breast composition in younger women and to avoid radiation exposure.
- If no mass is seen on ultrasound, surgical consultation may be considered, as some cancers may not be sonographically visible.
- If the mass meets all mammographic and sonographic criteria for a benign lesion than imaging, follow-up can be considered without biopsy.

REFERENCES

Cardenosa G. Breast imaging companion. 3rd ed. Philadelphia: Lippincott Williams and Wilkins; 2008. p. 112–3.

Harvey JA, Nicholson BT, LoRusso PT, et al. Short term follow-up of palpable breast lesions with benign imaging features: evaluation of 375 lesions in 320 women. AJR. 2009;193:1723–30.

Ikeda DM. Breast imaging the requisites. 2nd ed. Philadelphia: Elsevier, Mosby; 2011. p. 117–20.

Fig. 1.1

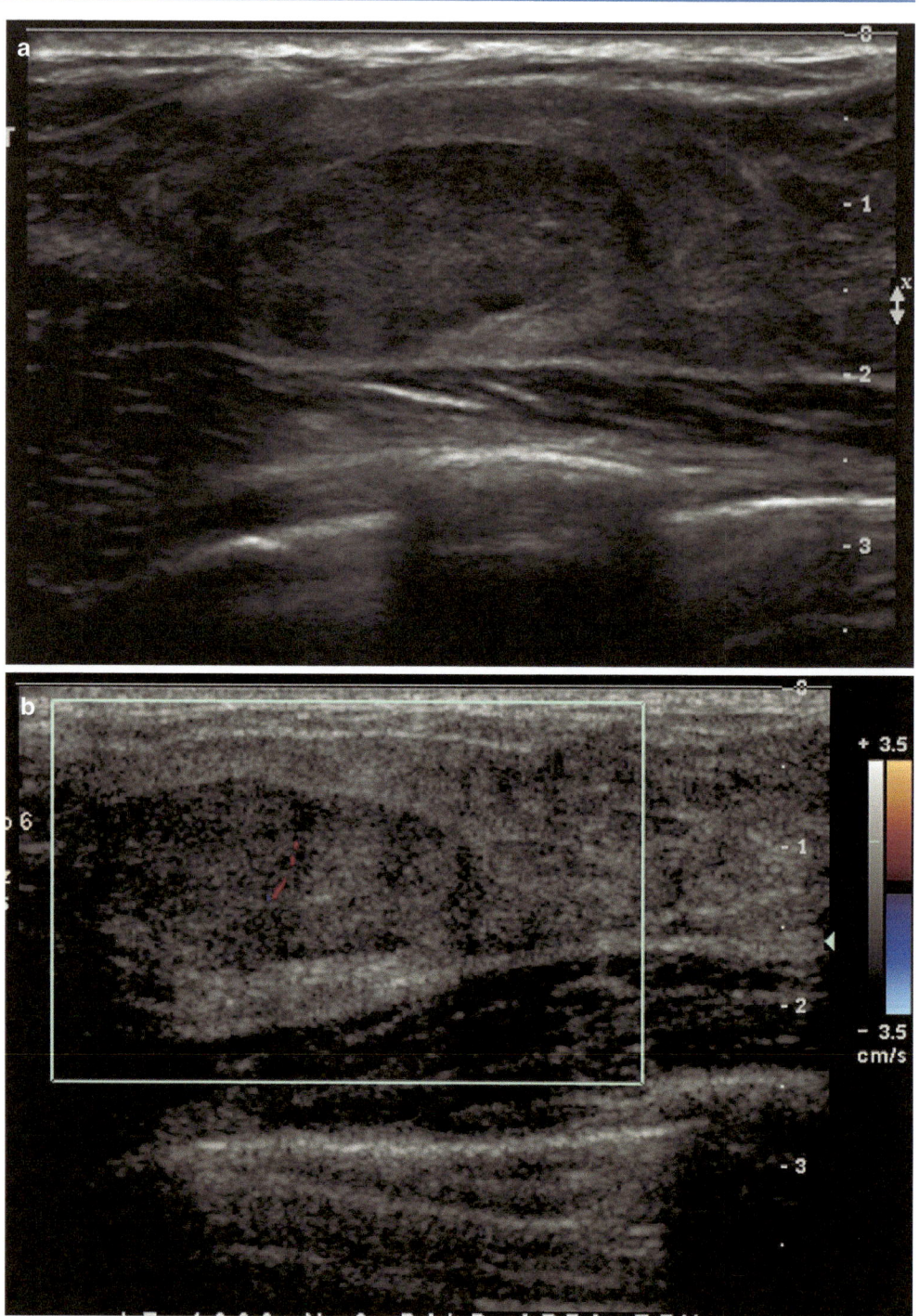

CASE 54
ARCHITECTURAL DISTORTION

PATIENT HISTORY

A 55-year-old female for a screening mammogram. No history of prior breast surgery or breast biopsy.

RADIOLOGY FINDINGS

Fig. 1.1 Spot-magnification (**a**) CC and (**b**) ML views show an area of architectural distortion in the upper outer left breast at middle depth.

Fig. 1.2 (**a**) Grayscale and (**b**) color Doppler images demonstrate an irregular hypoechoic mass with spiculated margins and posterior acoustic shadowing. There is vascular flow within the mass.

BI-RADS ASSESSMENT

BI-RADS 5. Highly suspicious for malignancy (following diagnostic workup, prior to biopsy).

DIAGNOSIS

Architectural distortion

DISCUSSION

- In the absence of clinical history of surgery or trauma, architectural distortion is suspicious for malignancy or radial scar, and therefore biopsy is recommended.
- Architectural distortion can be associated with a mass, asymmetry, or calcifications.
- On mammography, linear opacities radiating from a focal point or area with no definite central mass are seen.
- On ultrasound, an associated mass that is central to architectural distortion can be seen. There can also be thickening and tethering of Cooper ligaments.
- On MRI, an enhancing lesion with distortion or spiculated enhancement around the lesion is seen.
- Differential diagnosis includes:
  - Postsurgical scar
  - Radial scar
  - Fat necrosis
  - IDC
  - ILC

REFERENCES

American College of Radiology (ACR) BI-RADS® Atlas. ACR BI-RADS® atlas mammography. 5th ed. Reston: American College of Radiology; 2013. p. 79–80.

Berg WA, Birdwell RL, Gombos EC, et al. Diagnostic imaging breast. 1st ed. Salt Lake City: Amirsys; 2006. Section IV-1, p. 122–5.

Mandell J. Core radiology: a visual approach to diagnostic imaging. 1st ed. Cambridge: Cambridge University Press; 2013. p. 605.

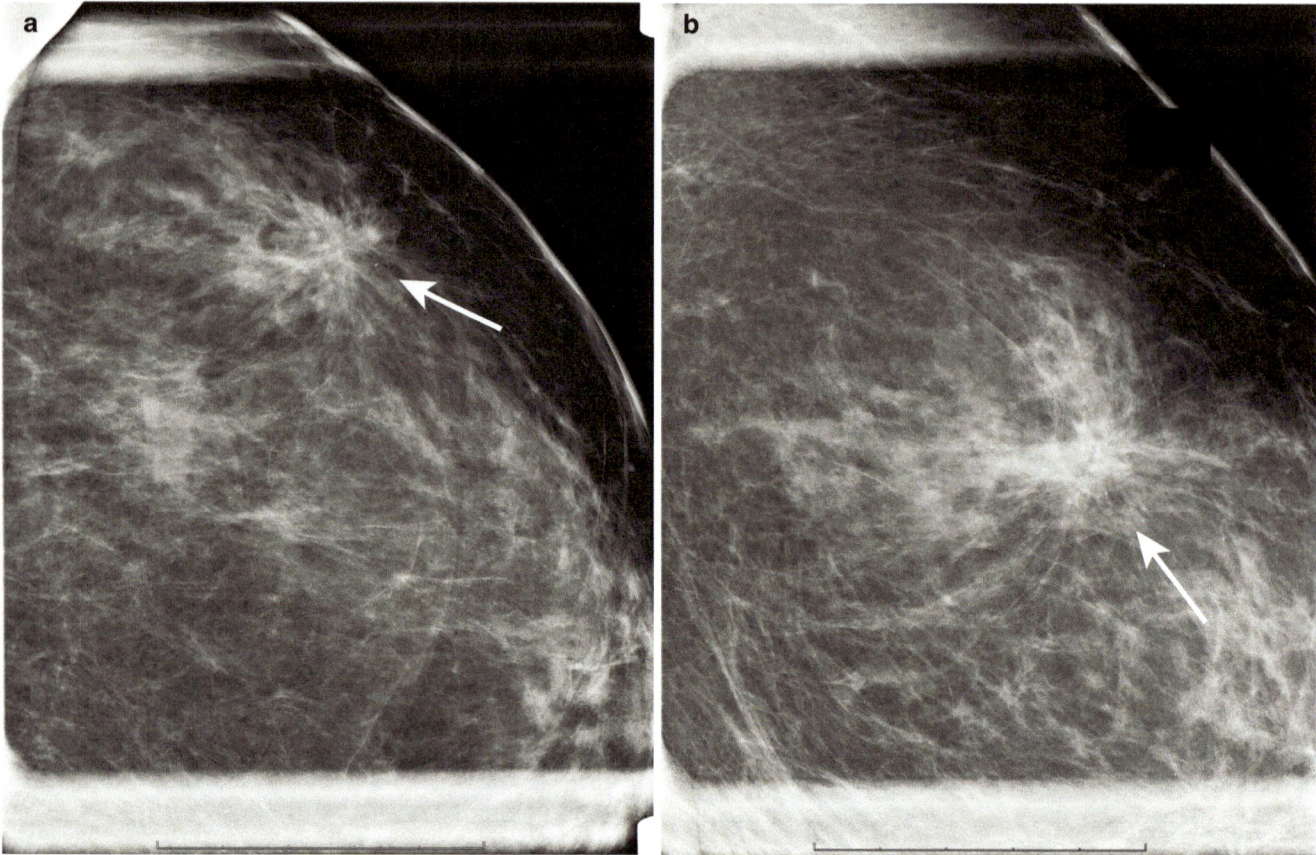

Fig. 1.1

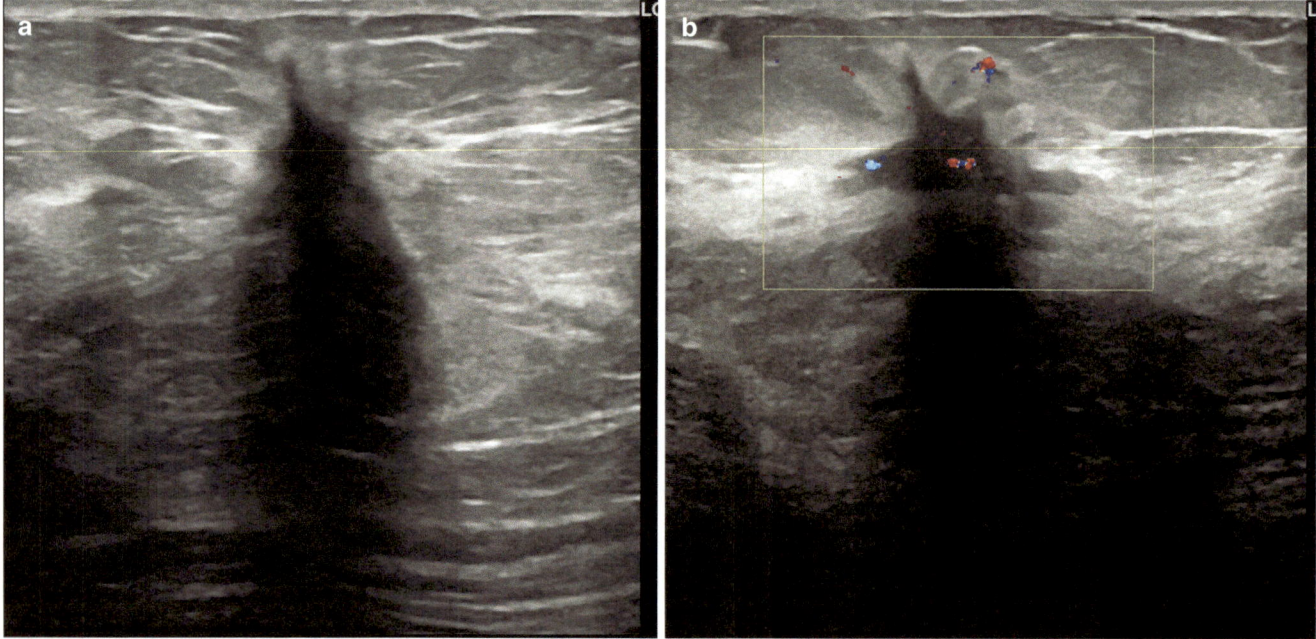

Fig. 1.2

CASE 55
PSEUDOANGIOMATOUS STROMAL HYPERPLASIA (PASH)

PATIENT HISTORY

A 51-year-old female for screening mammogram.

RADIOLOGY FINDINGS

Fig. 1.1 (**a**) CC, (**b**) ML, and (**c**) spot-compression CC views show a lobular mass at 6 o'clock in the right breast at middle depth.
Fig. 1.2 (**a**, **b**) Grayscale and (**c**) color Doppler ultrasound images show a circumscribed lobular mass with no vascular flow.

BI-RADS ASSESSMENT

BI-RADS 2. Benign finding (following diagnostic workup and biopsy).

DIAGNOSIS

Pseudoangiomatous stromal hyperplasia (PASH)

DISCUSSION

- PASH is a benign mesenchymal lesion.
- Most commonly occurs in premenopausal women.
- Typically seen as a circumscribed mass on mammogram, but spiculated, indistinct, or partially obscured margins can rarely be seen.
- Sonographically, PASH is seen as a solid hypoechoic circumscribed mass.
- PASH may clinically present as a firm palpable painless breast mass.
- Histologically, PASH needs to be distinguished from angiosarcoma.
- If imaging findings are concordant, excision is not indicated.

REFERENCES

Goel NB, Knight TE, Shilpa P, Riddick-Young M, Shaw de Paredes E, Trivedi A. Fibrous lesions of the breast: imaging-pathologic correlation. Radiographics. 2005;25:1547–59.

Harvey JA, March DE. Making the diagnosis: a practical guide to breast imaging. Philadelphia: Elsevier; 2013. p. 304.

Polger MR, Denison CM, Lester S, Meyer JE. Pseudoangiomatous stromal hyperplasia: mammographic and sonographic appearances. AJR. 1996;166:349–52.

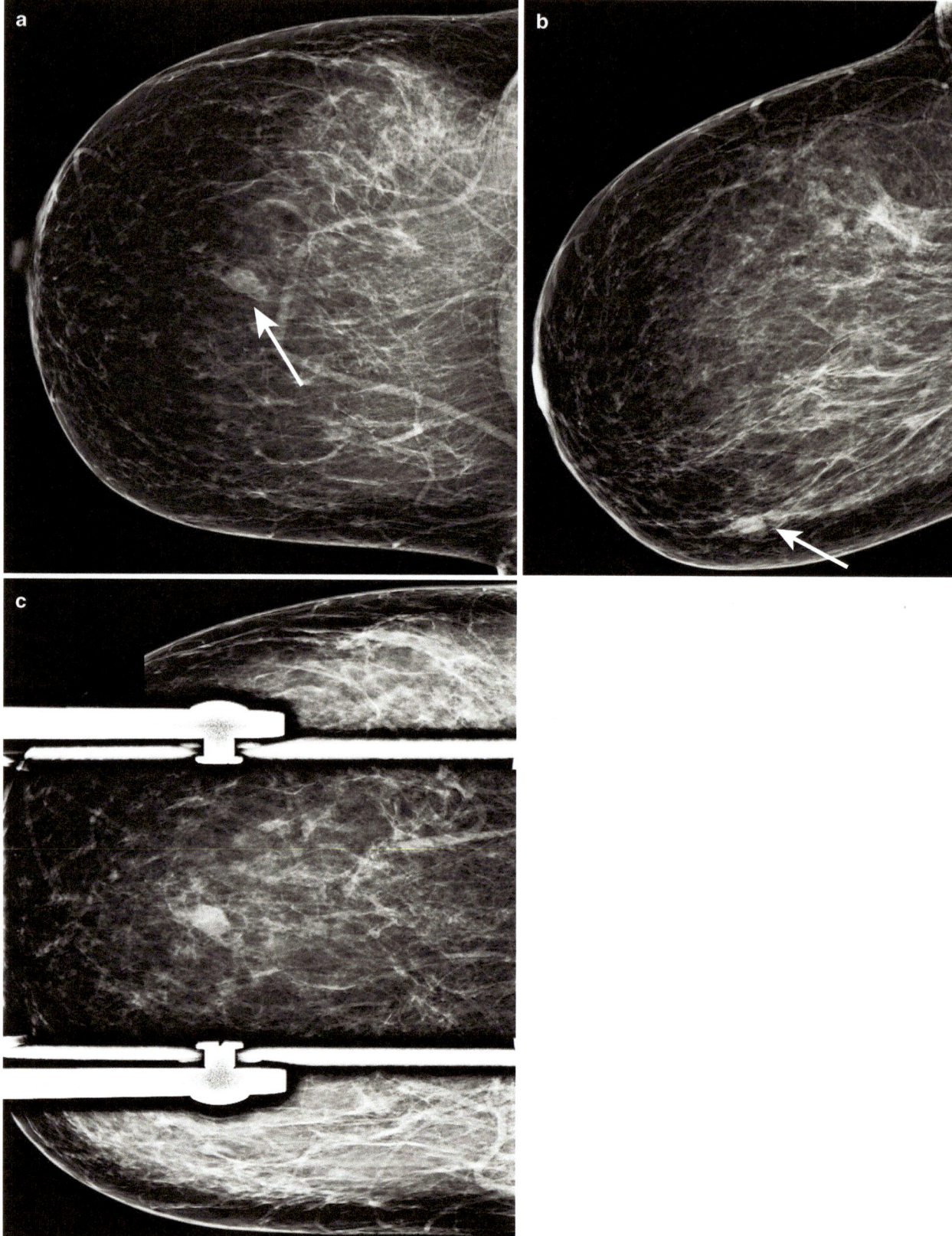

Fig. 1.1

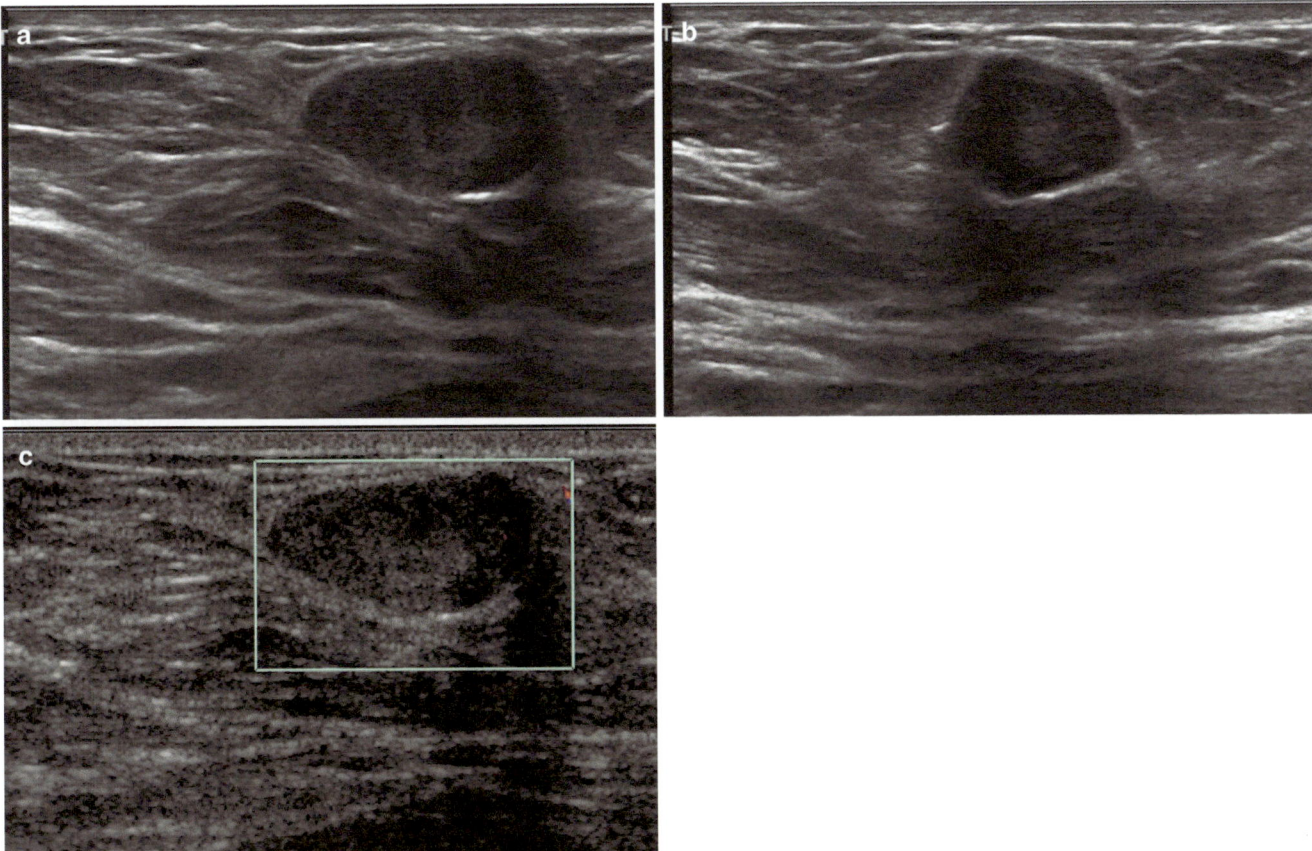

Fig. 1.2

Case 56
Sclerosing Adenosis

Patient History

A 44-year-old female for a screening mammogram.

Radiology Findings

Fig. 1.1 Spot magnification (**a**) CC and (**b**) ML views demonstrate two groups of amorphous and punctuate calcifications in the upper outer and upper inner left breast at anterior depth.

Fig. 1.2 MLO view in a different patient demonstrates a high-density, oval mass in the retroareolar region of the left breast.

BI-RADS Assessment

BI-RADS 2. Benign finding (following diagnostic workup and possible biopsy).

Diagnosis

Sclerosing adenosis

Discussion

- Sclerosing adenosis is a benign lesion caused by mammary lobular hyperplasia.
- Characterized by stromal sclerosis and adenosis.
- Most common mammographic finding is calcifications.
- Calcifications may be amorphous, round, or punctuate. Rarely, may appear pleomorphic.
- Less common presentations are spiculated (if associated with radial sclerosing lesion), circumscribed, or irregular masses.
- When sclerosing adenosis is diagnosed on core needle biopsy, excision is recommended for suspicious presentation such as:
  - Pleomorphic or linear branching calcifications
  - Spiculated mass
  - Architectural distortion
- Diagnosis of sclerosing adenosis increases the risk of invasive cancer by 1.7–2.5 times.

References

Berg WA, Birdwell RL, Gombos EC, et al. Diagnostic imaging breast. 1st ed. Salt Lake City: Amirsys; 2006. Section IV-2, p. 4–6.

Gill H, Ioffe O, Berg W. When is a diagnosis of sclerosing adenosis acceptable at core needle biopsy? Radiology. 2003;228:50–7.

Ikeda DM. Breast imaging the requisites. 2nd ed. Philadelphia: Elsevier, Mosby; 2011. p. 109–111.

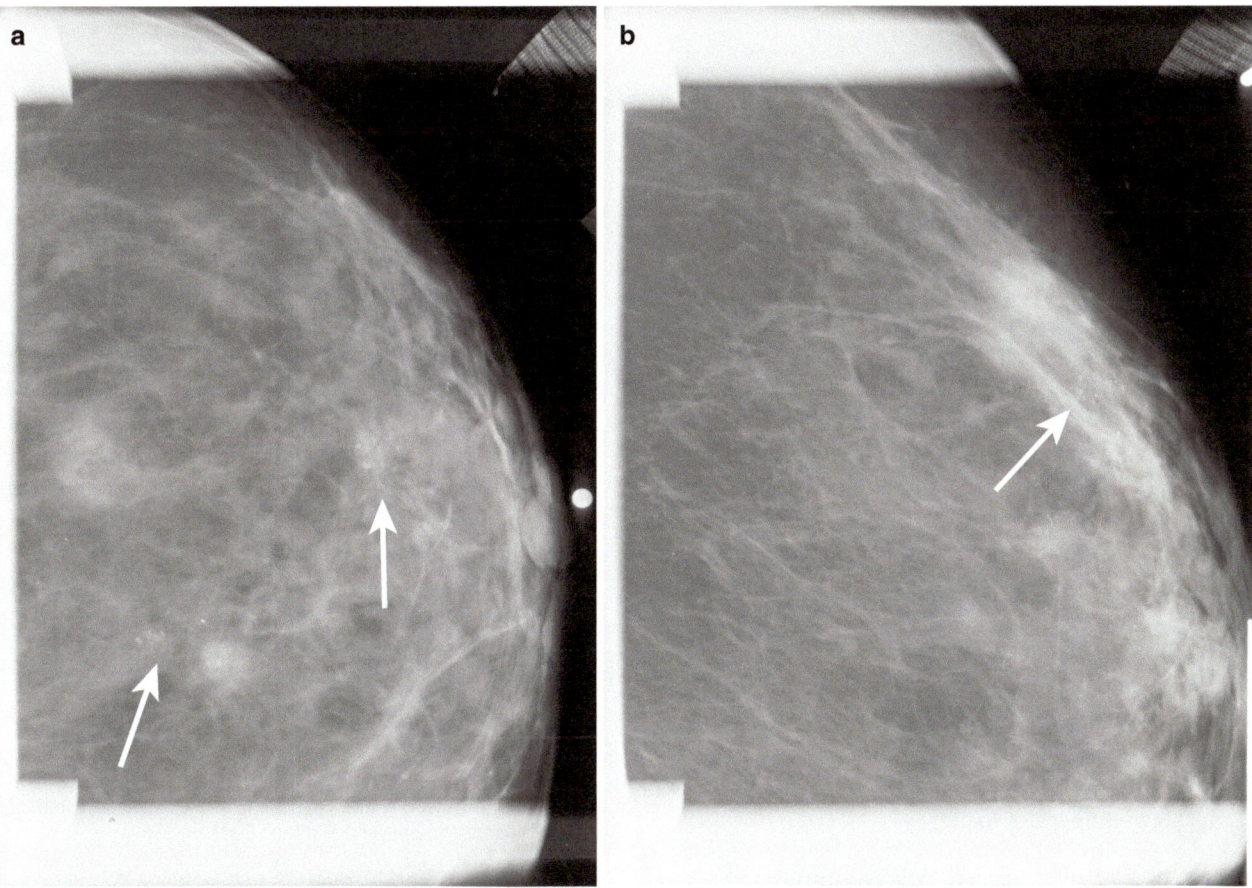

Fig. 1.1

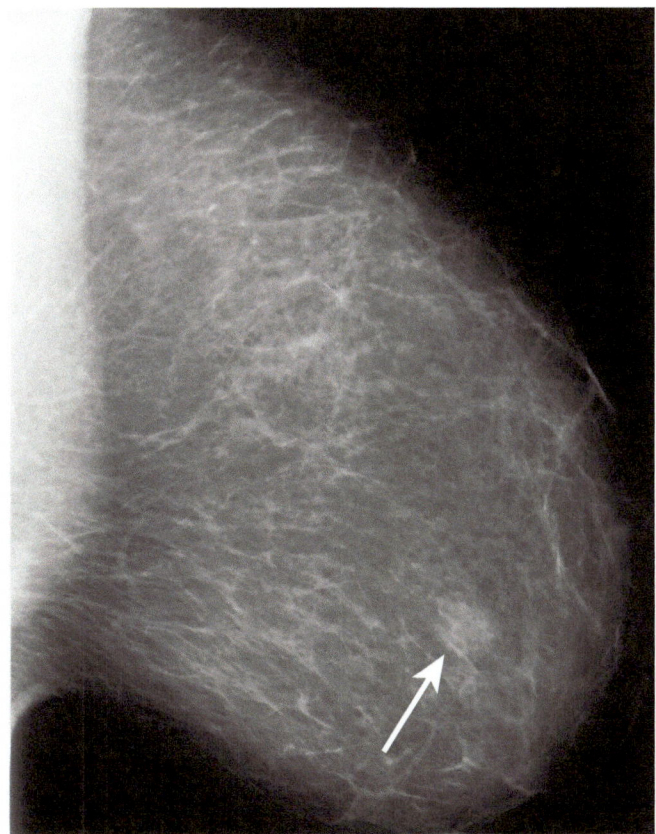

Fig. 1.2

CASE 57
MUCINOUS CARCINOMA

PATIENT HISTORY

A 62-year-old female for a screening mammogram. Family history of aunt with breast cancer.

RADIOLOGY FINDINGS

Fig. 1.1 (**a**) CC, (**b**) LM, (**c**) spot-compression CC, and (**d**) spot-compression MLO images show an irregular mass with spiculated margins in the upper inner right breast at posterior depth.

Fig. 1.2 (**a**) Grayscale and (**b**) color Doppler ultrasound images show a mass with heterogeneous echotexture and microlobulated margins. There is vascular flow within the mass.

BI-RADS ASSESSMENT

BI-RADS 5. Highly suggestive of malignancy (following diagnostic workup, prior to biopsy).

DIAGNOSIS

Mucinous carcinoma

DISCUSSION

- Mucinous carcinoma accounts for 2–3 % of all breast cancers.
- Most commonly seen in older postmenopausal women.
- Slow rate of growth.
- On mammography, mucinous carcinoma is typically seen as a circumscribed or ill-defined mass.
- A nonspecific hypoechoic mass with posterior acoustic shadowing is seen on ultrasound.
- On MRI, T1-weighted images demonstrate a low to high signal mass, while T2-weighted images demonstrate a high signal mass due to the large mucin component of the tumor.
- On MRI, mucinous carcinoma usually shows gradual persistent or plateau enhancement after the initial upstroke.
- Washout enhancement kinetics not readily seen with mucinous carcinoma.
- A core biopsy containing mucin can represent a benign mucocele or a mucinous carcinoma; thus, excision should be recommended.

REFERENCES

Cardenosa G. Breast imaging companion. 2nd ed. Philadelphia: Lippincott Williams and Wilkins; 2001. p. 256.

Harvey JA, March DE. Making the diagnosis: a practical guide to breast imaging. Philadelphia: Elsevier; 2013. p. 299.

Kawashima M, Tamaki Y, Nonaka T, et al. MR imaging of mucinous carcinoma of the breast. AJR. 2002;179:179–83.

Kopans DB. Breast imaging. 2nd ed. Philadelphia: Lippincott Williams and Wilkins; 1998. p. 587.

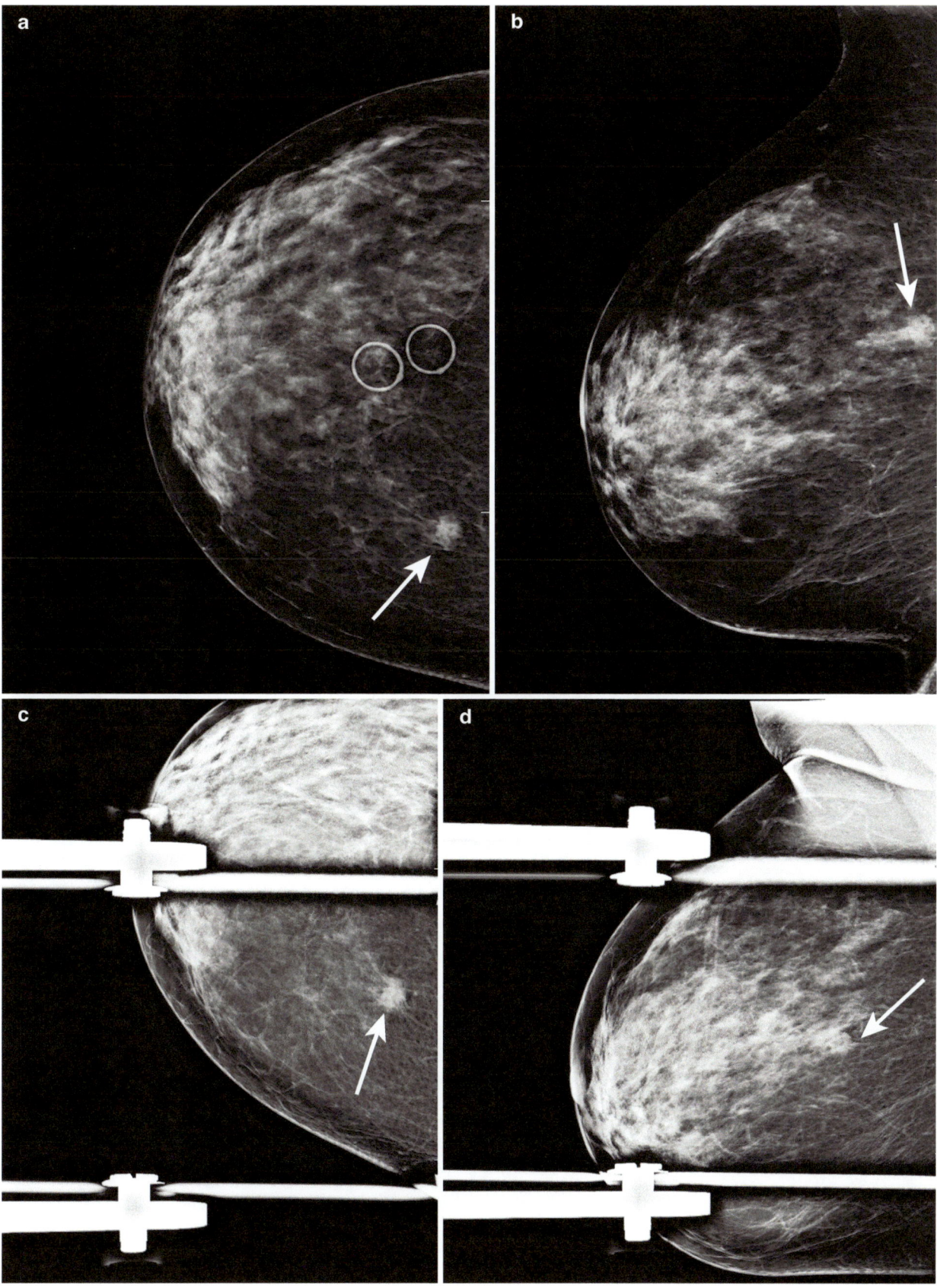

Fig. 1.1

Fig. 1.2

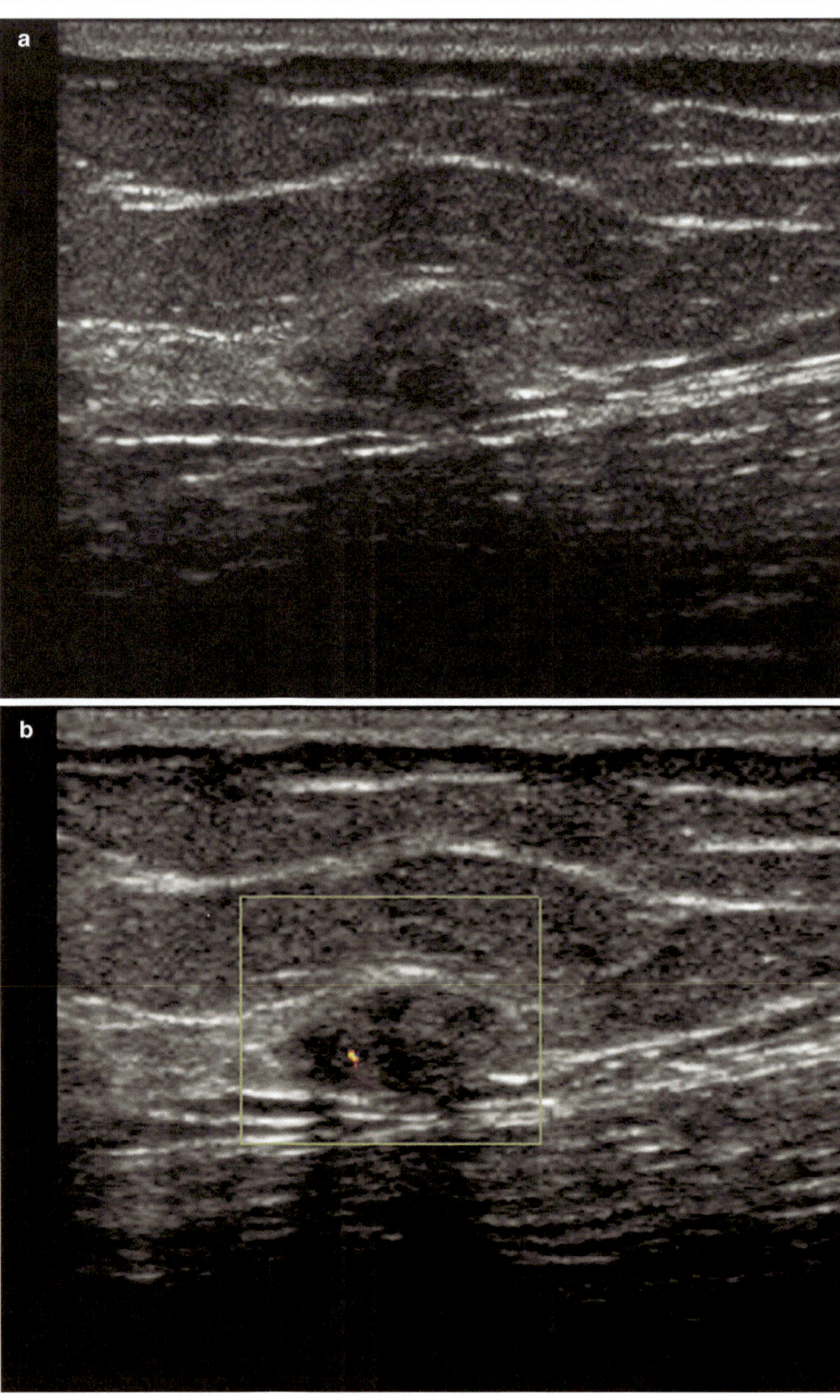

CASE 58
APOCRINE CYST CLUSTER

PATIENT HISTORY

A 43-year-old female for a screening mammogram.

RADIOLOGY FINDINGS

Fig. 1.1 Grayscale ultrasound image demonstrates multiple, small, adjacent anechoic masses with posterior acoustic enhancement.

Fig. 1.2 Color Doppler ultrasound image demonstrates no vascular flow within the masses.

BI-RADS ASSESSMENT

BI-RADS 2. Benign finding (following diagnostic workup and possible biopsy).

DIAGNOSIS

Apocrine cyst cluster

DISCUSSION

- Epithelial lining of the cysts is composed of columnar/cuboidal cells with granular eosinophilic cytoplasm, resembling the epithelium of apocrine sweat glands.
- On mammography, apocrine cyst cluster appears as lobulated, circumscribed masses or amorphous and punctuate calcifications.
- May contain milk of calcium.
- On T1-weighted postcontrast MRI, apocrine cyst cluster appears as lobulated masses with thin rim enhancement and enhanced internal septations.
- On ultrasound, if clustered microcysts demonstrate a classic appearance, then no intervention is needed.
- If appearance is not classic, then short-term (6 months) follow-up is required.
- Biopsy is recommended if a solid component is present or if mass is rapidly enlarging.

REFERENCES

Bassett LW, Jackson VP, Fu KL, Fu YS. Diagnosis of diseases of the breast. 2nd ed. Philadelphia: Elsevier; 2005. p. 436–8.

Berg WA, Birdwell RL, Gombos EC, et al. Diagnostic imaging breast. 1st ed. Salt Lake City: Amirsys; 2006. IV-2, p. 8–10.

Fig. 1.1

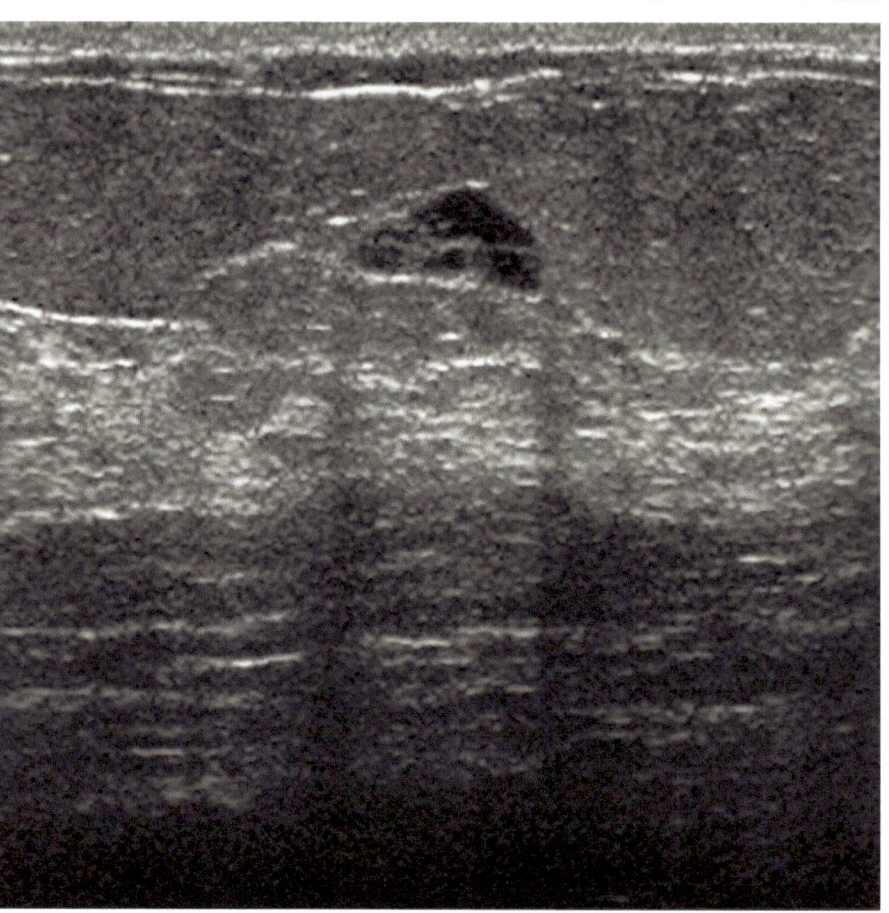

Fig. 1.2

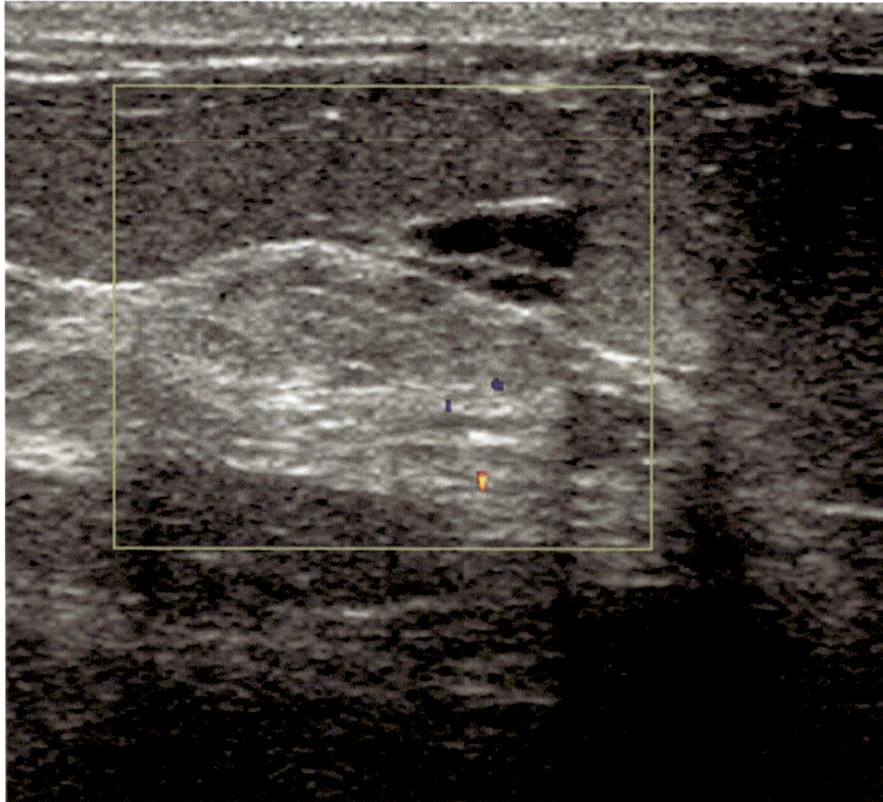

CASE 59
CALCIFICATIONS IN AXILLARY LYMPH NODES IN A PATIENT WITH SARCOIDOSIS

PATIENT HISTORY

A 41-year-old female for a bilateral screening mammogram.

RADIOLOGY FINDINGS

Fig. 1.1 Spot-magnification (**a**) XCCL and (**b**) ML images show amorphous calcifications within the left axillary lymph nodes.

BI-RADS ASSESSMENT

BI-RADS 2. Benign findings (following diagnostic workup and biopsy).

DIAGNOSIS

Calcifications in axillary lymph nodes in a patient with sarcoidosis

DISCUSSION

- Coarse calcifications within axillary lymph nodes are typically seen in the following:

  – Granulomatous disease (tuberculosis and histoplasmosis)
  – Sarcoidosis
  – Fat necrosis
- Amorphous and peripheral microcalcifications within axillary lymph nodes are typically from metastatic disease, including:
  – Breast
  – Ovarian
  – Thyroid cancer
- Punctate or amorphous calcifications within axillary lymph nodes can be seen from:
  – Gold deposits in patients who have undergone long-term treatment with intramuscular gold therapy for rheumatoid arthritis
  – Silicone deposition in patients with a ruptured or previously ruptured silicone breast implant
- Correlation with clinical history and possible workup for metastatic disease or systemic process is necessary.

REFERENCES

Berg WA, Birdwell RL, Gombos EC, et al. Diagnostic imaging breast. 1st ed. Salt Lake City: Amirsys; 2006. Section IV-3, p. 36–7.

Ikeda DM. Breast imaging the requisites. 2nd ed. Philadelphia: Elsevier, Mosby; 2011. p. 396.

Fig. 1.1

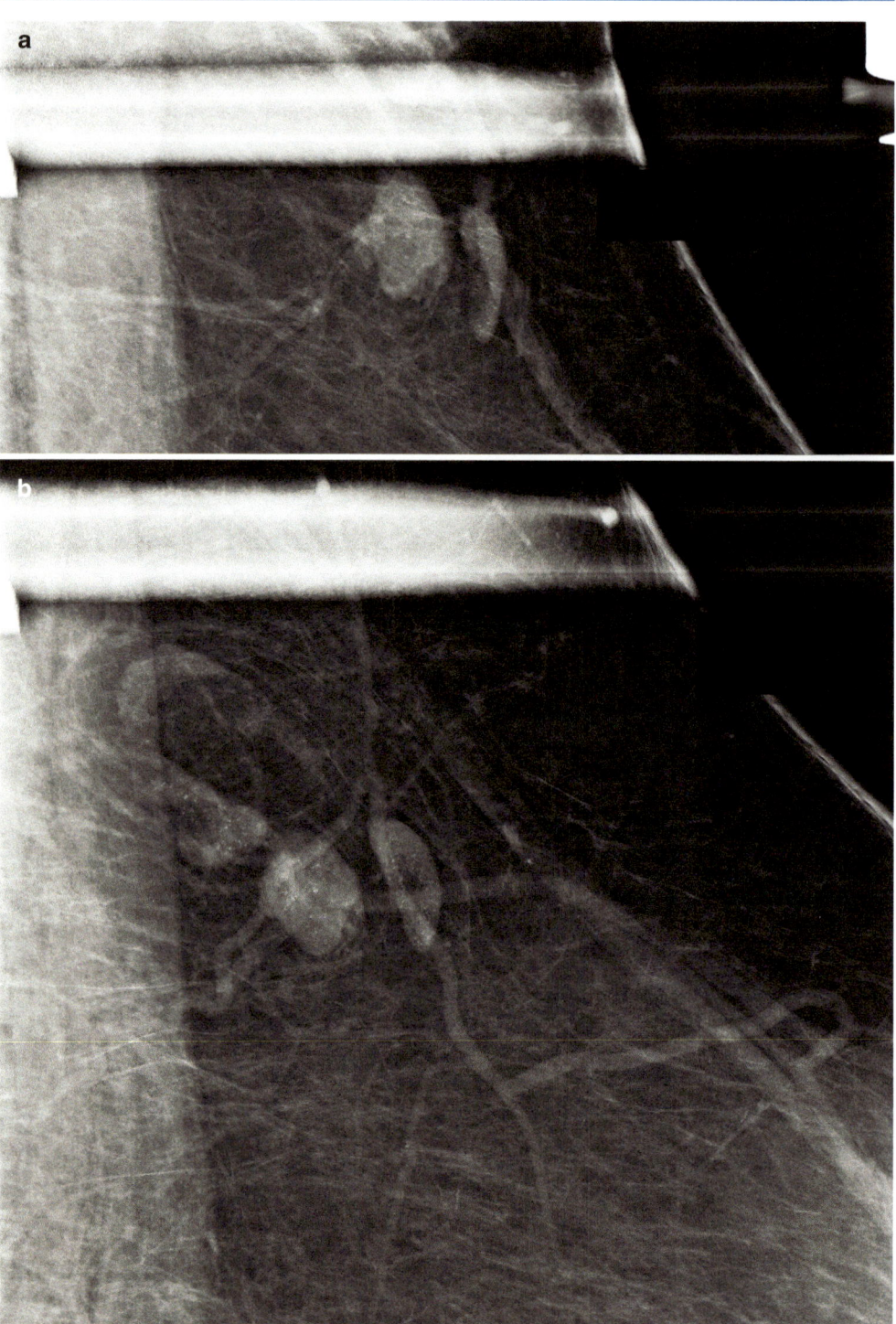

CASE 60
FIBROADENOLIPOMA (HAMARTOMA)

PATIENT HISTORY

A 44-year-old female for a bilateral screening mammogram.

RADIOLOGY FINDINGS

Fig. 1.1 (**a**) CC and (**b**) MLO views show an oval circumscribed mass in the lower inner right breast at anterior depth containing fat and fibroglandular tissue within it, surrounded by a thin capsule.

BI-RADS ASSESSMENT

BI-RADS 2. Benign finding.

DIAGNOSIS

Fibroadenolipoma (hamartoma)

DISCUSSION

- Pathognomonic appearance of a hamartoma on mammogram is a "breast within a breast" appearance.
- Classic appearance of a hamartoma is an oval or round circumscribed mass containing fat and fibroglandular tissues. Benign calcifications may be present.
- Can occur anywhere in the breast and may be multiple.
- Typically asymptomatic and no intervention is necessary.
- Very rare for breast cancer to develop in a hamartoma.

REFERENCES

Ikeda DM. Breast imaging the requisites. 2nd ed. Philadelphia: Elsevier, Mosby; 2011. p. 135–7.

Mandell J. Core radiology: a visual approach to diagnostic imaging. 1st ed. Cambridge: Cambridge University Press; 2013. p. 623.

Wahner-Roedler DL, Sebo TJ, Gisbold JJ. Hamartomas of the breast: clinical, radiologic, and pathologic manifestations. Breast J. 2001;7(2):101–5.

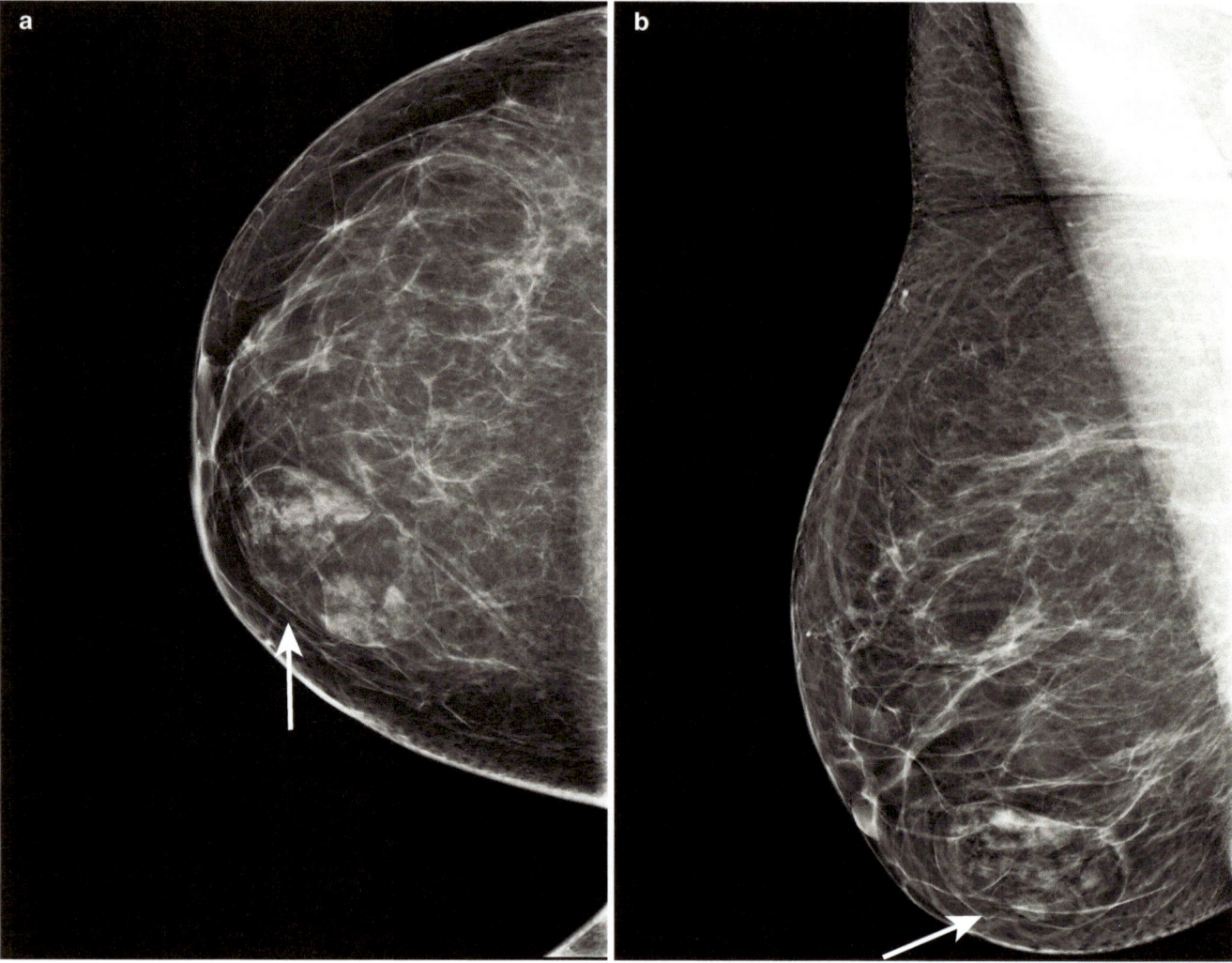

Fig. 1.1

CASE 61
ATYPICAL DUCTAL HYPERPLASIA (ADH)

PATIENT HISTORY

A 45-year-old female for a screening mammogram.

RADIOLOGY FINDINGS

Fig. 1.1 Spot-magnification (**a**) CC and (**b**) ML images reveal pleomorphic calcifications that are grouped at 6 o'clock in the right breast at middle depth.

BI-RADS ASSESSMENT

High-risk lesion.

DIAGNOSIS

Atypical ductal hyperplasia (ADH)

DISCUSSION

- ADH is considered as a high-risk lesion, which should be surgically excised.
- Most common presentation is amorphous calcifications.
- Grouped distribution occurs more often than regional distribution.
- Four to five times increased risk for developing invasive breast cancer in either breast.

REFERENCES

Berg WA, Birdwell RL, Gombos EC, et al. Diagnostic imaging: breast. 1st ed. Salt Lake City: Amirsys. Section IV-2, 2006, p. 70–3.

Brem RT, Behrndt VS, Sanow L, Gatewood OM. Atypical ductal hyperplasia: histologic underestimation of carcinoma in tissue harvested from impalpable breast lesions using 11-gauge stereotactically guided directional vacuum-assisted biopsy. Am J Roentgenol. 1999;172:1405–7.

Ikeda DM. Breast imaging the requisites. 2nd ed. Philadelphia: Elsevier, Mosby; 2011. p. 230–1.

Fig. 1.1

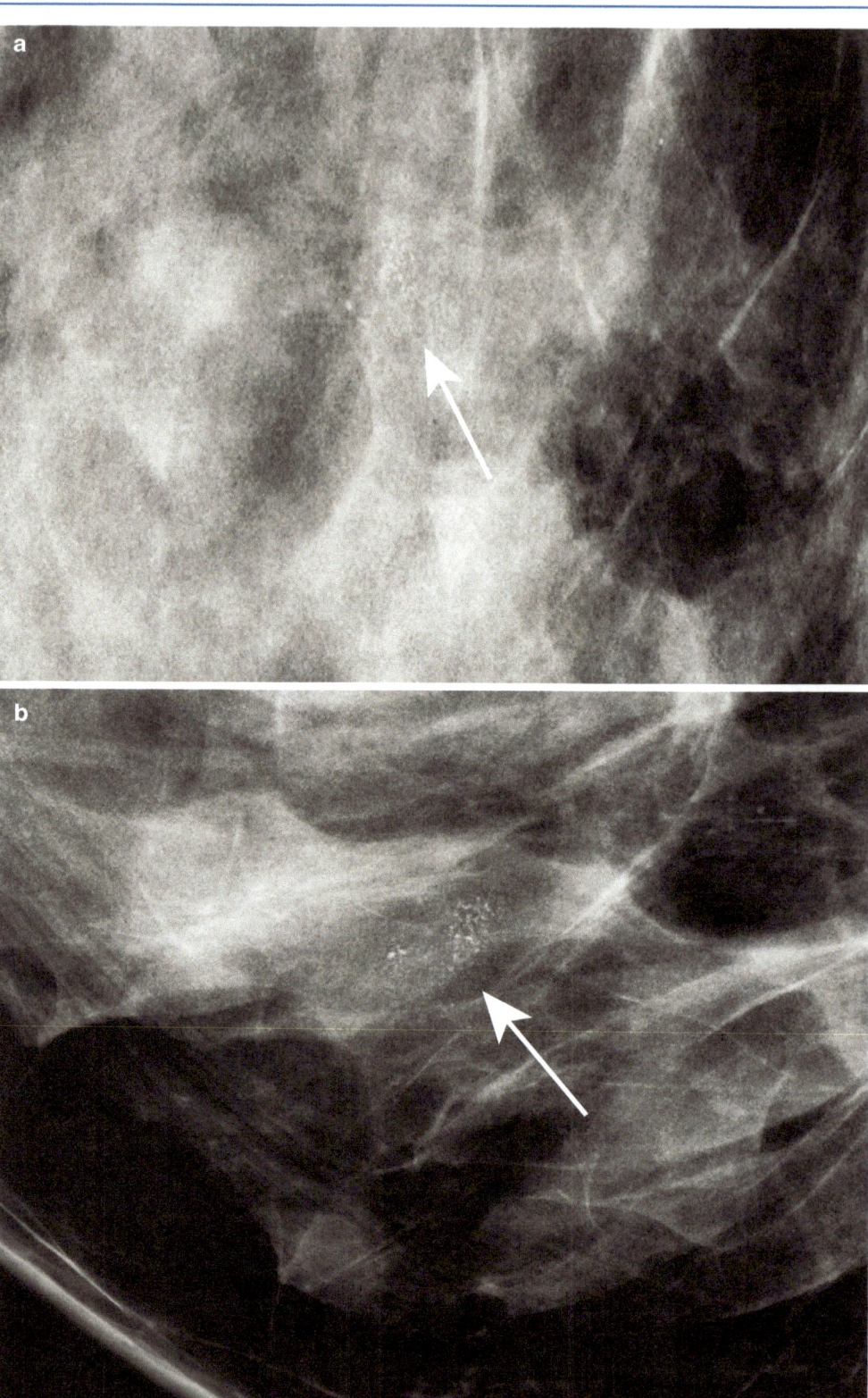

CASE 62
ANGIOLIPOMA

PATIENT HISTORY

A 54-year-old female with a history of a palpable mass at 9 o'clock in the left breast.

RADIOLOGY FINDINGS

Fig. 1.1 Spot-compression (**a**) CC and (**b**) MLO images show a predominately fatty breast with no mammographic finding corresponding to the triangular marker.
Fig. 1.2 (**a**) Grayscale and (**b**) color Doppler images of the left breast corresponding to the palpable mass reveal a homogeneously hyperechoic oval avascular mass with circumscribed margins.

BI-RADS ASSESSMENT

BI-RADS 2. Benign finding (following diagnostic workup and biopsy).

DIAGNOSIS

Angiolipoma

DISCUSSION

- Angiolipoma typically presents as a painless mass.
- Pathologically, the hallmark of an angiolipoma is scattered microthrombi in small blood vessels.
- There is no typical mammographic appearance of an angiolipoma. Mammogram may be negative and show an asymmetry or a mass.
- The key to diagnosis is suggested by the homogeneous echogenic ultrasound appearance.
- Differential diagnosis for a hyperechoic mass includes the following:
  - Acute hemorrhage
  - Acute hematoma
  - Focal fibrosis
  - Hemangioma
  - Angiolipoma
  - Lipoma
  - Malignancy
- Angiolipoma of the breast is noninfiltrative, and thus treatment is surgical excision.

REFERENCE

Weinstein SP, Conant EF, Acs G. Case 59: angiolipoma of the breast. Radiology. 2003;227:773–5.

a

b

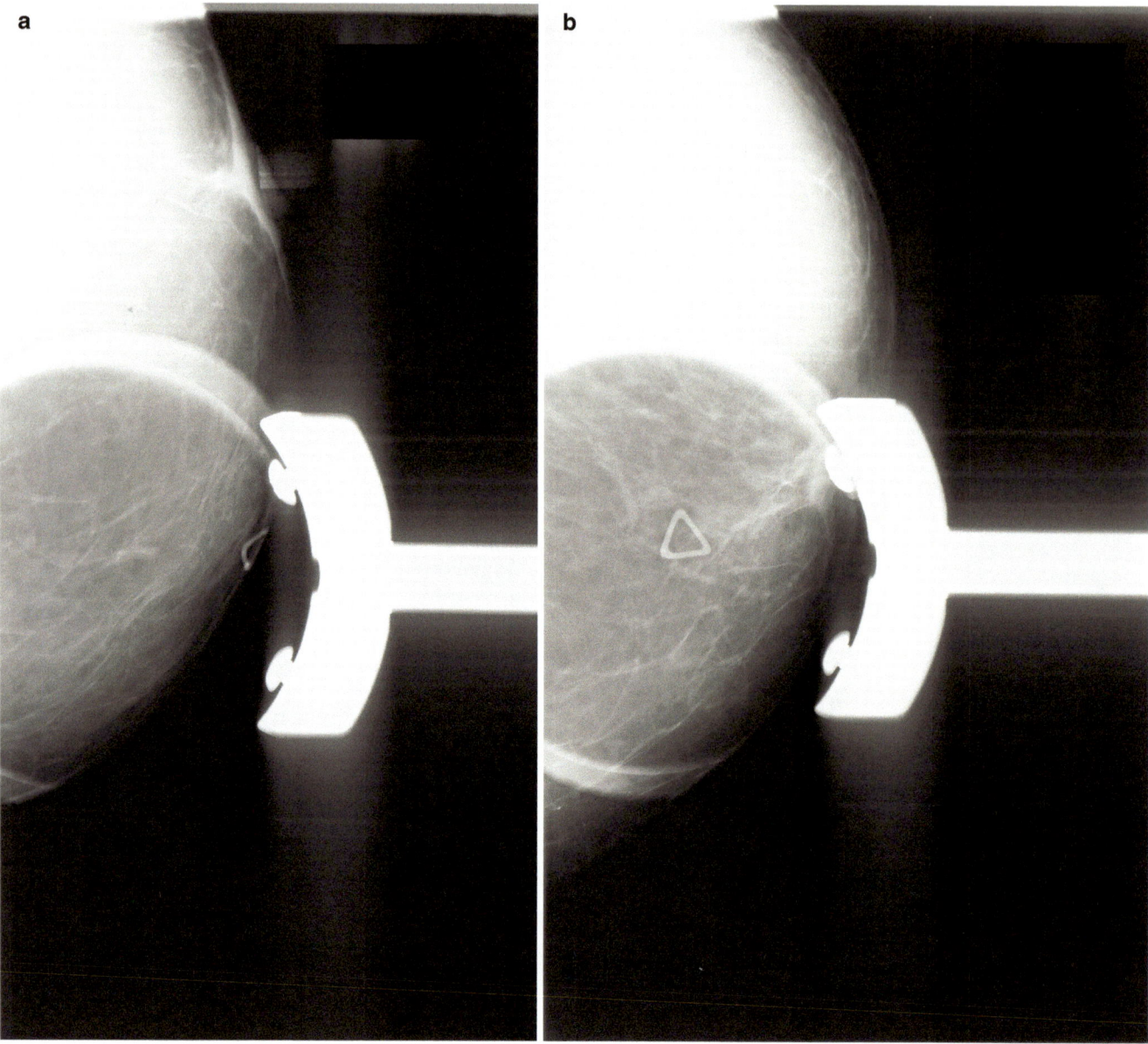

Fig. 1.1

Fig. 1.2

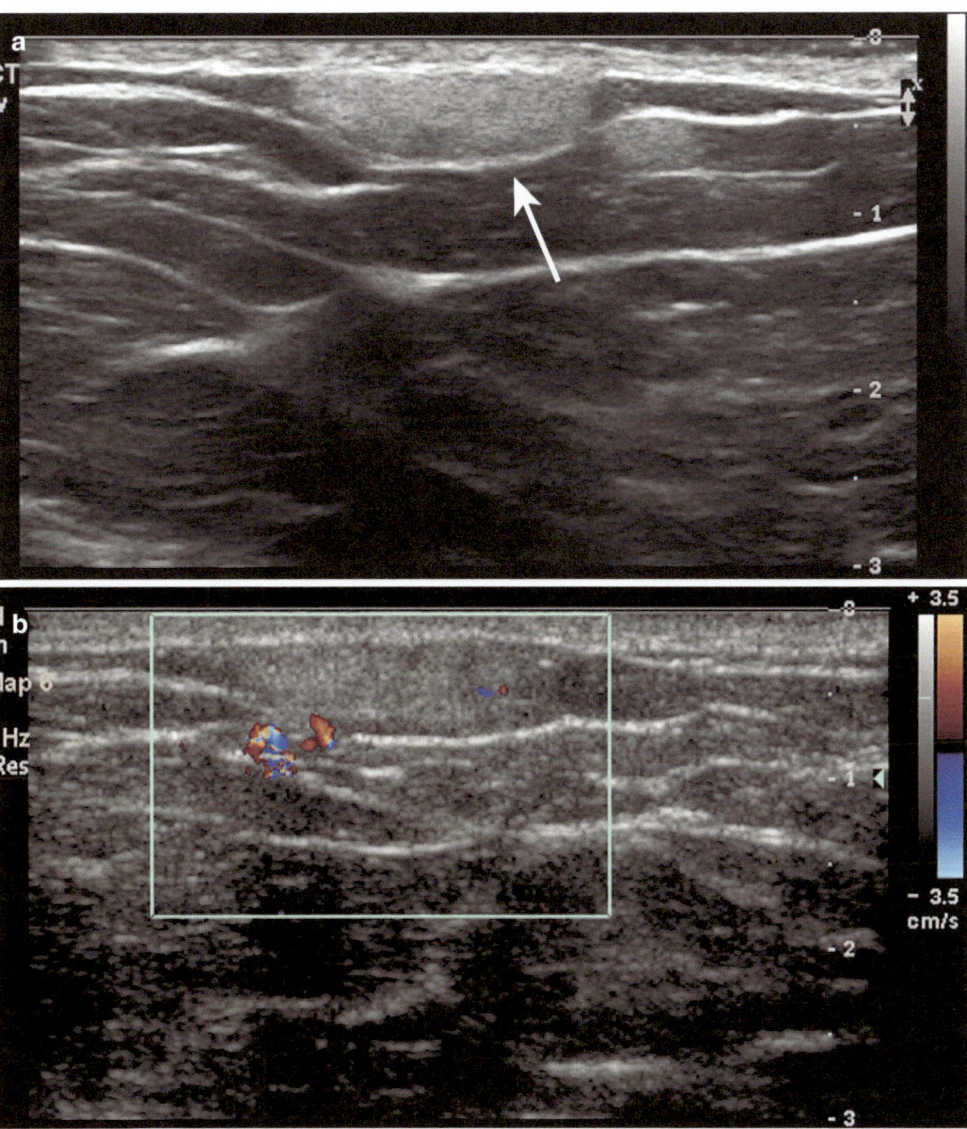

CASE 63
MICROPAPILLARY CARCINOMA

PATIENT HISTORY

A 31-year-old female with a history of right breast DCIS status postbilateral mastectomies with reconstruction; patient for screening MRI.

RADIOLOGY FINDINGS

Fig. 1.1 Sagittal (**a**) contrast-enhanced T1-weighted and (**b**) subtracted T1-weighted images demonstrate adjacent enhancing masses posterior to the implant.
Fig. 1.2 (**a**) Grayscale and (**b**) color Doppler ultrasound images show an irregular hypoechoic mass with indistinct margins and vascular flow.

BI-RADS ASSESSMENT

BI-RADS 4. Suspicious abnormality (following diagnostic workup, prior to biopsy).

DIAGNOSIS

Micropapillary carcinoma

DISCUSSION

- Micropapillary carcinoma accounts for 0.7–3 % of all breast cancers.
- Metastasis to axillary lymph nodes is common.
- Micropapillary carcinoma is an aggressive tumor with poor prognosis.
- On mammography, a high-density irregular mass with spiculated margins is seen, commonly with associated microcalcifications.
- Sonographically seen as an irregular solid hypoechoic mass with indistinct margins.
- On MRI, an enhancing mass or area of non-mass-like enhancement is seen.

REFERENCES

Adrada B, Árribas E, Gilcrease M, Yang WT. Invasive micropapillary carcinoma of the breast: mammographic, sonographic and MRI features. AJR. 2009;190:W58–63.
Gunhan-Bilgen I, Zekioglu O, Ustun EE, Memis A, Erhan Y. Invasive micropapillary carcinoma of the breast: clinical, mammographic and sonographic findings with histopathologic correlation. AJR. 2002;179:927–31.

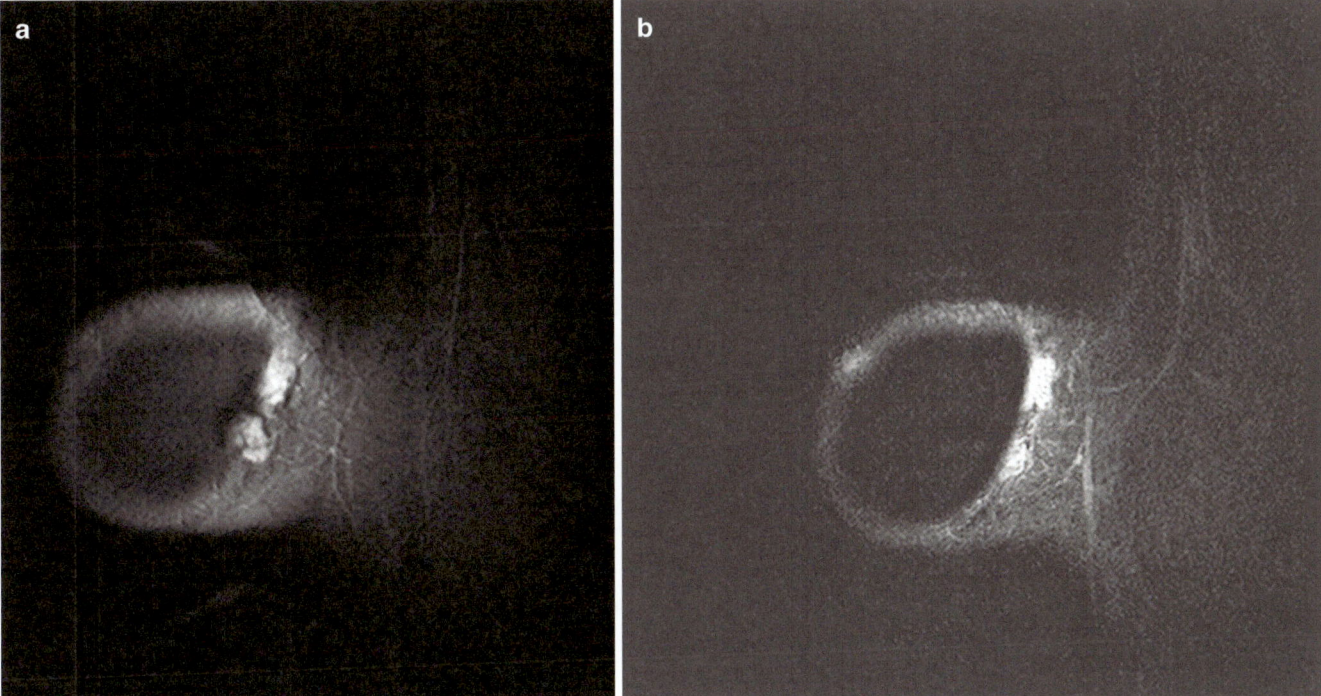

Fig. 1.1

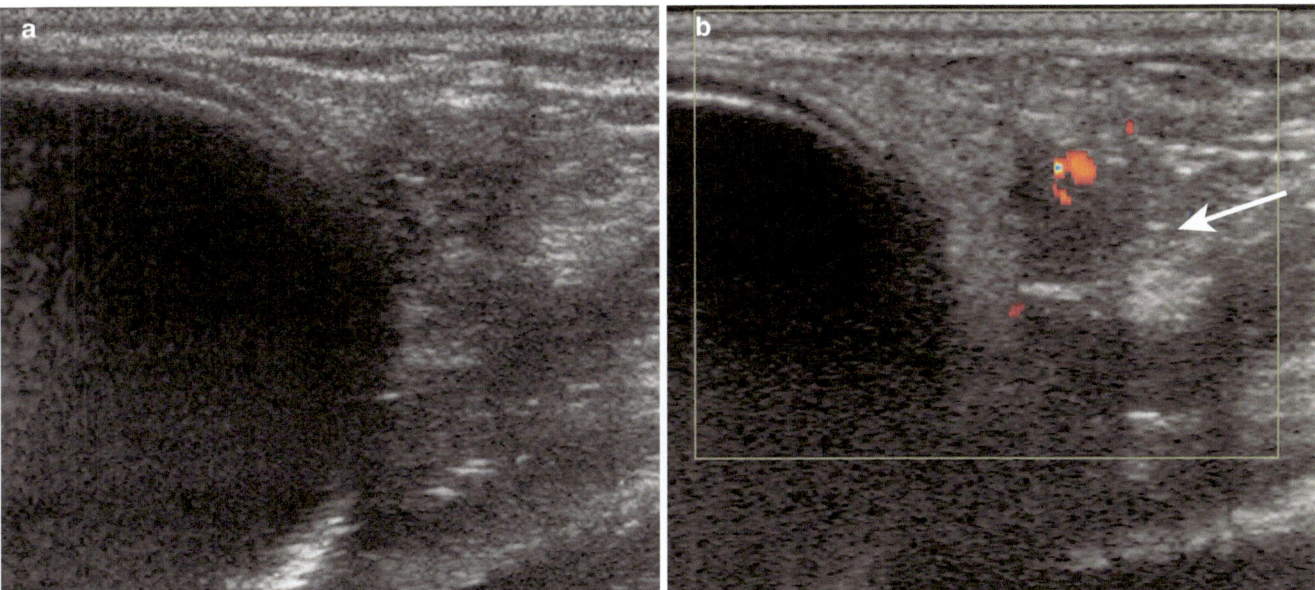

Fig. 1.2

Case 64
Intraductal Papilloma on Galactography

Patient History

A 45-year-old female with unilateral spontaneous clear nipple discharge.

Radiology Findings

Fig. 1.1 (**a**) CC and (**b**) ML views after contrast administration demonstrate a frond-like filling defect in a retroareolar central duct in the right breast.
Fig. 1.2 CC view in a different patient demonstrates an oval filling defect in a retroareolar duct.

Assessment

High-risk lesion.

Diagnosis

Intraductal papilloma on galactography

Discussion

- Galactography is an examination to visualize lesions in mammary ducts using contrast.
- Once an intraductal lesion is visualized, image-guided biopsy or wire localization and excision can be performed.
- Bloody nipple discharge whether spontaneous or with stimulation is an indication for galactography.
- Spontaneous, clear, or serous nipple discharges from a single duct are also indications for galactography.
- Patient may experience increased discharge for several days after the procedure.
- Complications include the following:
  - Ruptured duct
  - Mastitis
  - Vasovagal reaction

References

Berg WA, Birdwell RL, Gombos EC, et al. Diagnostic imaging breast. 1st ed. Salt Lake City: Amirsys; 2006. Section V-2, p. 4–5.
Slawson SH, Johnson B. Ductography: how to and what if? Radiographics. 2001;21:133–50.

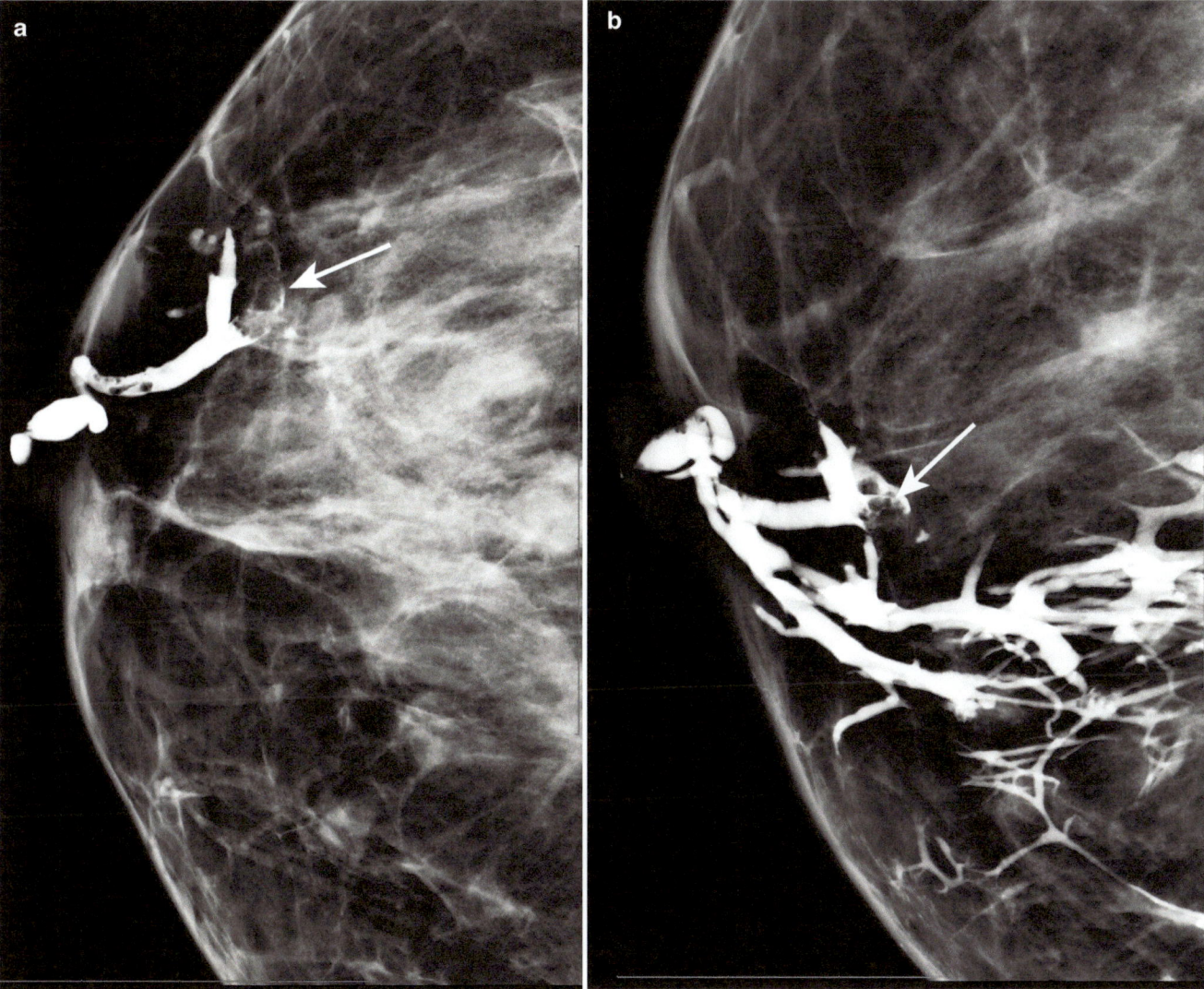

Fig. 1.1

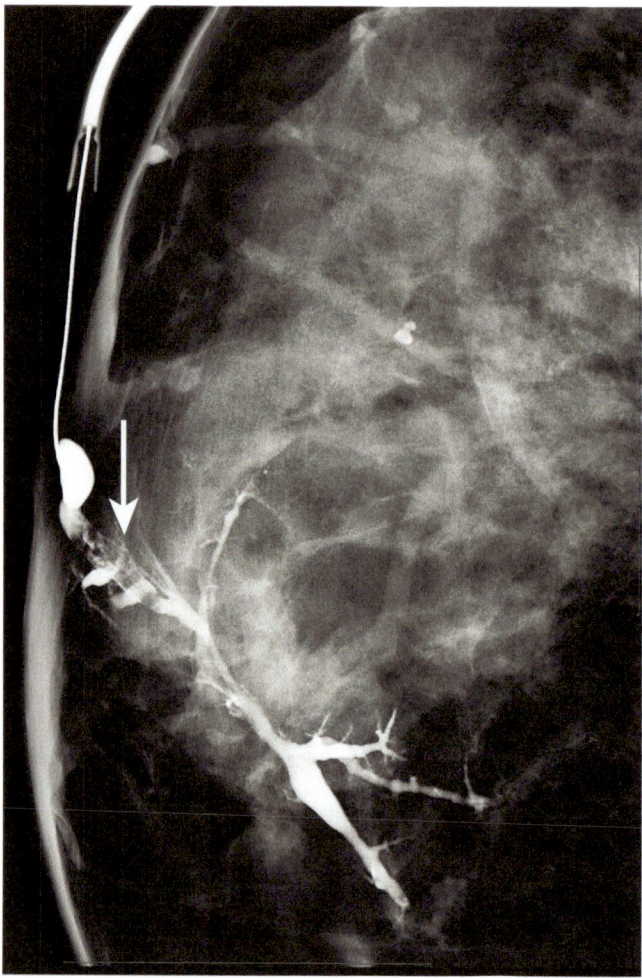

Fig. 1.2

CASE 65
TUBULAR CARCINOMA

PATIENT HISTORY

A 42-year-old female for a screening mammogram.

RADIOLOGY FINDINGS

Fig. 1.1 CC view demonstrates an irregular, high-density mass with spiculated margins in the inner left breast at anterior depth.

Fig. 1.2 Sagittal subtracted T1-weighted image in a different patient demonstrates an enhancing irregular spiculated mass. Central part of the mass does not enhance.

Fig. 1.3 Kinetic curve demonstrates rapid initial enhancement followed by washout (type III).

BI-RADS ASSESSMENT

BI-RADS 4. Suspicious abnormality (following diagnostic workup, prior to biopsy).

DIAGNOSIS

Tubular carcinoma

DISCUSSION

- Tubular carcinoma accounts for 2% of female breast cancers.
- It is slow growing and small in size at detection.
- Most are detected mammographically as a small spiculated mass.
- Can be associated with pleomorphic calcifications in up to 50 % of the cases.
- Tubular carcinoma is a type of well-differentiated IDC usually smaller than 2 cm in size.
- Composed of well-differentiated tubular structures.
- Low rates of axillary node metastases and recurrence.
- May be false-negative on MRI or PET.
- Histologically, it can mimic a radial scar.
- Actin stain is used to detect myoepithelial cells in the basement membrane of tubules in a radial scar. These cells are not present in tubular carcinoma.
- Generally can be treated with breast conservation surgery and sentinel node biopsy. Radiation therapy is controversial.

REFERENCES

Bassett LW, Jackson VP, Fu KL, Fu YS. Diagnosis of diseases of the breast. 2nd ed. Philadelphia: Elsevier; 2005. p. 506–7.

Berg WA, Birdwell RL, Gombos EC, et al. Diagnostic imaging breast. 1st ed. Salt Lake City: Amirsys; 2006. Section IV-2, p. 178–81.

Harvey JA, March DE. Making the diagnosis: a practical guide to breast imaging. Philadelphia: Elsevier; 2013. p. 297–8.

Leonard CE, Howell K, Shapiro H, Ponce J, Kercher J. Excision only for tubular carcinoma of the breast. Breast J. 2005;11(2):129–33.

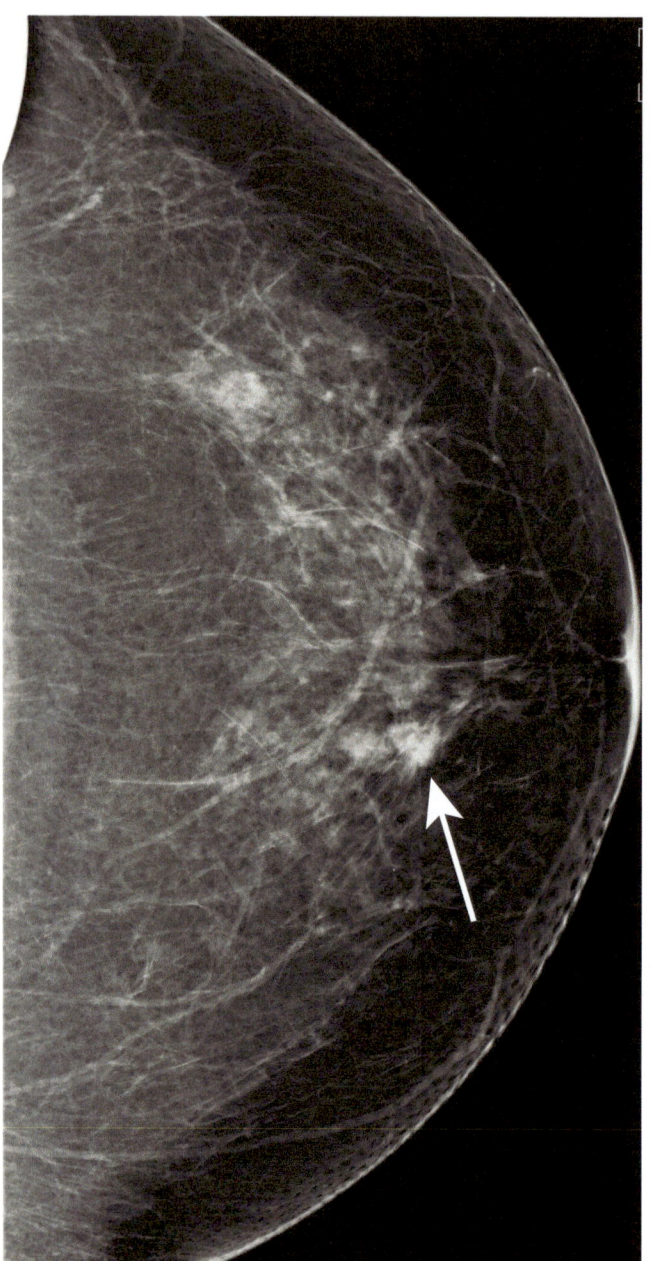

Fig. 1.1

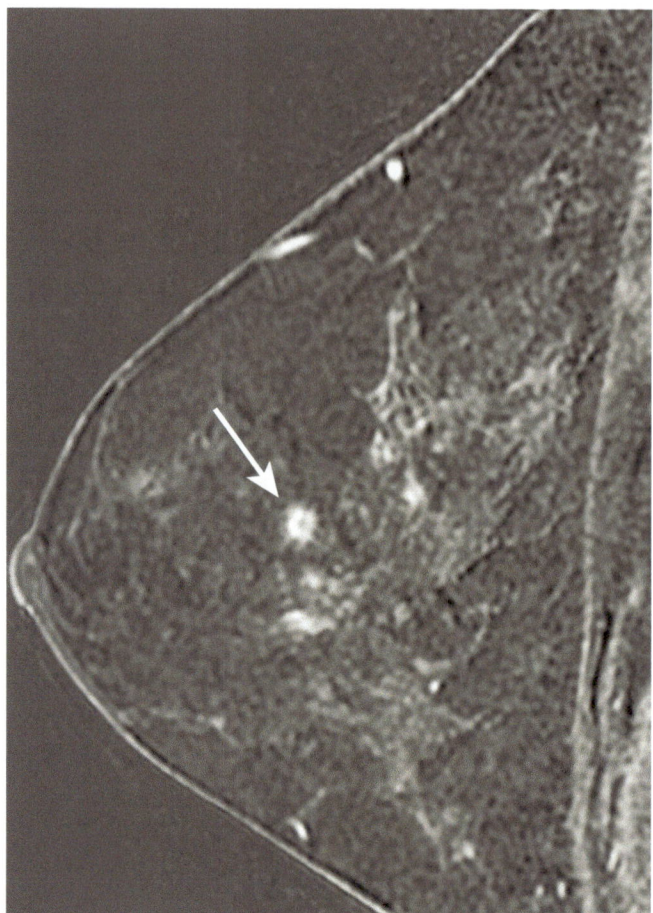

Fig. 1.2

Fig. 1.3

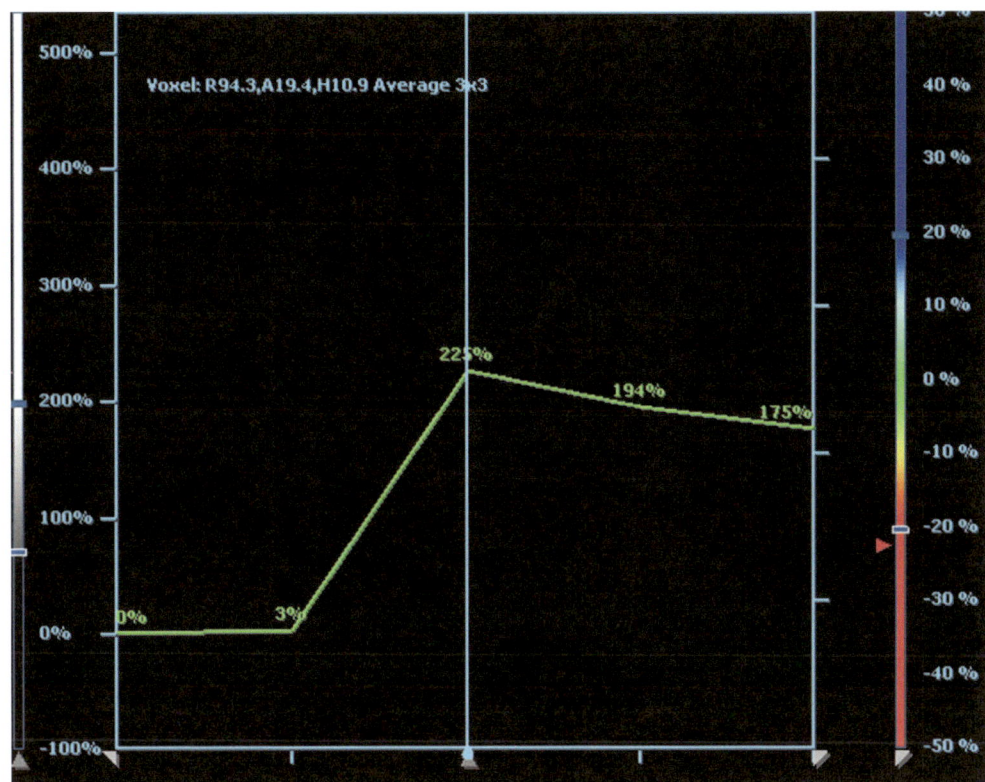

CASE 66
RECURRENT INVASIVE DUCTAL CARCINOMA
IN A TRAM FLAP

PATIENT HISTORY

A 44-year-old female with a history of left breast cancer status postmastectomy and TRAM (transverse rectus abdominis myocutaneous) flap reconstruction for screening mammogram.

RADIOLOGY FINDINGS

Fig. 1.1 (**a**) CC and (**b**) MLO images show an irregular mass with spiculated margins in the upper outer left TRAM flap at posterior depth. There is a microclip from a prior biopsy in the upper TRAM flap at posterior depth.
Fig. 1.2 (**a**) Grayscale and (**b**) color Doppler ultrasound images show a hypoechoic irregular mass with spiculated margins and vascular flow.
Fig. 1.3 (**a**) Sagittal subtracted T1-weighted and (**b**) axial contrast-enhanced delayed T1-weighted images show a heterogeneously enhancing irregular mass with spiculated margins in the left TRAM flap at posterior depth.

BI-RADS ASSESSMENT

BI-RADS 5. Highly suggestive of malignancy (following diagnostic workup, prior to biopsy).

DIAGNOSIS

Recurrent invasive ductal carcinoma in a TRAM flap

DISCUSSION

- TRAM flap is an autologous means of breast reconstruction following mastectomy.
- A TRAM flap appears radiolucent on mammogram; predominantly fatty appearance with variable density depending on muscle component and postoperative scarring.
- Controversy exists about whether routine screening mammogram is indicated to detect nonpalpable recurrent breast cancer in a TRAM flap.
- Mammographic presentation of cancer in a TRAM flap has an appearance similar to that of primary breast cancer.

REFERENCES

Helvie MA, Bailey JE, Roubidoux MA, et al. Mammographic screening of TRAM flap breast reconstructions for detection of nonpalpable recurrent cancer. Radiology. 2002;224:211–6.

Hogge J, Zuurbier RA, de Paredes ES. Mammography of autologous myocutaneous flaps. Radiographics. 1999;19:S63–72.

Lee JM, Georgian-Smith D, Gazelle GS, et al. Detecting nonpalpable recurrent breast cancer: the role of routine mammographic screening of transverse rectus abdominis myocutaneous flap reconstructions. Radiology. 2008;248:398–405.

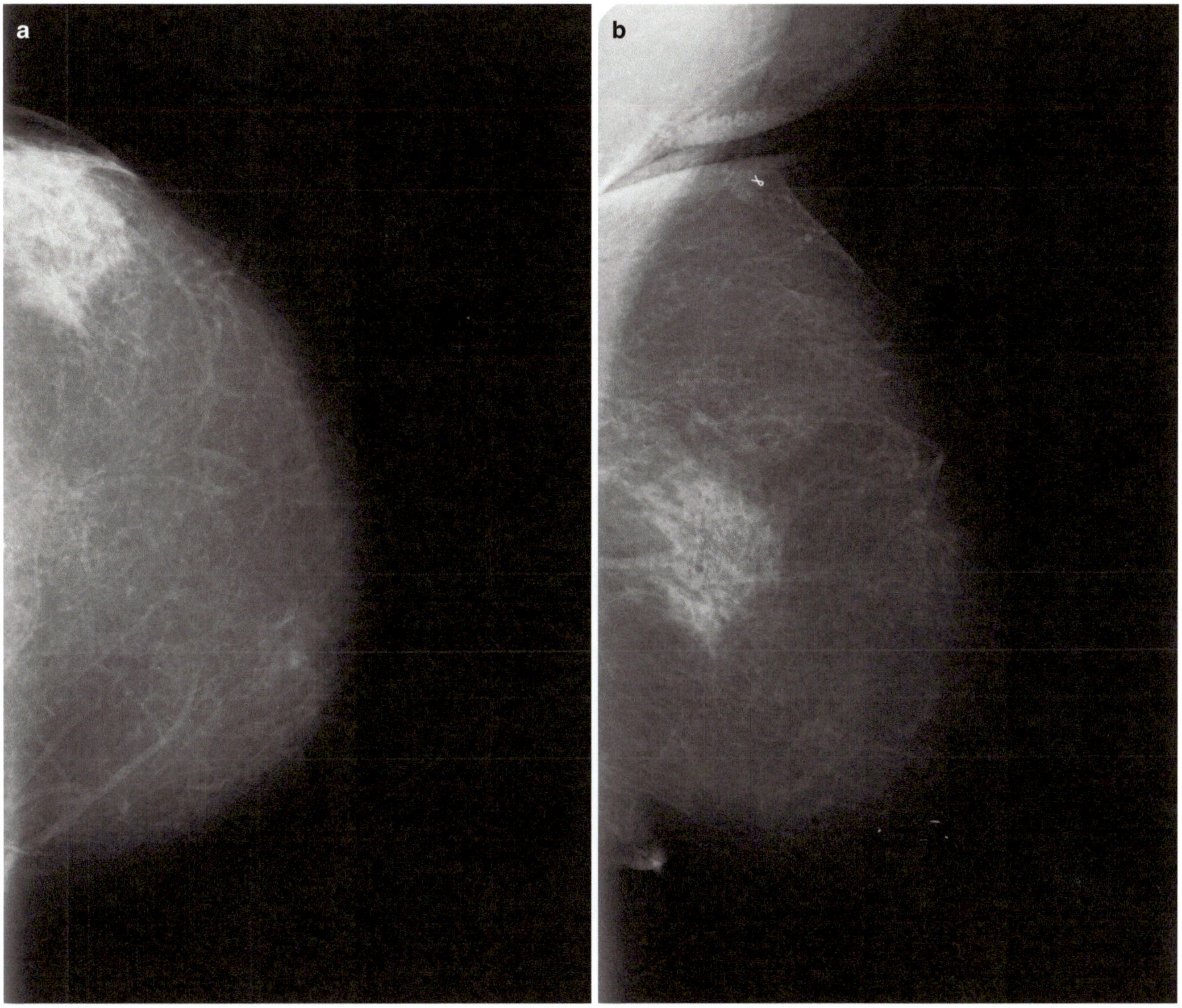

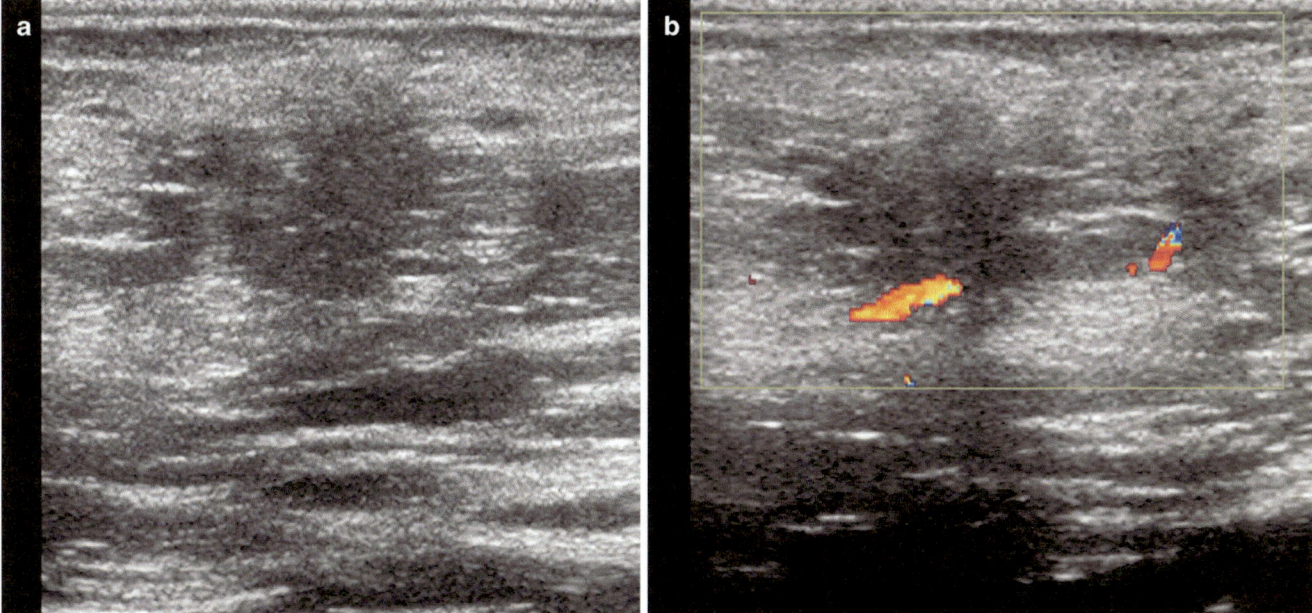

Fig. 1.1

Fig. 1.2

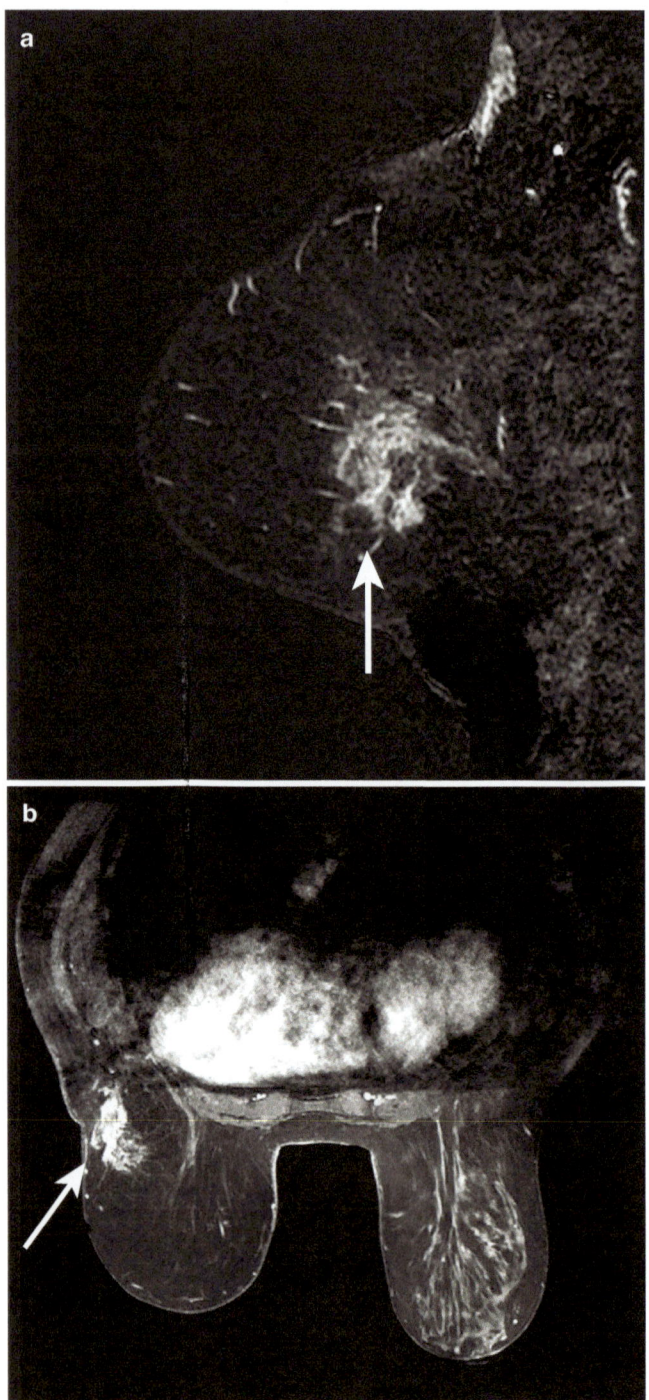

Fig. 1.3

Case 67
Nonpuerperal Abscess of the Breast

Patient History

A 41-year-old female with a history of a painful lump in the retroareolar right breast.

Radiology Findings

Fig. 1.1 Spot-compression (**a**) CC and (**b**) ML images show an irregular mass with indistinct margins in the retroareolar right breast with associated thickening of adjacent skin.

Fig. 1.2 (**a**) Grayscale and (**b**) color Doppler ultrasound images show an irregular fluid collection with mobile internal echoes and posterior enhancement in the retroareolar right breast corresponding to the mammographic finding. There is no vascular flow within the mass.

BI-RADS Assessment

BI-RADS 2. Benign finding (following diagnostic workup).

Diagnosis

Abscess of the breast (nonpuerperal abscess)

Discussion

- An abscess of the breast is a walled-off purulent collection within the breast tissue.
- Often retroareolar or periareolar in location.

- Most common in premenopausal females.
- Common symptoms include the following:
  - Painful lump
  - Erythema
  - Induration
  - Nipple retraction
  - Nipple discharge
- Usually caused by Staphylococcus or Streptococcus.
- In a nursing mother, an infection is caused by bacterial entry from a cracked nipple (puerperal abscess).
- Increase risk factors for abscess include the following:
  - Diabetes
  - HIV
  - Steroids
  - Recent surgery
  - Postradiation
- Systemic antibiotics are the method of treatment.
- Although systemic antibiotics are required for treatment, an abscess of <3 cm is usually successfully aspirated. On the other hand, an abscess of >3–4 cm may require catheter drainage or surgical incision and drainage.
- Differential diagnosis includes the following:
  - Hematoma
  - Seroma
  - Mastitis
  - Inflammatory breast cancer
  - Necrotic tumor (such as invasive ductal carcinoma, not otherwise specified)

References

Ikeda DM. Breast imaging the requisites. 2nd ed. Philadelphia: Elsevier, Mosby; 2011. p. 140–1.

Berg WA, Birdwell RL, Gombos EC, et al. Diagnostic imaging breast. 1st ed. Salt Lake City: Amirsys; 2006. Section IV-6, p. 2–5.

Mandell J. Core radiology: a visual approach to diagnostic imaging. 1st ed. Cambridge: Cambridge University Press; 2013. p. 596.

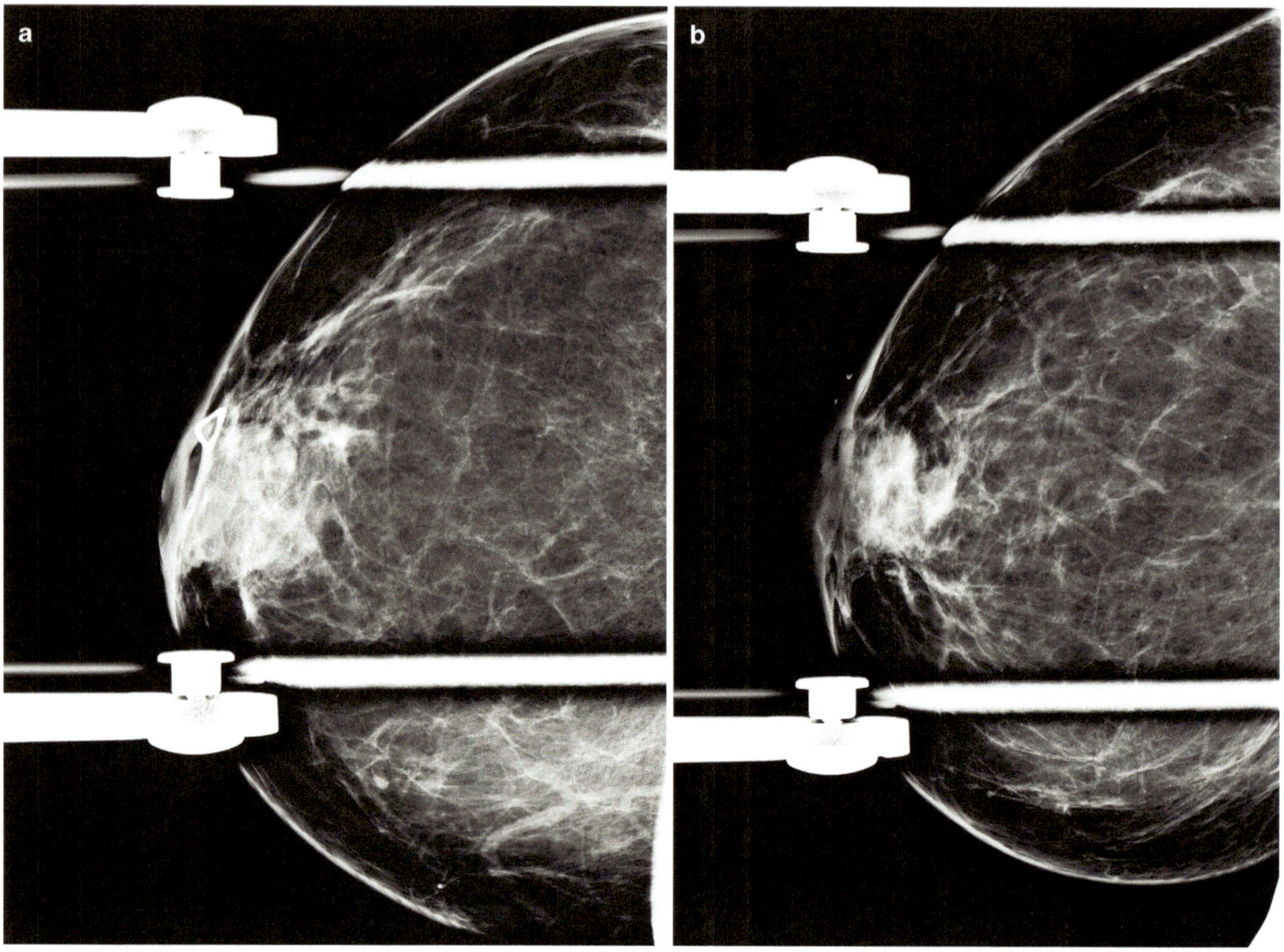

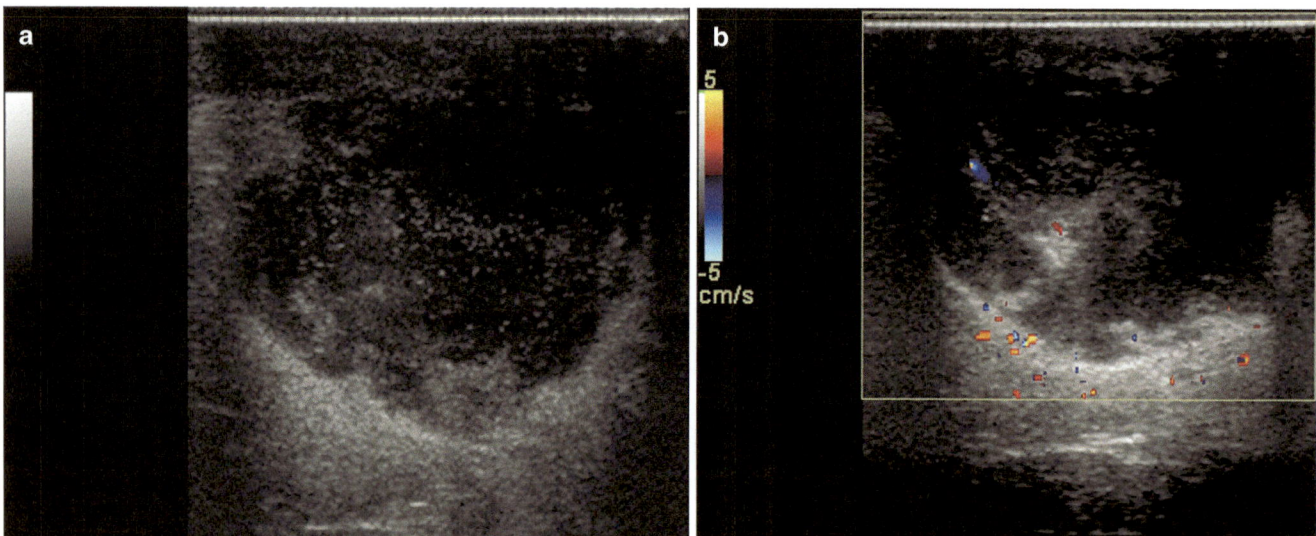

Fig. 1.1

Fig. 1.2

CASE 68
SMALL CELL CARCINOMA METASTASIS

PATIENT HISTORY

A 67-year-old male with shortness of breath.

RADIOLOGY FINDINGS

Fig. 1.1 PA view of the chest shows right perihilar fullness.
Fig. 1.2 Contrast-enhanced CT scan shows (**a**) right hilar adenopathy and (**b**) a mass in the right breast adjacent to the pectoralis muscle.
Fig. 1.3 A portion of a dense mass is seen in the retroareolar plane at posterior depth only on MLO view.
Fig. 1.4 (**a**) Grayscale and (**b**) color Doppler ultrasound images show a hypoechoic mass with indistinct margins and no vascular flow.

BI-RADS ASSESSMENT

BI-RADS 5. Highly suggestive of malignancy (following diagnostic workup, prior to biopsy).

DIAGNOSIS

Small cell carcinoma rarely metastasizes to the breast

DISCUSSION

- Small cell carcinoma is an aggressive neuroendocrine tumor, which most commonly occurs in the lung.
- Small cell carcinoma has been seen ranging from a circumscribed to an ill-defined marginated mass on mammogram.
- On ultrasound, small cell carcinoma has been seen as a hypoechoic mass with microlobulated borders.
- Most common metastatic lesion to the breast is metastasis from a contralateral breast cancer.
- Most common extramammary metastatic diseases to the breast include:
  - Melanoma
  - Non-Hodgkin's lymphoma
  - Lung carcinoma
- Metastatic disease to the breast is more likely to be bilateral or multiple when compared with primary breast cancers.
- Usually metastatic diseases to the breast present as round masses with circumscribed or ill-defined margins.

REFERENCES

Feder JM, Shaw de Paredes E, Hogge JP, Wilken JJ. Unusual breast lesions: radiologic and pathologic correlation. Radiographics. 1999;19:S11–26.
Irshad A, Ackerman SJ, Pope TL, Moses CK, Rumboldt T, Panzegrau B. Rare breast lesions: correlation of imaging and histologic features with WHO classification. Radiographics. 2008;28:1399–414.
Mariscal A, Balliu E, Diaz R, Casas JD, Gallant AM. Primary oat cell carcinoma of the breast: imaging features. AJR. 2004;183:1169–71.

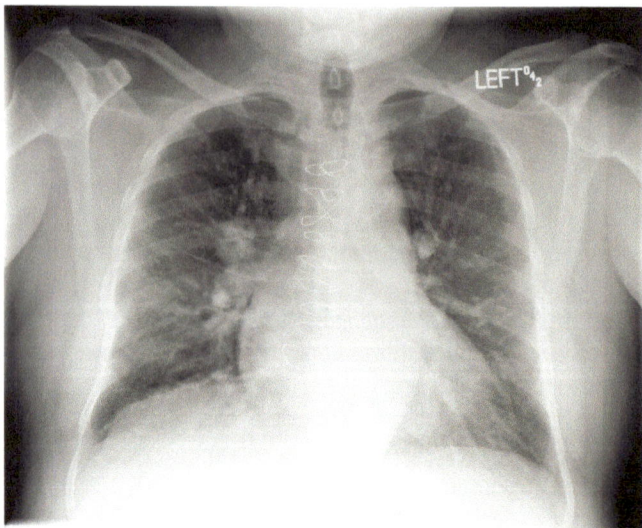

Fig. 1.1

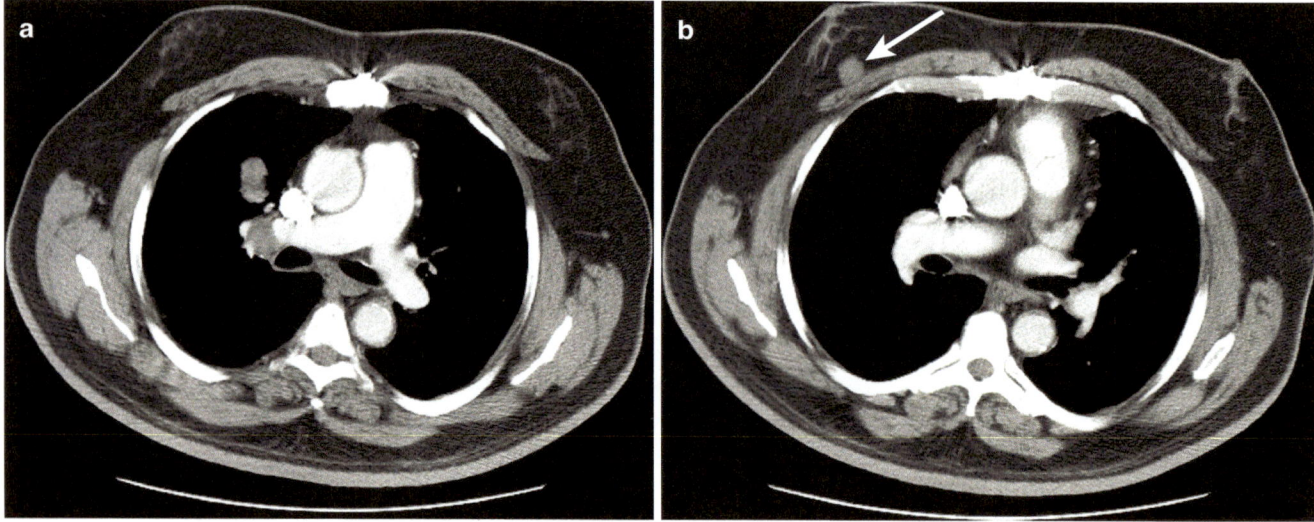

Fig. 1.2

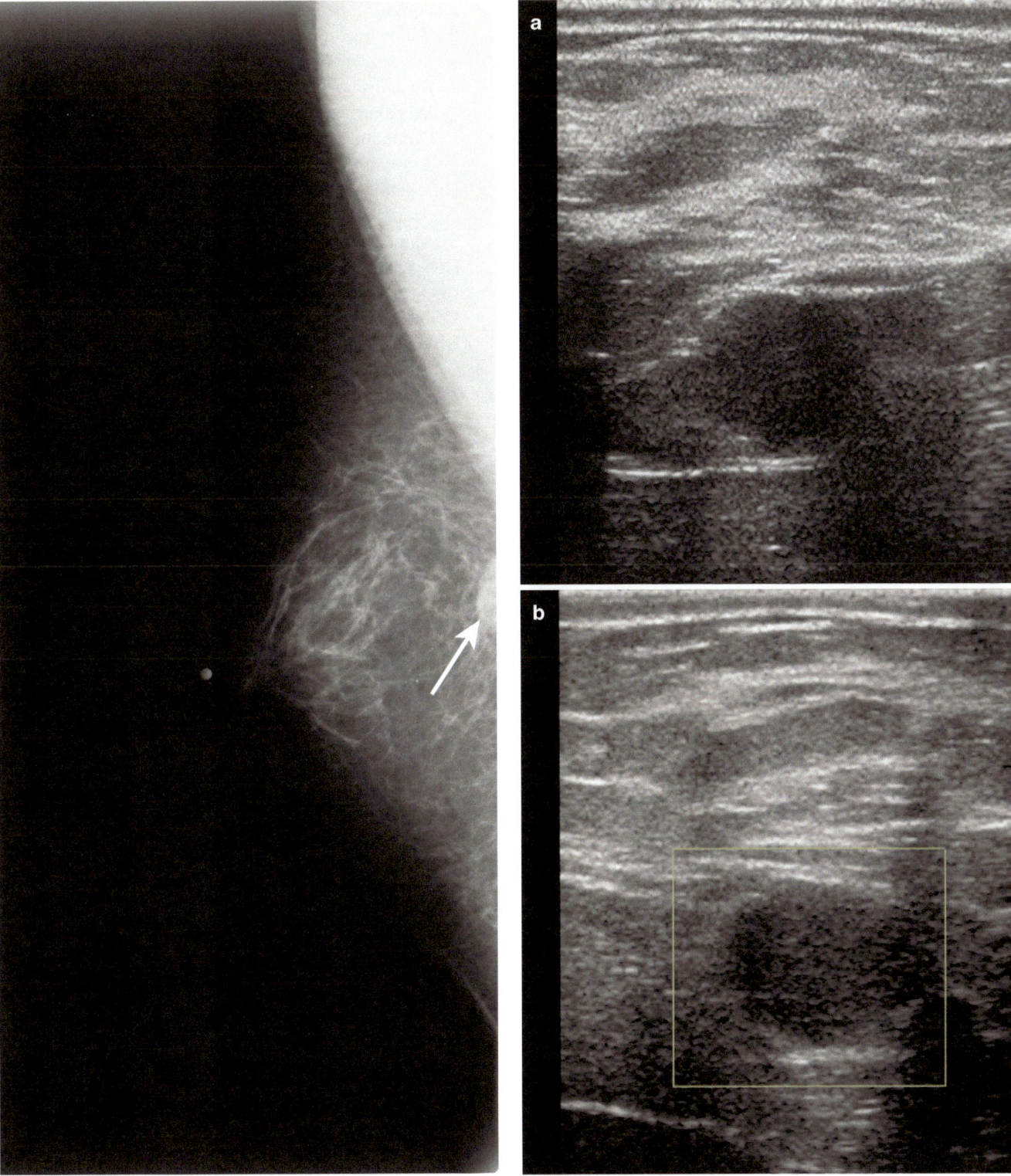

Fig. 1.3

Fig. 1.4

CASE 69
BILATERAL AXILLARY LYMPHADENOPATHY

PATIENT HISTORY

A 51-year-old female for a bilateral screening mammogram.

RADIOLOGY FINDINGS

Fig. 1.1 (**a, b**) CC and (**c, d**) MLO views demonstrate multiple, bilateral, dense axillary lymph nodes of varying sizes.

BI-RADS ASSESSMENT

BI-RADS 4. Suspicious abnormality (following diagnostic workup, prior to biopsy).

DIAGNOSIS

Bilateral axillary lymphadenopathy in a patient with chronic lymphocytic leukemia

DISCUSSION

- Axillary lymphadenopathy is defined as an axillary lymph node of >2 cm.

- Abnormal appearance of axillary lymph nodes include the following:
  - Increased density
  - Round shape
  - Irregular shape
  - Diminutive or complete loss of the fatty hilum
  - Asymmetric cortical thickening of the lymph node
- Differential diagnosis of bilateral axillary lymphadenopathy includes the following:
- Systemic infection
- HIV
- Rheumatoid arthritis
- Collagen vascular disease
- Lymphoma
- Leukemia
- Metastatic cancer

REFERENCES

Berg WA, Birdwell RL, Gombos EC, et al. Diagnostic imaging breast. 1st ed. Salt Lake City: Amirsys; 2006. Section IV-3, p. 30–3.

Ikeda DM. Breast imaging the requisites. 2nd ed. Philadelphia: Elsevier, Mosby; 2011. p. 395–7.

Mandell J. Core radiology: a visual approach to diagnostic imaging. 1st ed. Cambridge: Cambridge University Press; 2013. p. 633.

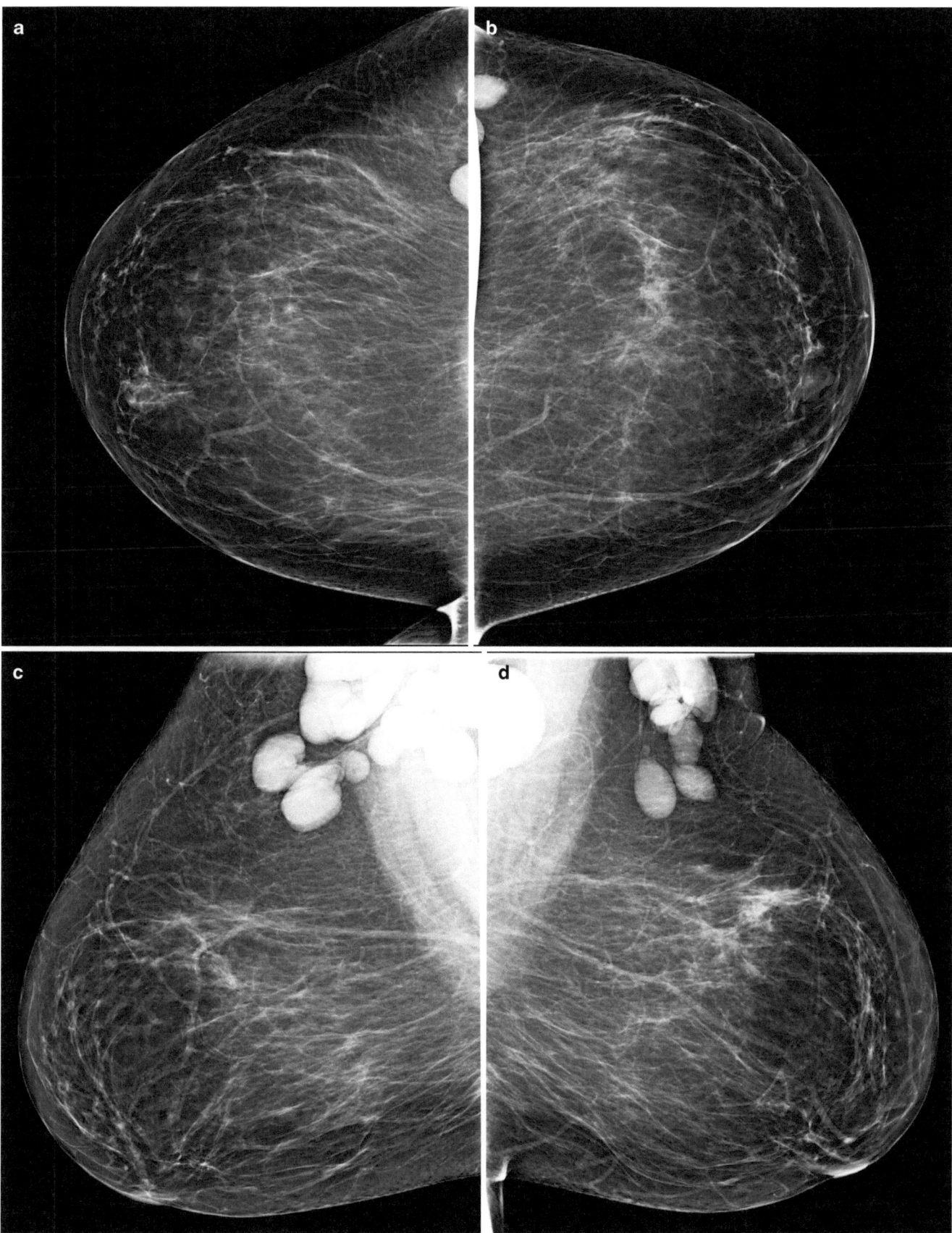

Fig. 1.1

Case 70
Calcified Fibroadenoma (Involuting Fibroadenoma)

Patient History

A 57-year-old female for a bilateral screening mammogram.

Radiology Findings

Fig. 1.1 (**a**) CC and (**b**) MLO views show an oval mass with associated coarse calcifications in the lower outer left breast at middle depth. There is a microclip incidentally seen in the upper outer left breast at middle depth.

BI-RADS Assessment

BI-RADS 2. Benign findings.

Diagnosis

Calcified fibroadenoma

Discussion

- Fibroadenomas are the most common benign breast mass.
- Fibroadenomas are oval masses that can occasionally present with coarse or "popcorn-like" calcifications.
- Usually, calcified fibroadenomas are seen after menopause.
- Calcifications within a fibroadenoma typically start at its periphery, moving toward the center. Fibroadenomas can often become completely calcified.
- Coarse or popcorn calcifications are pathognomonic of a fibroadenoma that has undergone involution and hyaline degeneration.

References

American College of Radiology (ACR) BI-RADS® Atlas. ACR BI-RADS® atlas-mammography. 5th ed. Reston: American College of Radiology; 2013. p. 42–3.

Cole-Beuglet C, Soriano RZ, Curtz AB, Goldberg BB. Fibroadenoma of the breast: sonomammography correlated with pathology in 122 patients. AJR. 1983;140(2):369–75.

Ikeda DM. Breast imaging the requisites. 2nd ed. Philadelphia: Elsevier, Mosby; 2011. p. 83.

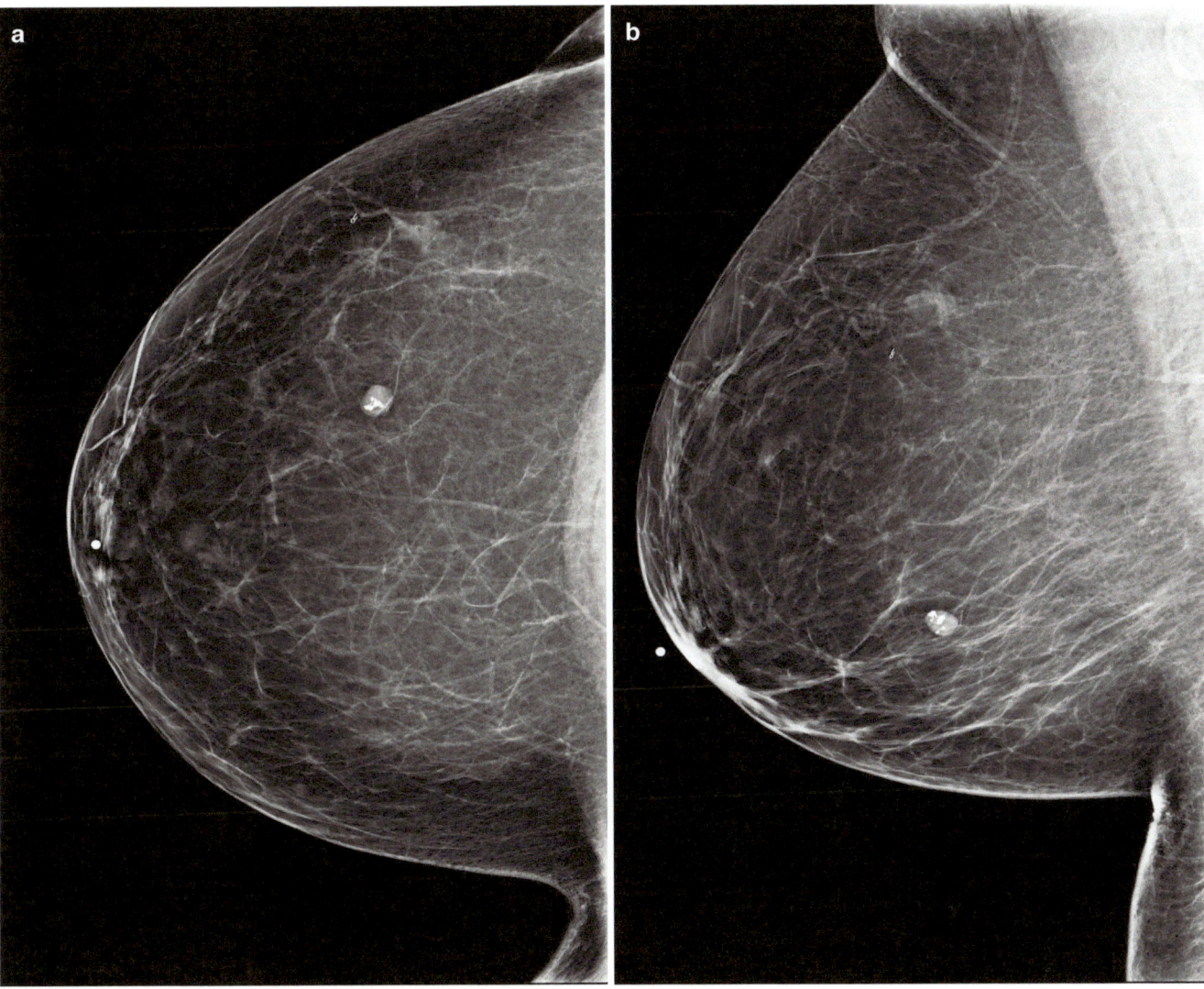

Fig. 1.1

CASE 71
GRANULAR CELL TUMOR

PATIENT HISTORY

A 50-year-old female with a palpable lump in the right breast.

RADIOLOGY FINDINGS

Fig. 1.1 (**a**) CC, (**b**) MLO, and spot-compression (**c**) CC and (**d**) MLO views show an irregular spiculated mass in the lower inner quadrant of the right breast posteriorly.
Fig. 1.2 (**a**, **b**) Grayscale and (**c**) color Doppler ultrasound show an irregular avascular hypoechoic mass with angular margins.

BI-RADS ASSESSMENT

BI-RADS 4. Suspicious abnormality (following diagnostic workup, prior to biopsy).

DIAGNOSIS

Granular cell tumor

DISCUSSION

- A granular cell tumor is composed of a nest or sheets of cells that contain eosinophilic cytoplasmic granules.
- Usually benign; malignant in approximately 2 %.
- On mammography, a high-density mass without calcifications is seen.
- On ultrasound, an irregular, hypoechoic mass is seen, which may have posterior acoustic shadowing.
- Imaging appearance may mimic a breast cancer.
- Although granular cell tumor is most commonly benign, surgical excision is recommended.

REFERENCES

Berg WA, Birdwell RL, Gombos EC, et al. Diagnostic imaging: breast. 1st ed. Salt Lake City: Amirsys; 2006. Section IV-2, p. 94–5.
Gogas J, Markopoulos C, Kouskos E, et al. Granular cell tumor of the breast: a rare lesion resembling breast cancer. Eur J Gynaecol Oncol. 2002;23(4):333–4.

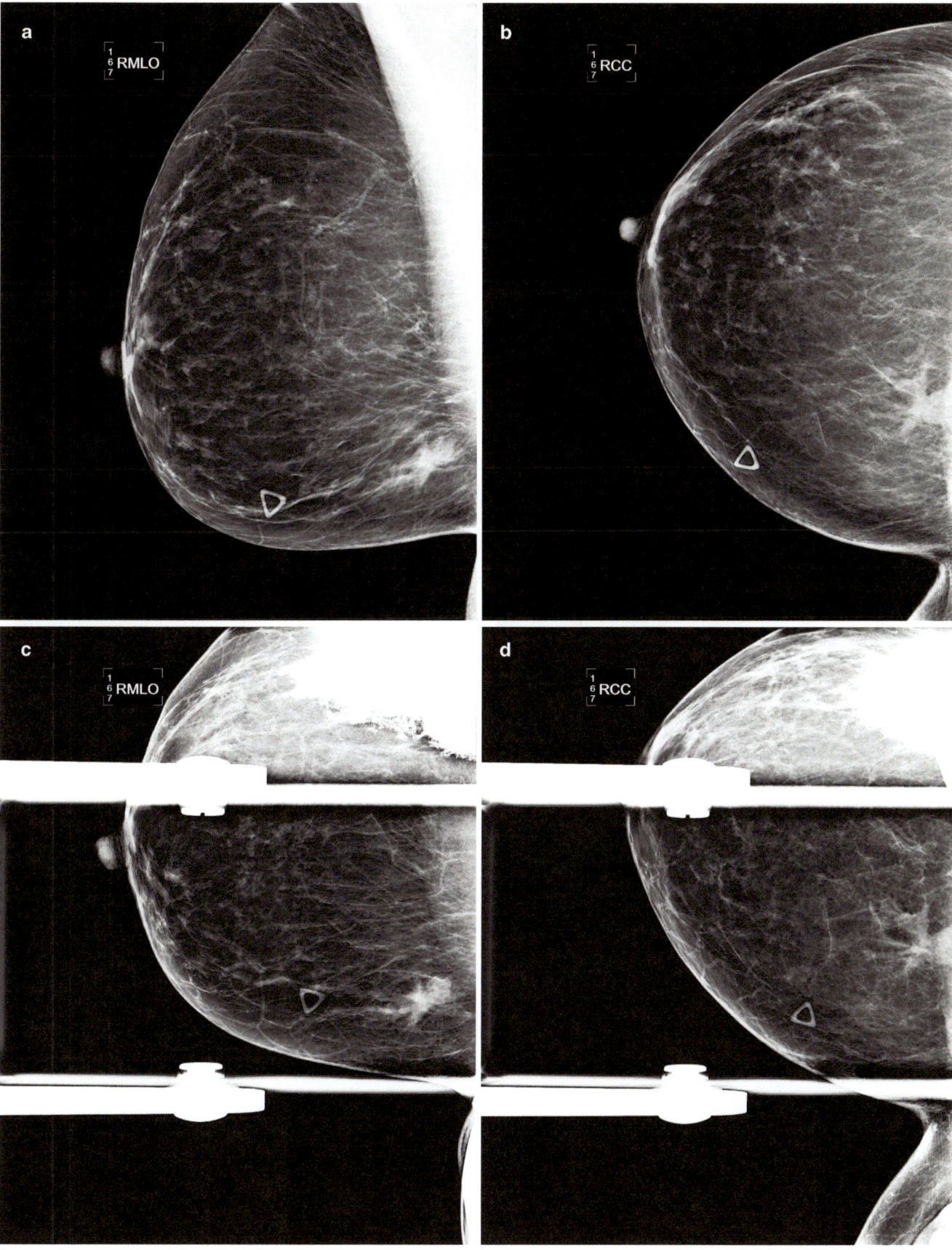

Fig. 1.1

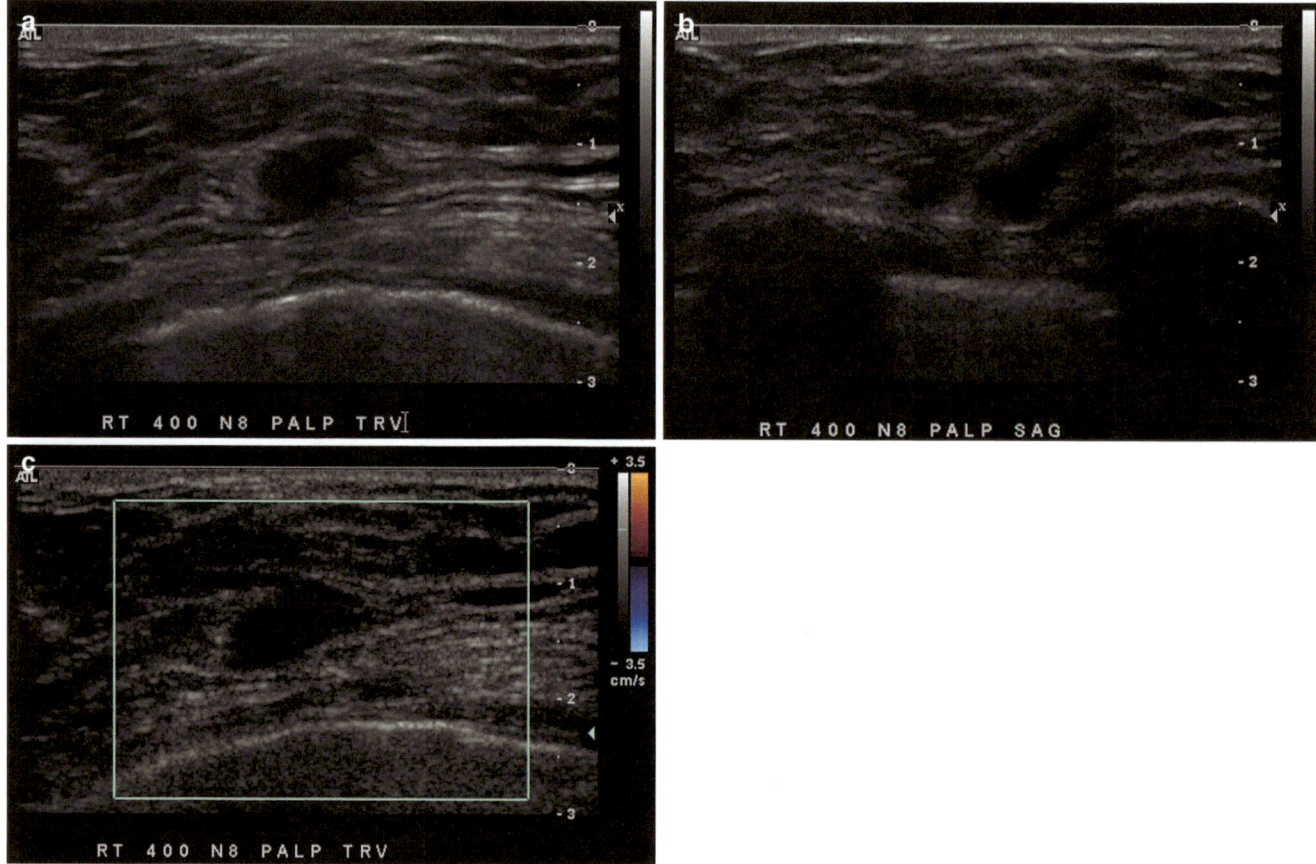

RT 400 N8 PALP TRV

RT 400 N8 PALP SAG

RT 400 N8 PALP TRV

Fig. 1.2

CASE 72
HEMATOMA

PATIENT HISTORY

A 62-year-old female who takes 81 mg of aspirin daily noticed bruising on her skin but denies trauma or injury to her breasts.

RADIOLOGY FINDINGS

Fig. 1.1 (**a**) Grayscale and (**b**) color Doppler ultrasound images show a oval hyperechoic avascular mass containing a sonolucent area at 12 o'clock in the right breast.

BI-RADS ASSESSMENT

BI-RADS 2. Benign findings (following diagnostic workup).

DIAGNOSIS

Hematoma of the breast

DISCUSSION

- A hematoma is a collection of extravasated blood; a mixture of serum and clot.
- Clinical history is important to avoid unnecessary intervention.
- Findings often mimic a malignancy.
- Hematoma is avascular. Any internal vascular flow should increase suspicion for a malignancy.
- Most hematomas resolve rapidly.
- Differential diagnosis includes the following:
  - Seroma
  - Hemorrhagic cyst
  - Intracystic carcinoma
  - Galactocele
  - Fibroadenolipoma (hamartoma)
  - Abscess

REFERENCES

Berg WA, Birdwell RL, Gombos EC, et al. Diagnostic imaging breast. 1st ed. Salt Lake City: Amirsys; 2006. Section IV-2, p. 50–5.

Harish MG, Konda SD, MacMahon H, Newstead GM. Breast lesions incidentally detected with CT: what the general radiologist needs to know. Radiographics. 2007;27:S37–51.

Ikeda DM. Breast imaging the requisites. 2nd ed. Philadelphia: Elsevier, Mosby; 2011. p. 139.

Fig. 1.1

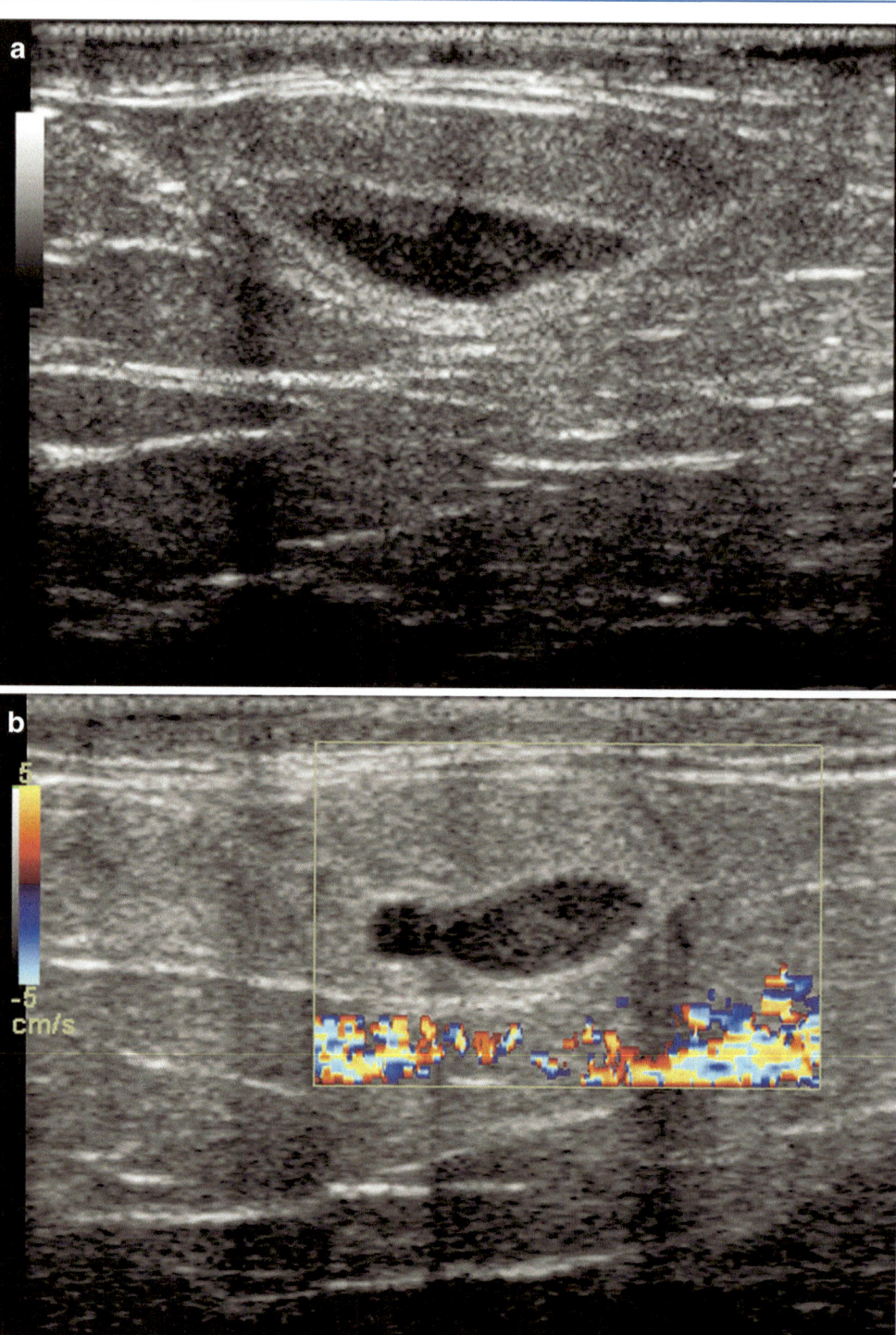

CASE 73
ANGIOSARCOMA

PATIENT HISTORY

An 83-year-old female with complaints of palpable mass with associated breast pain and tenderness in the right breast; history of right lumpectomy in 1998.

RADIOLOGY FINDINGS

Fig. 1.1 (**a**) CC, (**b**) ML, and spot-compression (**c**) CC and (**d**) MLO views show a contour deformity in the retroareolar right breast, compatible with history of right lumpectomy. Adjacent to this area, there is a focal asymmetry with associated architectural distortion on the CC view.

Fig. 1.2 (**a**, **b**) There is also skin thickening and increased trabecular pattern when compared to the prior mammogram 1 year ago. Targeted ultrasound was negative.

BI-RADS ASSESSMENT

BI-RADS 4. Suspicious abnormality (following diagnostic workup, prior to biopsy).

DIAGNOSIS

Angiosarcoma

DISCUSSION

- Angiosarcoma is a malignant stromal breast neoplasm.
- Mean age at diagnosis is 35 years.
- Increased risk of developing angiosarcoma following radiation exposure.
- Usually a palpable rapidly enlarging mass. May have associated overlying bluish skin discoloration.
- On mammography, angiosarcoma appears as a mass with microlobulated or indistinct margins.
- On ultrasound, angiosarcoma appears as a hypoechoic circumscribed or spiculated mass.
- On MRI, angiosarcoma is low signal on T1-weighted images, is higher signal on T2-weighted images, and demonstrates enhancement of the mass with a low-intensity central region.

REFERENCES

Berg WA, Birdwell RL, Gombos EC, et al. Diagnostic imaging: breast. 1st ed. Salt Lake City: Amirsys; 2006. Section IV-2, p. 176–7.

Ikeda DM. Breast imaging the requisites. 2nd ed. Philadelphia: Elsevier, Mosby; 2011. p. 399.

Lilaia C, Pereira F, Andre S, Cabrita B. Breast angiosarcoma. Internet J Gynecol Obstet. 2007;6(2).

Fig. 1.1

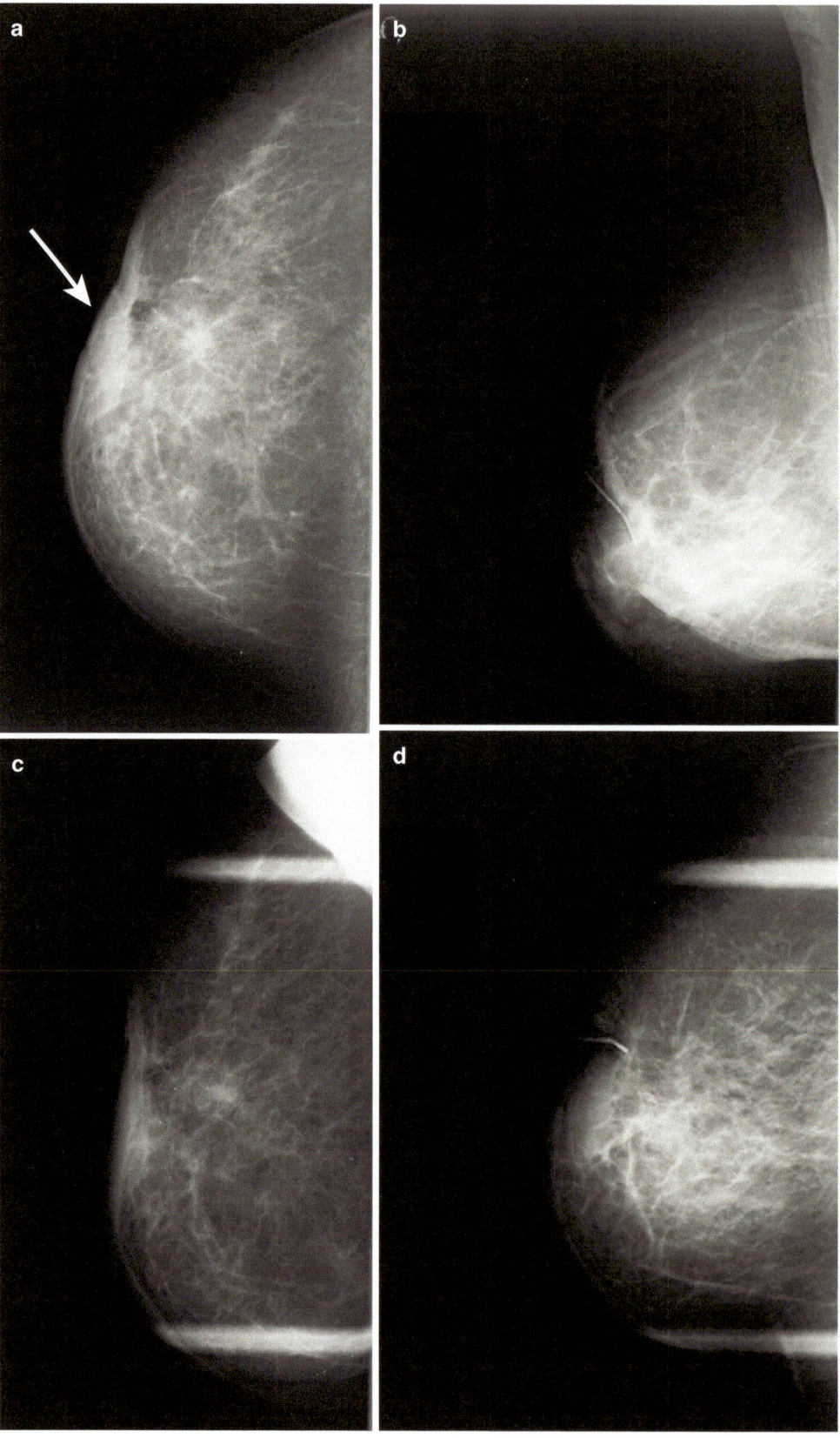

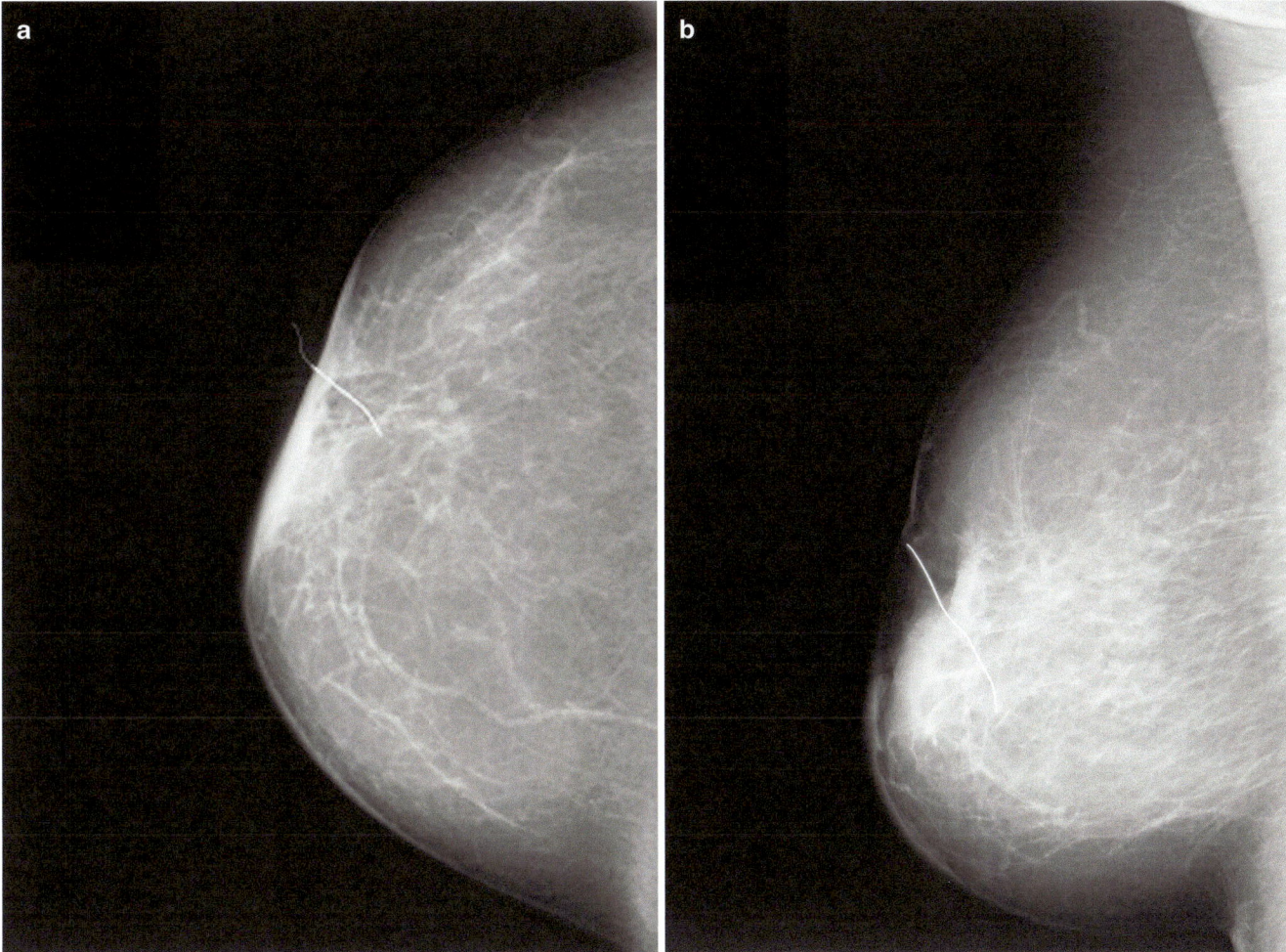

Fig. 1.2

Case 74
Free Silicone Oil Injections

Patient History

A 46-year-old female for a bilateral screening mammogram.

Radiology Findings

Fig. 1.1 (**a**, **b**) CC and (**c**, **d**) MLO views demonstrate multiple, diffuse, bilateral, innumerable, round, and oval dense masses with rim calcifications.

BI-RADS Assessment

BI-RADS 2. Benign findings.

Diagnosis

Free silicone oil injections

Discussion

- Silicone oil injections into breast parenchyma are performed for cosmetic augmentation.
- The procedure is most frequently performed in China.
- Patients can complain of focal or diffuse lumps, pain, or discomfort.
- Typically, mammography and ultrasound are not sensitive for breast cancer detection following free silicone injection.
- Postcontrast MRI of the breast may be more useful for breast cancer detection.

References

Ikeda DM. Breast imaging the requisites. 2nd ed. Philadelphia: Elsevier, Mosby; 2011. p. 84–5, 349–50.

Scaranelo AM, de Fatima Ribeiro Maia M. Sonographic and mammographic findings of breast liquid silicone injection. J Clin Ultrasound. 2006;34(6):273–7.

Yang WT, Suen M, Ho WS, Metreweli C. Paraffinomas of the breast: mammographic, ultrasonographic and radiographic appearances with clinical and histopathological correlation. Clin Radiol. 1996;51:130–3.

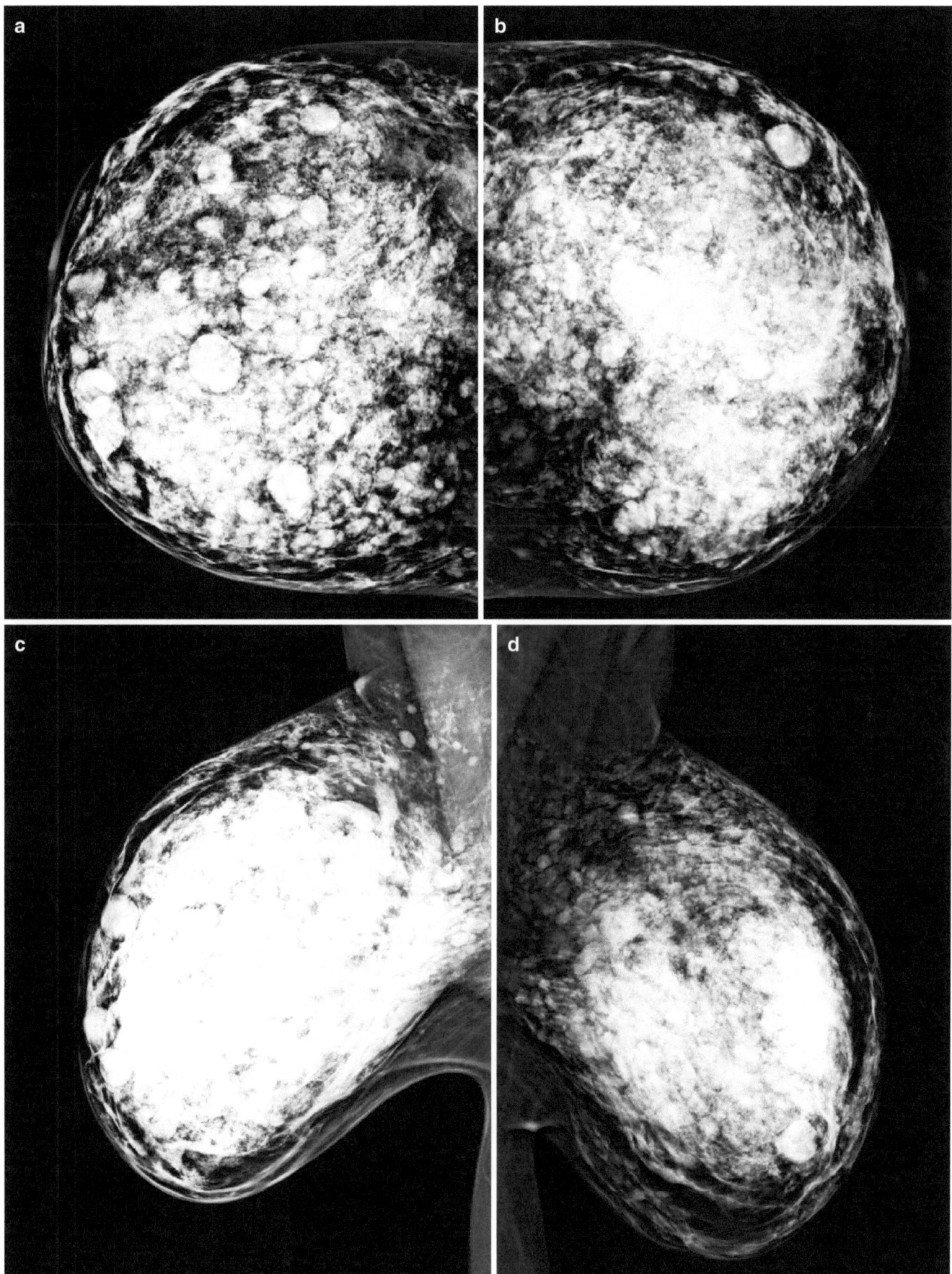

Fig. 1.1

Case 75
Phyllodes Tumor

Patient History

A 52-year-old female with a palpable mass in the upper inner left breast.

Radiology Findings

Fig. 1.1 (**a**) CC and (**b**) MLO views show an oval circumscribed mass in the upper inner left breast at posterior depth corresponding to the triangular marker indicating a palpable mass.
Fig. 1.2 (**a**) Grayscale and (**b**) color Doppler ultrasound images show an oval circumscribed hypoechoic avascular mass.

BI-RADS Assessment

BI-RADS 4. Suspicious abnormality (following diagnostic workup, prior to biopsy).

Diagnosis

Phyllodes tumor

Discussion

- Phyllodes tumor is a large rapidly growing circumscribed mass without calcifications.
- Phyllodes tumor contains papillary growths of epithelial-lined stroma in a leaflike configuration.
- Has both stromal and epithelial elements.
- Median age is 45–49 years.
- About 25 % of phyllodes tumors are malignant and 20 % of the malignant subtype may metastasize.
- Complete surgical excision is recommended and often curative.
- Twenty-one percent risk of recurrence, most within 2 years.

References

Berg WA, Birdwell RL, Gombos EC, et al. Diagnostic imaging breast. 1st ed. Salt Lake City: Amirsys; 2006. Section IV-2, p. 96–8.
Ikeda DM. Breast imaging the requisites. 2nd ed. Philadelphia: Elsevier, Mosby; 2011. p. 120, 126.
Mandell J. Core radiology: a visual approach to diagnostic imaging. 1st ed. Cambridge: Cambridge University Press; 2013. p. 627.

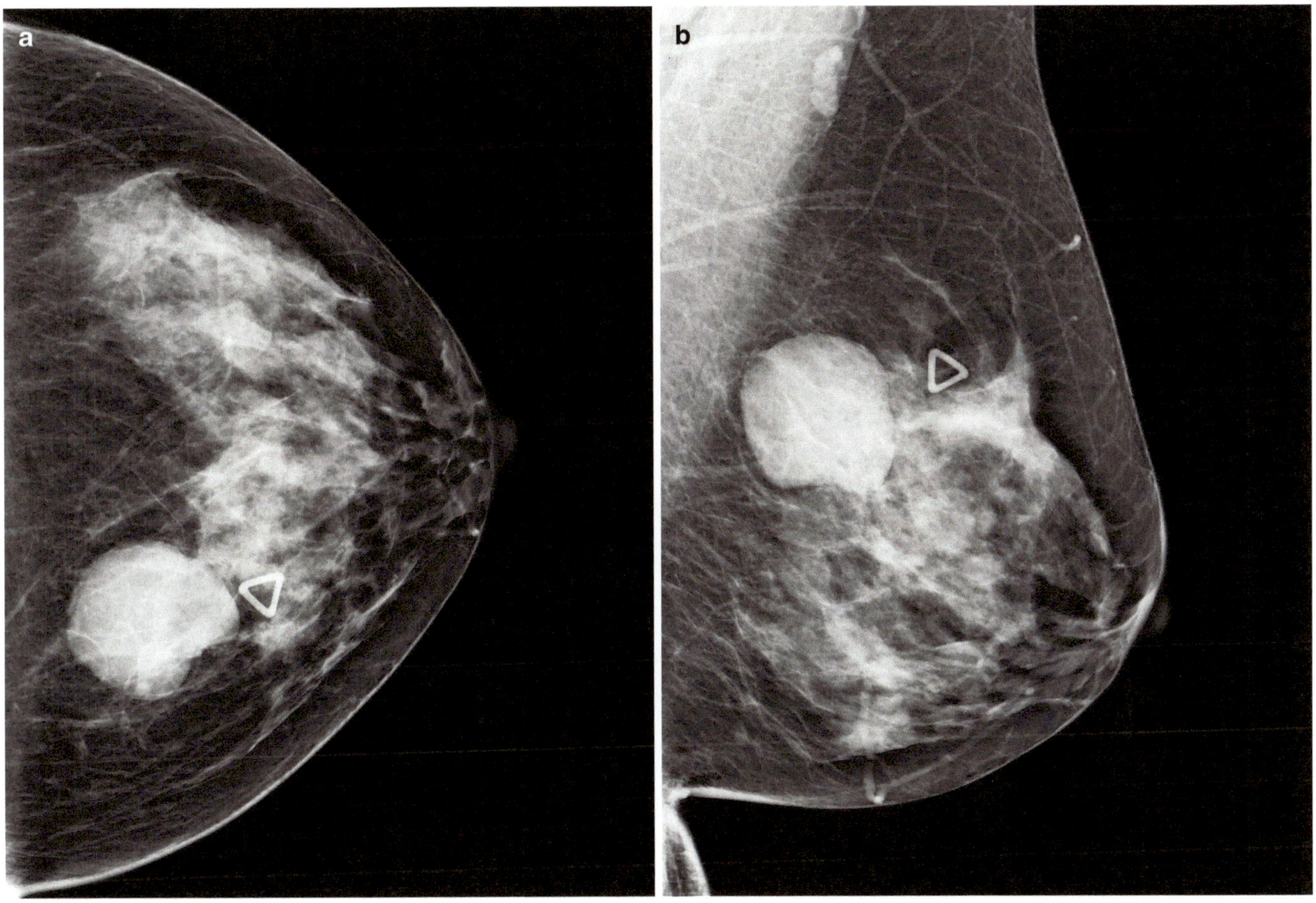

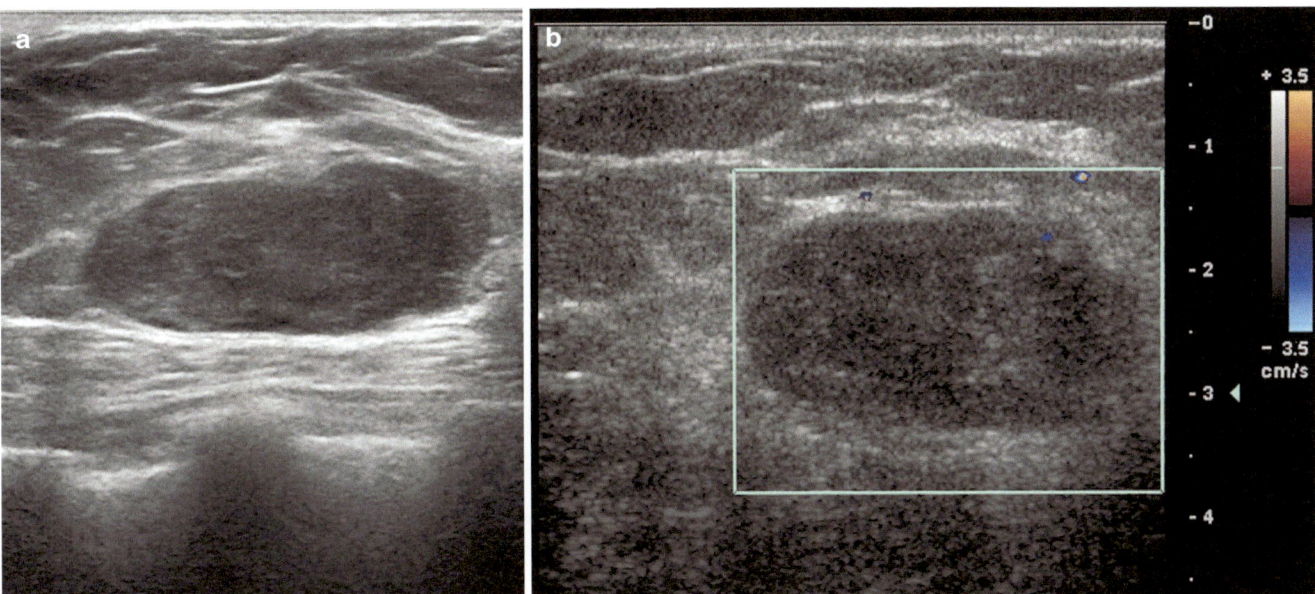

Fig. 1.1

Fig. 1.2

CASE 76
DCIS COMEDONECROSIS

PATIENT HISTORY

A 43-year-old female for a screening mammogram.

RADIOLOGY FINDINGS

Fig. 1.1 (**a**) CC, (**b**) LM, and spot-magnification (**c**) CC view and (**d**) LM views demonstrate a segmental area of fine linear branching calcifications at 12 o'clock in the right breast at anterior to middle depth.

BI-RADS ASSESSMENT

BI-RADS 5. Highly suggestive for malignancy (following diagnostic workup, prior to biopsy).

DIAGNOSIS

DCIS comedonecrosis

DISCUSSION

- DCIS comedonecrosis is a high-grade type of DCIS.
- It is associated with rapid growth and necrosis of the central duct.
- Calcifications are the hallmark of DCIS comedonecrosis.
- Classic appearance is fine, linear branching-type calcifications, in either a linear or segmental distribution.
- Majority of patients are asymptomatic at time of presentation.
- Associated with higher rate of recurrence than other subtypes of DCIS due to high nuclear grade and radiation resistance of the tumor.

REFERENCE

Berg WA, Birdwell RL, Gombos EC, et al. Diagnostic imaging breast. 1st ed. Salt Lake City: Amirsys; 2006. Section IV-2, p. 118–21.

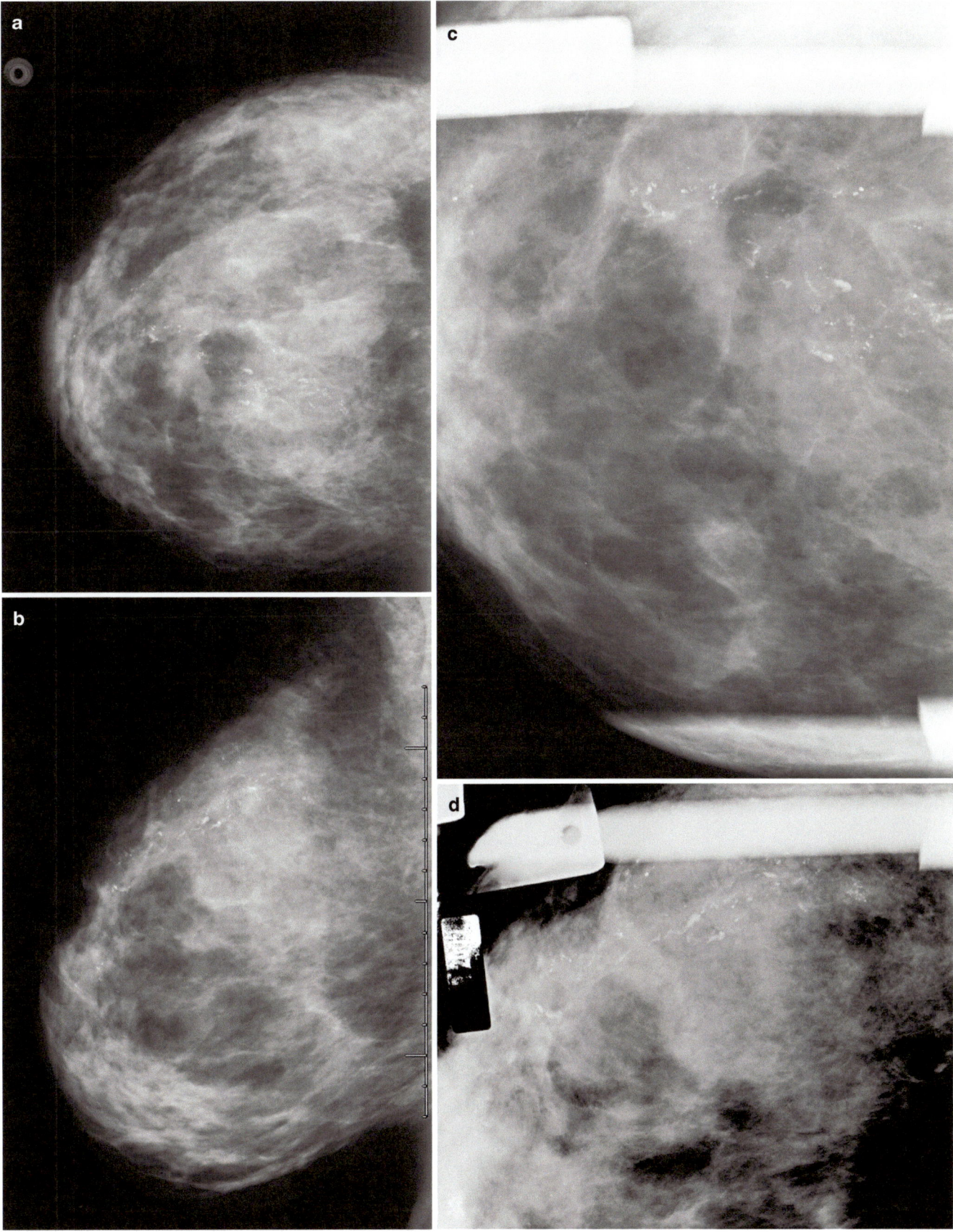

Fig. 1.1

Case 77
Bilateral Breast Cancer

Patient History

A 90-year-old female with a history of palpable masses in both breasts.

Radiology Findings

Fig. 1.1 (**a, b**) CC and (**c, d**) MLO images show an oval mass with angular margins and associated coarse calcifications at 12 o'clock in the right breast at middle depth. There is also an irregular mass with spiculated margins and associated coarse calcifications at 3 o'clock in the left breast at middle depth.

Fig. 1.2 (**a**) Grayscale and (**b**) color Doppler ultrasound images show an oval hypoechoic mass with angular margins that has internal vascularity in the right breast.

Fig. 1.3 (**a**) Grayscale and (**b**) color Doppler ultrasound images show an irregular spiculated hypoechoic mass that is avascular and demonstrates posterior acoustic shadowing in the left breast.

BI-RADS Assessment

BI-RADS 5. Highly suspicious for malignancy (following diagnostic workup, prior to biopsy).

Diagnosis

Bilateral invasive ductal carcinoma (IDC)

Discussion

- There is a one in eight lifetime probability of developing breast cancer.
- Breast cancer is the second leading cause of cancer mortality (15 % of all cancer deaths).
- Risk factors for breast cancer include the following:
  - Higher incidence in women
  - Increasing age
  - Personal history of breast cancer
  - First-degree relative with breast cancer
  - Early menarche
  - Late menopause
  - Nulliparous
  - First birth after the age of 30 years
  - Atypical ductal hyperplasia (ADH)
  - Atypical lobular hyperplasia (ALH)
  - Lobular carcinoma in situ (LCIS)
  - Juvenile papillomatosis
  - BRCA-1, BRCA-2 gene mutations
  - History of radiation exposure to the chest wall
- Patients with breast cancer have increased risk of developing either synchronous or metachronous breast cancer, which ranges between 0.5 and 0.8 % each year.

References

Cardenosa G. Breast imaging companion. 3rd ed. Philadelphia: Lippincott Williams and Wilkins; 2008. p. 1–2.

Tousimis E. Synchronous bilateral invasive breast cancer. Breast Cancer Online. 2008;8(4).

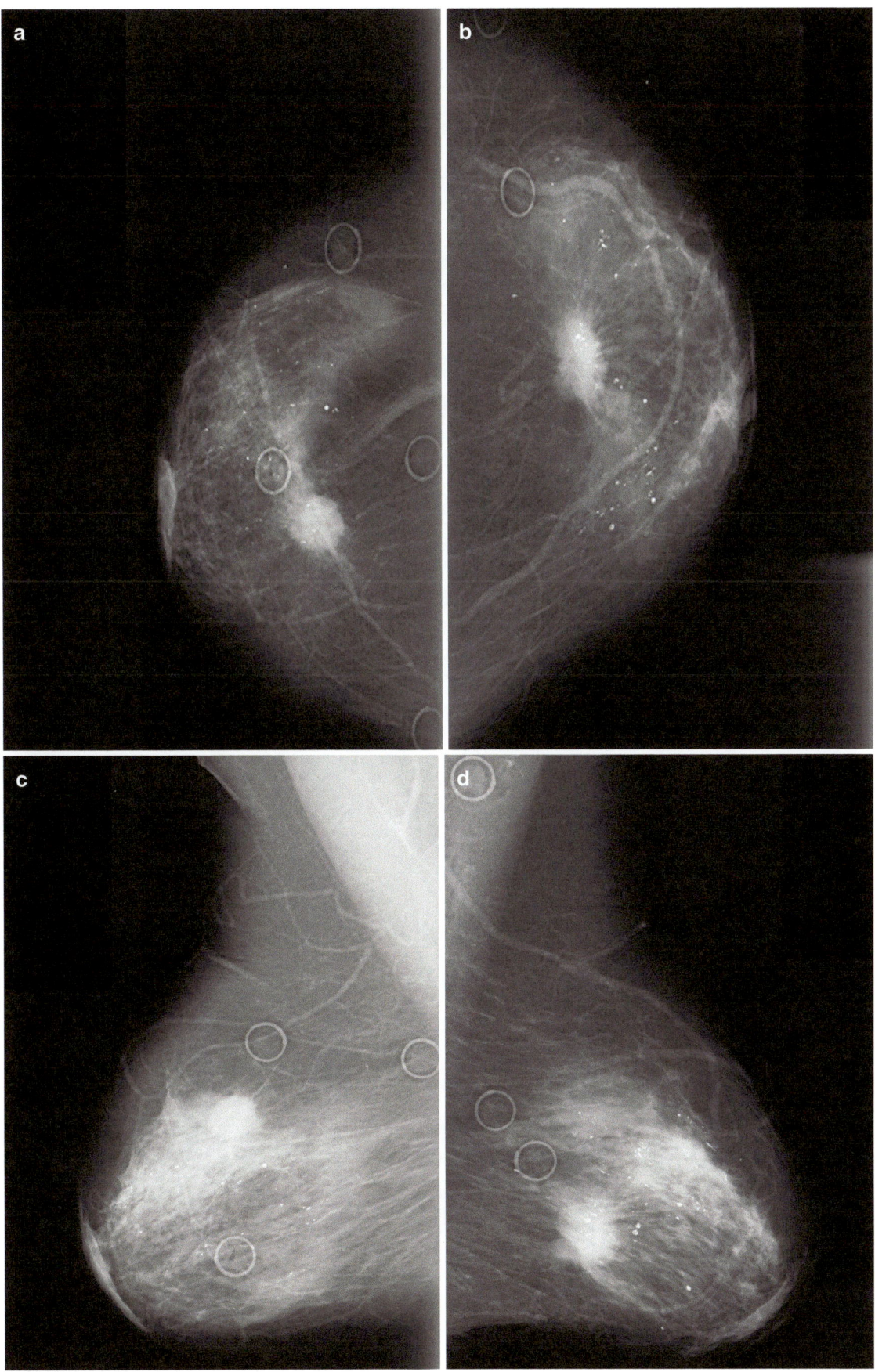

Fig. 1.1

Fig. 1.2

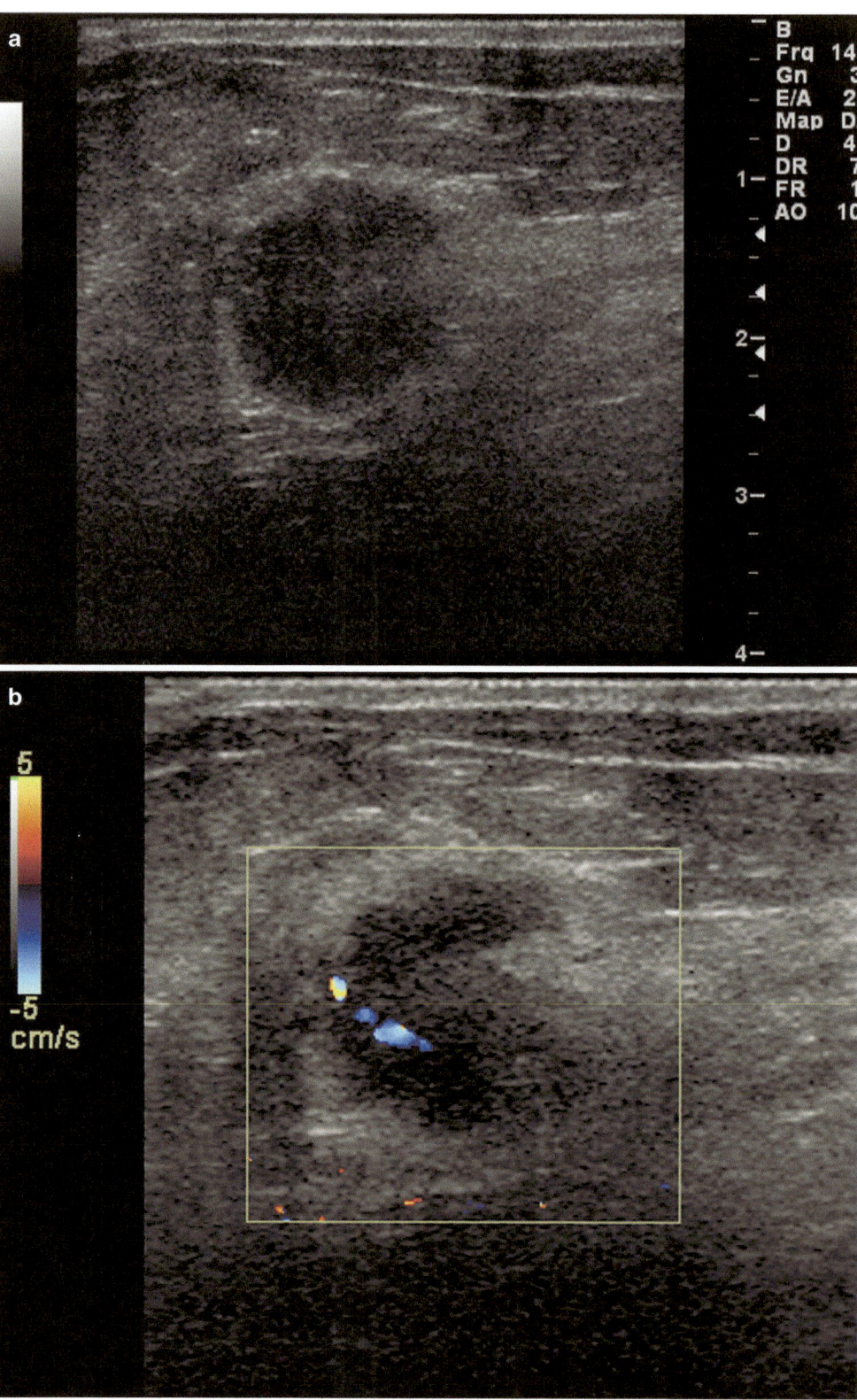

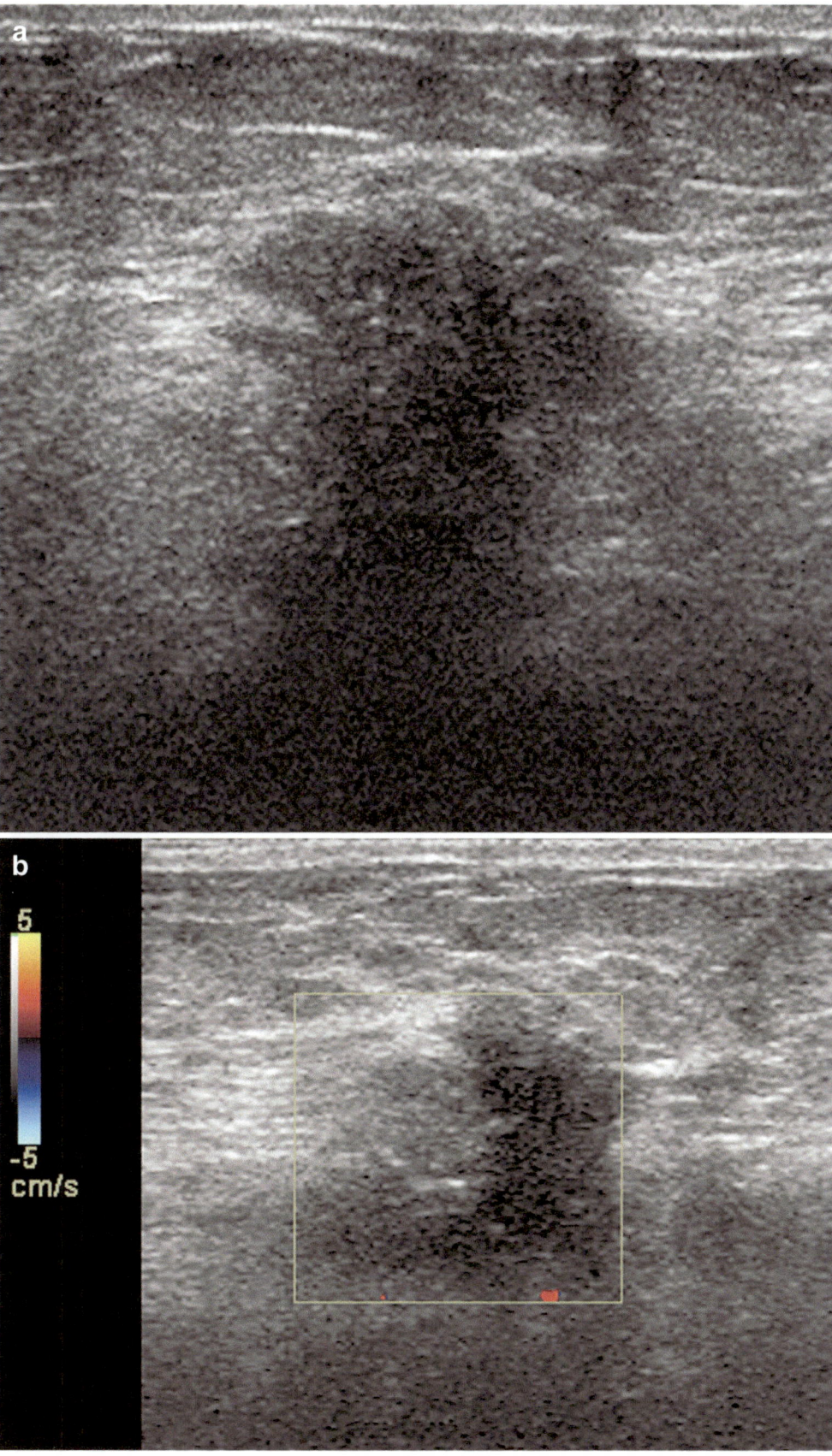

Fig. 1.3

Case 78
Sebaceous Cyst/Epidermal Inclusion Cyst

Patient History

A 52-year-old female with a palpable finding in the left breast for 2 months.

Radiology Findings

Fig. 1.1 (**a**) MLO and (**b**) spot-compression CC views demonstrate a partially visualized circumscribed, high-density oval mass in the upper outer left breast at posterior depth, at the site of the palpable finding.
Fig. 1.2 Grayscale ultrasound image demonstrates an oval, hypoechoic mass with posterior acoustic enhancement. Hypoechoic line is seen extending from the mass to the skin.
Fig. 1.3 MLO view in a different patient demonstrates an oval mass with circumscribed margins containing punctuate calcifications in the upper left breast.

BI-RADS Assessment

BI-RADS 2. Benign finding (following diagnostic workup).

Diagnosis

Sebaceous cyst/epidermal inclusion cyst

Discussion

- Cutaneous or subcutaneous masses arising from the sebaceous glands (sebaceous cysts) or from obstructed hair follicles (epidermal inclusion cysts).

- Can arise anywhere in the skin of the breast and axilla.
- Clinically and on imaging, sebaceous cysts and epidermal inclusion cysts are indistinguishable from each other.
- Equally seen in males and females.
- Clinically, sebaceous and epidermal inclusion cysts present as elevated, palpable, smooth, and firm skin lesions.
- The claw sign on ultrasound is an echogenic line representing the skin which wraps around the lesion. It helps determine the dermal location of these lesions.
- There is no malignant potential for sebaceous cysts, and it is extremely rare in epidermal inclusion cysts.
- Biopsy of sebaceous cysts and epidermal inclusion cysts should be avoided, as it may incite an inflammatory response.
- Excision is for symptomatic relief.
- Calcifications are present in 20 % of epidermal inclusion cysts.

References

Bassett LW, Jackson VP, Fu KL, Fu YS. Diagnosis of diseases of the breast. 2nd ed. Philadelphia: Elsevier; 2005. p. 399–400.
Berg WA, Birdwell RL, Gombos EC, et al. Diagnostic imaging breast. 1st ed. Salt Lake City: Amirsys; 2006. Section IV-3, p. 16.
Bergmann-Koester CU, Kolberg HC, Rudolf I, Krueger S, Gellissen J, Stoeckelhuber BM. Epidermal cyst of the breast mimicking malignancy: clinical, radiological, and histological correlation. Arch Gynecol Obstet. 2006;273(5):312–4.
Harvey JA, March DE. Making the diagnosis: a practical guide to breast imaging. Philadelphia: Elsevier; 2013. p. 189.

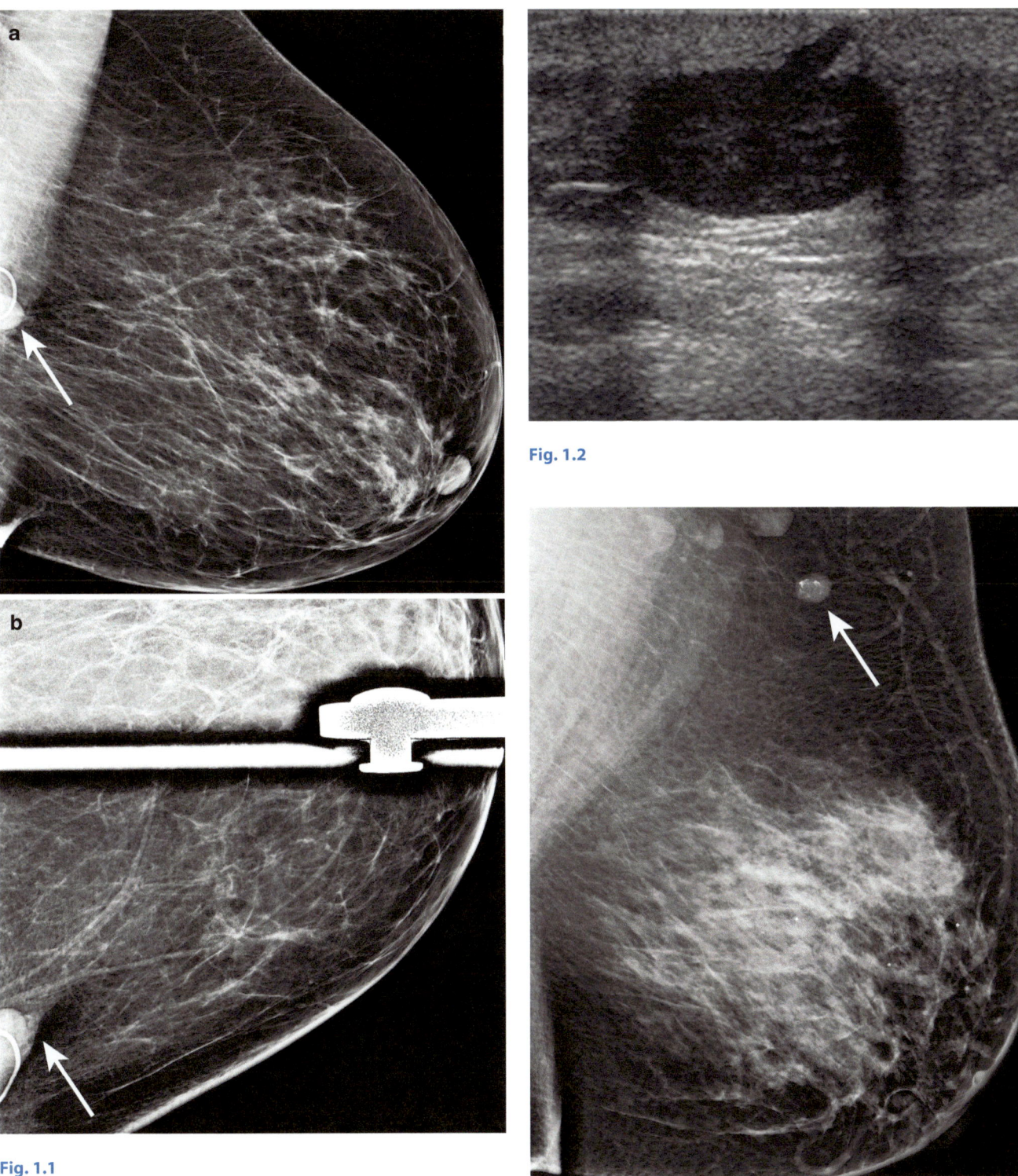

Fig. 1.2

Fig. 1.1

Fig. 1.3

CASE 79
DISPLACED BIOPSY SITE MARKER AFTER STEREOTACTIC CORE NEEDLE BIOPSY

PATIENT HISTORY

A 48-year-old female who recently underwent a left breast stereotactic core needle biopsy.

RADIOLOGY FINDINGS

Fig. 1.1 Postprocedure (**a**) CC and (**b**) ML views show a biopsy site marker that is located medial to the biopsy cavity.

DIAGNOSIS

Displaced biopsy site marker after stereotactic core needle biopsy

DISCUSSION

- The primary reason for deploying a biopsy site marker is to provide a visible marker at the site of the excised biopsy target, so that wire localization can be performed if indicated.

- To be effective, a biopsy site marker should be deployed at the intended site and must remain close to the intended target site.
- Although a biopsy site marker may initially appear to be deployed within the biopsy cavity when the breast is in compression, as the compression is released, small discrepancies in the location of the marker and the biopsy cavity may become magnified (the accordion effect). This occurs particularly perpendicular to the plane of compression used during stereotactic core needle biopsy.
- Careful correlation between the biopsy site and marker location on two orthogonal mammographic views should be routinely performed after biopsy to reveal any discrepancies and allow accurate needle localization, if required.

REFERENCES

Esserman LE, Cura MA, DaCosta D. Recognizing pitfalls in early and late migration of clip markers after imaging-guided directional vacuum-assisted biopsy. Radiology. 2004;24:147–56.
Rosen EL, Vo TT. Metallic clip deployment during stereotactic breast biopsy: retrospective analysis. Radiology. 2001;218:510–6.

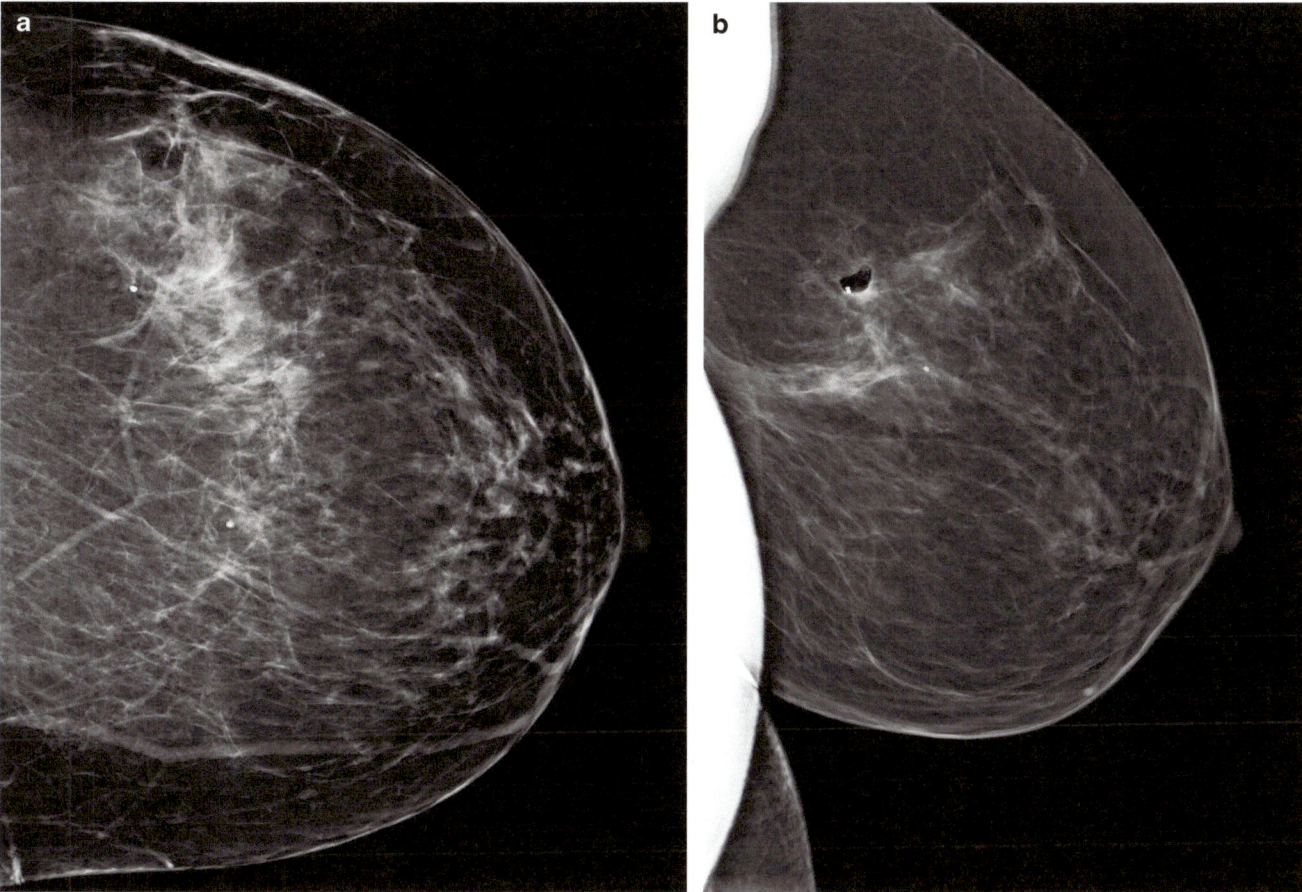

Fig. 1.1

MRI Case Review

2

B.A. Shah et al., *Breast Imaging Review: A Quick Guide to Essential Diagnoses*,
DOI 10.1007/978-3-319-07791-8_2, © Springer International Publishing Switzerland 2015

CASE 1
MRI ARTIFACTS

PATIENT HISTORY

MR images in multiple patients.

RADIOLOGY FINDINGS

Fig. 2.1 Axial subtracted T1-weighted image demonstrates a mirror image of the aorta seen in the soft tissue of the left chest wall. This finding is consistent for a ghosting artifact from motion from the aorta.

Fig. 2.2 Axial nonfat-suppressed T2-weighted image demonstrates too wide of a field of view due to poor technique.

Fig. 2.3 Sagittal fat-suppressed T2-weighted image demonstrates a signal void with surrounding increased signal from a tissue marker clip in the upper breast. This artifact is called a susceptibility artifact.

Fig. 2.4 Sagittal water-suppressed FSTIR image demonstrates incorrect water suppression. Instead, the silicone is suppressed. Findings are consistent for silicone saturation artifact.

Fig. 2.5 Axial subtracted T1-weighted image postcontrast image demonstrates ghosting artifact in the phase-encoding direction due to the patient coughing.

Fig. 2.6 Axial subtracted T1-weighted image postcontrast image demonstrates inhomogeneous fat saturation.

Fig. 2.7 Sagittal nonfat-suppressed T1-weighted localizer image shows portion of the spine seen on the left aspect of the image consistent with a phase-wrap artifact.

DIAGNOSIS

MRI artifacts

DISCUSSION

- Artifacts from metallic artifacts are also called black hole artifacts or susceptibility artifacts.
- Susceptibility artifacts manifest as signal voids on gradient echo sequences. On spin echo sequences, a signal

flare void component may be seen in addition to the signal void.
- Small lesions in the region of the susceptibility artifact from tissue markers may not be visible due to the signal void. This can limit the MRI assessment for the extent of the disease, surgical margins, or size of lesion.
- Motion artifact, or also called ghosting, is always in the phase-encoding direction. The phase-encoding direction should be left to right for axial sequences and superior to inferior for sagittal sequences to reduce the effect of cardiac and respiratory motion.
- Ghosting can arise from patient motion or cardiac, respiratory, or great vessel motion. Motion can result in blurring of moving tissues but can cause a structured noise pattern, resulting in ghosting of brighter moving tissues in the phase-encoding direction.
- Phase wrap, also known as aliasing artifact or wraparound artifact, occurs when tissue extends beyond the field of view (FOV), causing signal from tissues outside the FOV to be superimposed on structures within the FOV.
- Enlarging the FOV can correct phase-wrap artifact.
- Silicone saturation artifact is caused by saturation of silicone signal, which can occur when silicone is selected for saturation rather than fat.
- Inhomogeneous fat saturation artifact may be due to unexpected variation in the magnetic field for which protons in fat tissue are precessing out of range of frequencies included in the suppression pulse. These protons will not be suppressed, and the fat containing these protons will maintain its brighter signal.
- Shimming the magnet (optimizing field homogenicity) of an MRI unit can sometimes correct inhomogeneous fat saturation.
- MRI technologists may not be used to positioning the breasts, and training by mammography technologists may be helpful.

REFERENCES

Genson CC, Blane CE, Helvie MA, Waits SA, Chenevert TL. Effects on breast MRI of artifacts caused by metallic tissue marker clips. Am J Roentgoenol. 2007;188:372–76.
Harvey JA, Hendrick RE, Coll JM, Nicholson BT, Burkholde BT, Cohen MA. Breast MR imaging artifacts. How to recognize and fix them. Radiographics. 2007;27:S137–45.

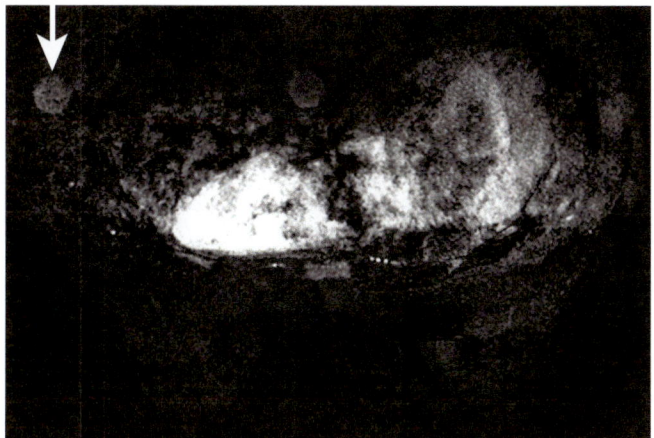

Fig. 2.1

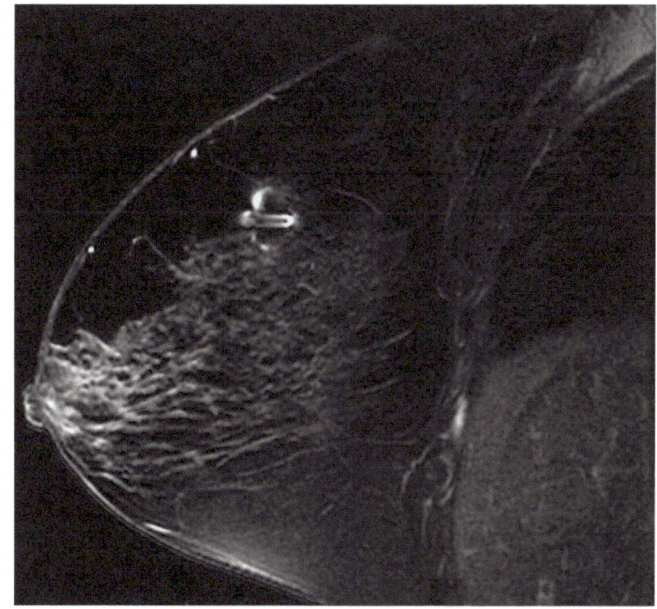

Fig. 2.3

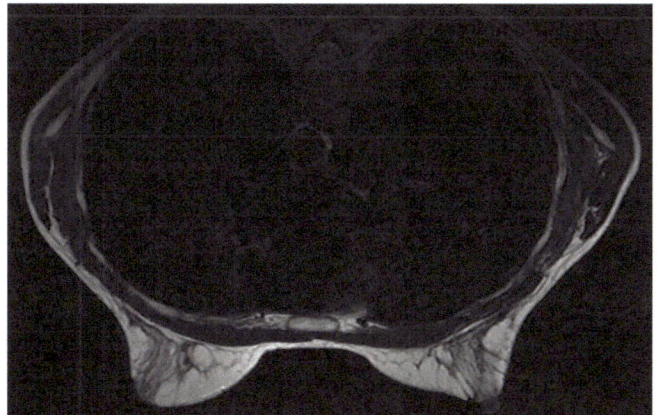

Fig. 2.2

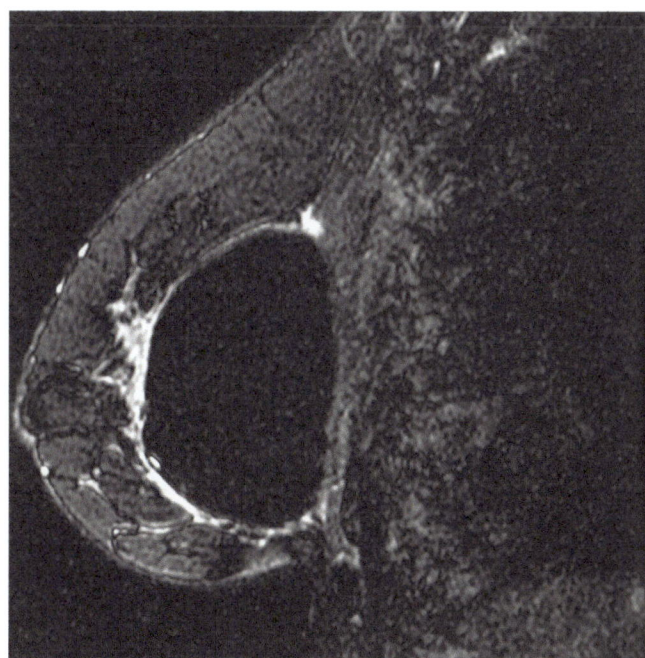

Fig. 2.4

Fig. 2.5

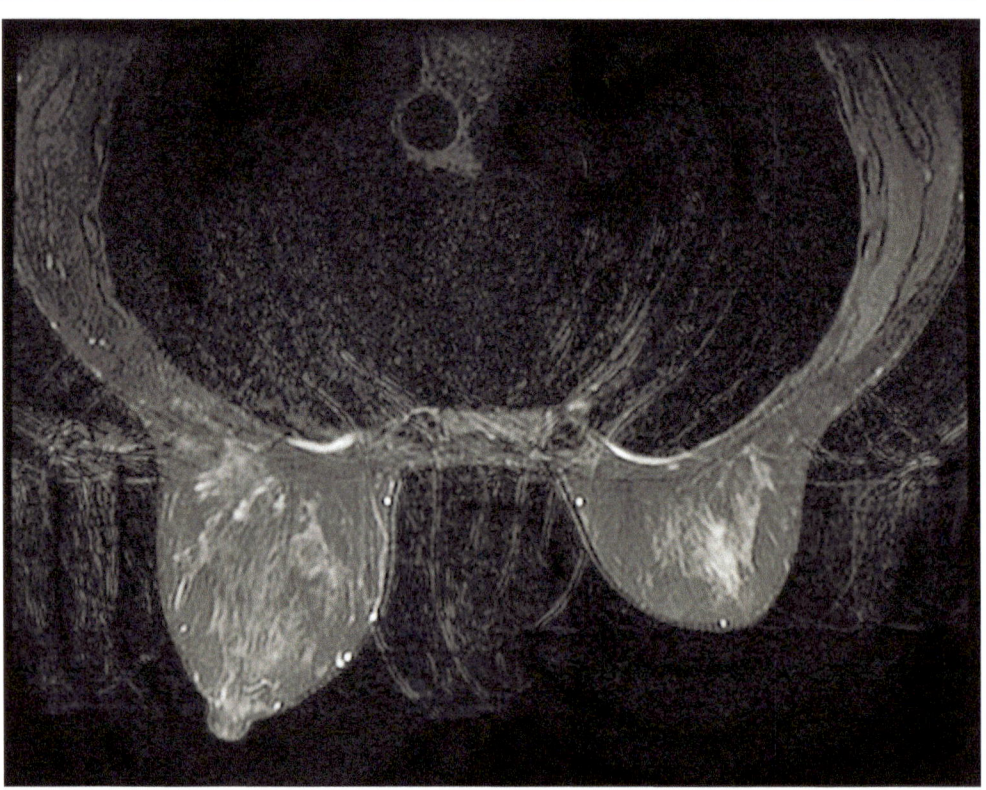

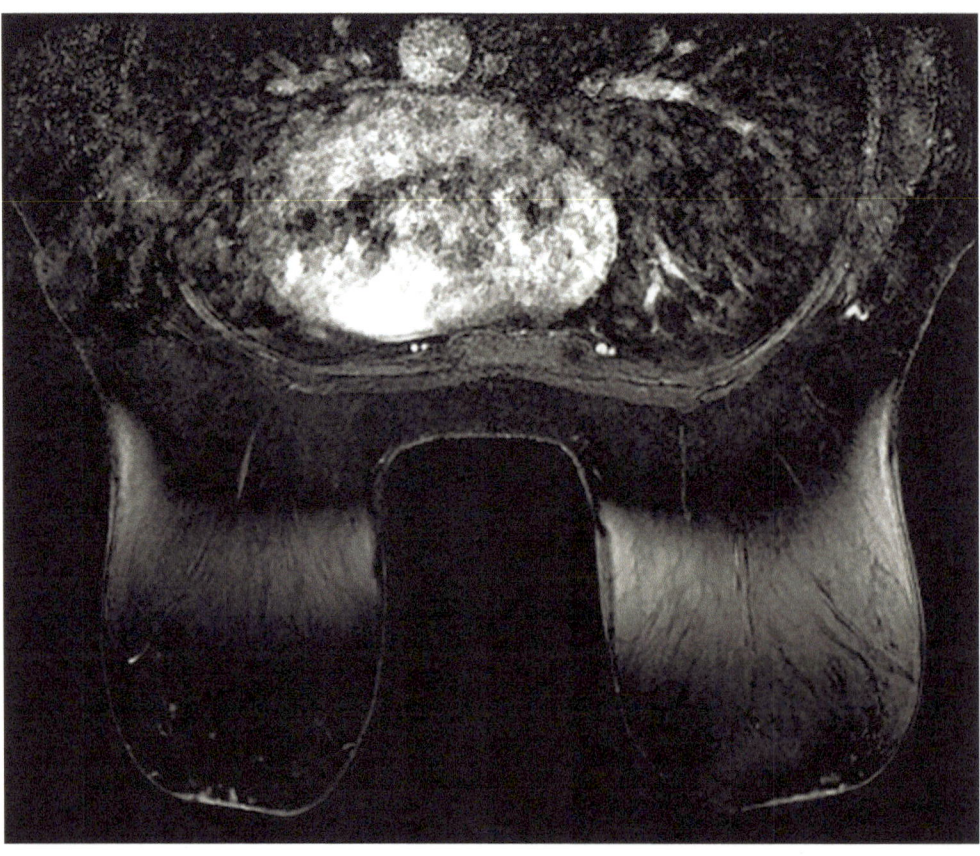

Fig. 2.6

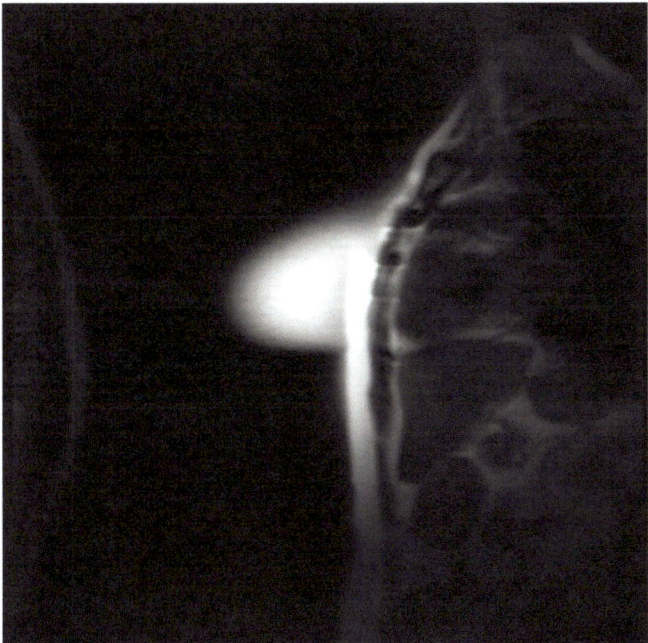

Fig. 2.7

CASE 2
RIM ENHANCEMENT

PATIENT HISTORY

Breast MRI studies in multiple patients.

RADIOLOGY FINDINGS

Fig. 2.1 Axial subtracted T1-weighted image demonstrates an enhancing mass in the outer left breast posteriorly. The mass shows thin, irregular rim enhancement.

Fig. 2.2 Sagittal (**a**) T2-weighted image in a different patient demonstrates multiple oval high-signal-intensity masses in the left breast. There is skin thickening. Sagittal (**b**) contrast-enhanced T1-weighted image demonstrates multiple thin rim-enhancing masses.

Fig. 2.3 (**a**) Axial nonfat-suppressed T1-weighted image demonstrates a lobular area isointense to fat in the inner right breast at anterior depth. (**b**) Sagittal fat-suppressed contrast-enhanced T1-weighted image demonstrates the mass to have a thin rim of peripheral enhancement consistent with fat necrosis.

Fig. 2.4 (**a**) Axial nonfat-suppressed T2-weighted image demonstrates a high-signal-intensity area in the inner right breast at posterior depth. (**b**) Sagittal fat-suppressed contrast-enhanced T1-weighted image demonstrates the area in the lower breast with thin peripheral rim enhancement consistent with a seroma.

DIAGNOSIS

Rim enhancement (edge enhancement)

DISCUSSION

- Rim enhancement is defined as enhancement at the periphery of a mass on MRI.

- Morphology of the enhancement is variable based on lesion characteristics.
- Benign lesions typically have a uniform and smooth rim.
- Malignant lesions and infections typically have an irregular rim.
- Rim enhancement is caused by peripheral vascularization of lesions.
- If present in invasive cancer, the prognosis is worse.
- Differential diagnosis includes:
  - Invasive ductal carcinoma (IDC)
    Margin is irregular and thin.
  - Seroma
    Margin is thin and smooth (<4 mm).
    High in signal on T2-weighted image and STIR.
    Becomes smaller on later examinations.
  - Inflammatory cyst
    Margin is thin and smooth.
    High in signal on T2-weighted image and STIR.
  - Abscess
    High in signal on T2-weighted image and STIR.
    May be associated with edema and skin thickening.
    May be palpable and tender.
  - Fat necrosis
    High in signal on nonfat-suppressed T1-weighted images.
- Any solid mass with rim enhancement should be biopsied.

REFERENCES

Berg WA, Birdwell RL, Gombos EC, et al. Diagnostic imaging breast. 1st ed. Salt Lake City: Amirsys; 2006. Section IV 1, p. 174–77.

Morris EA, Liberman L, editors. Breast MRI diagnosis and intervention. 1st ed. New York: Springer; 2005. p. 61–4.

Fig. 2.1

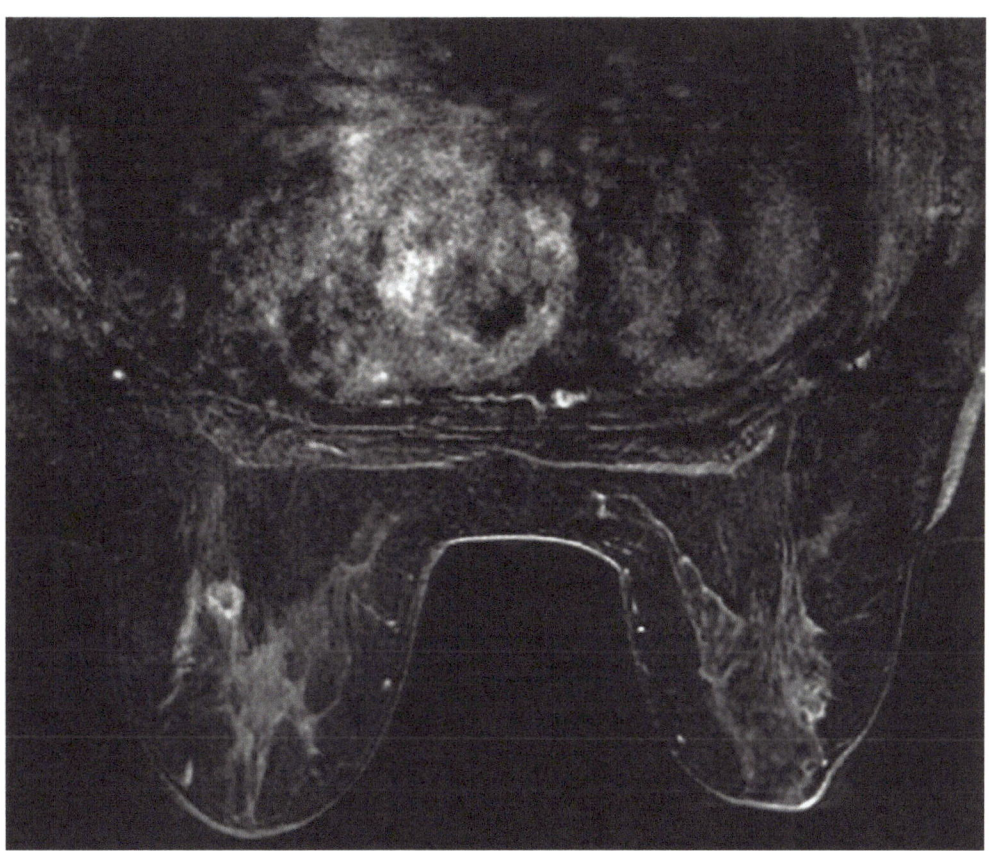

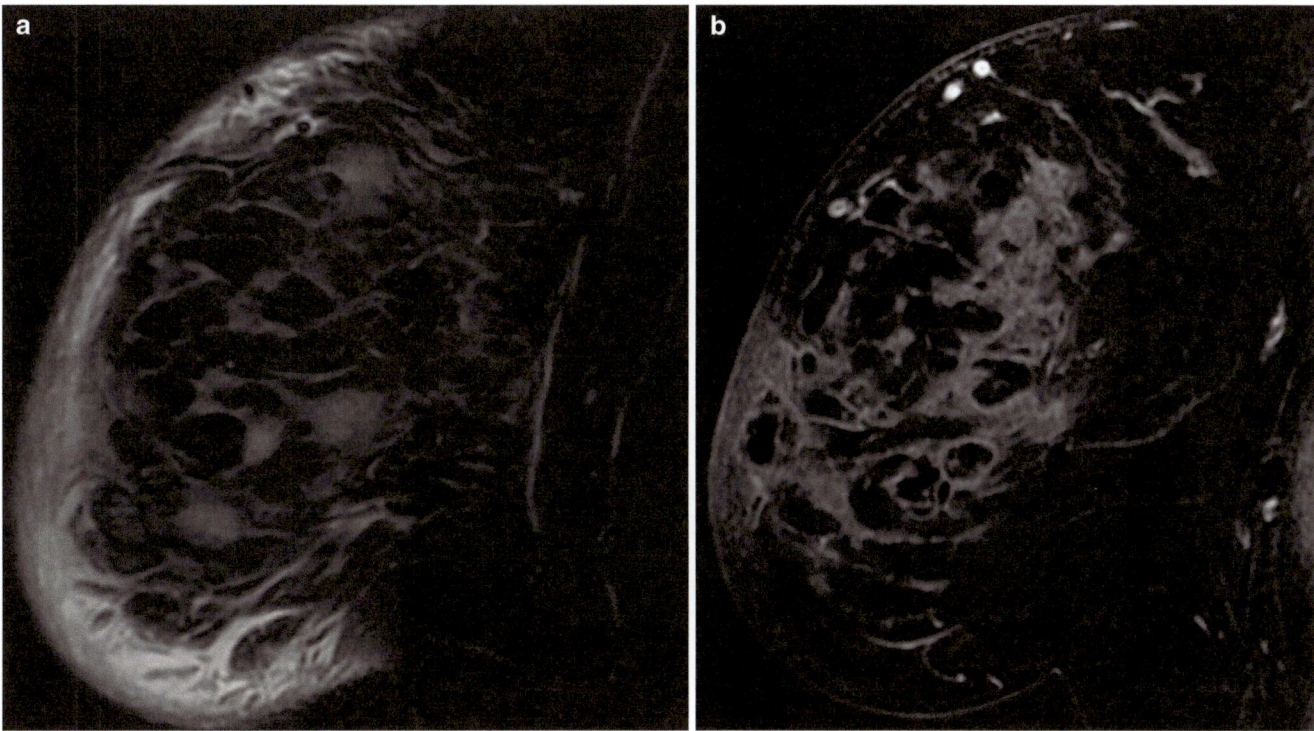

Fig. 2.2

Fig. 2.3

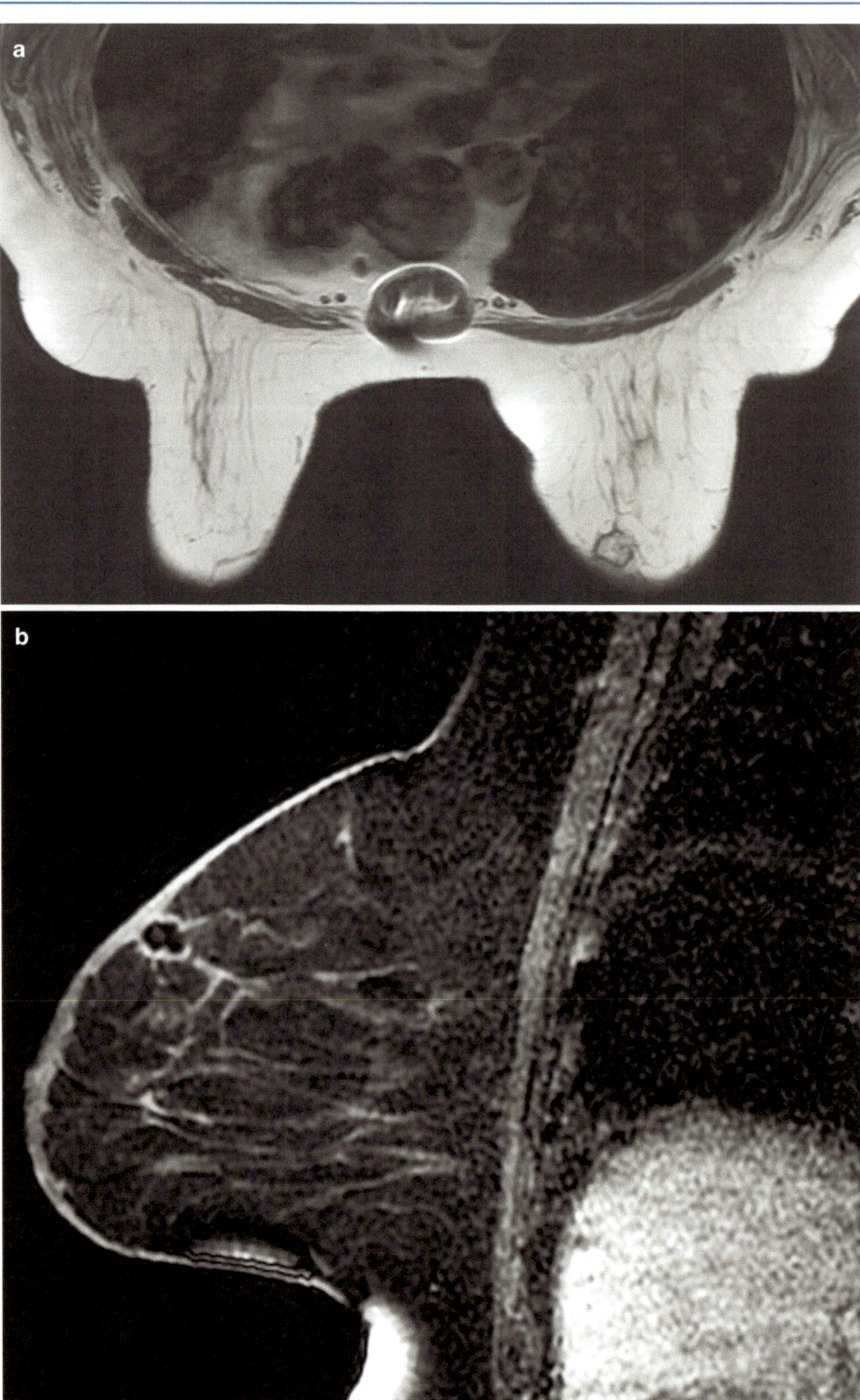

Fig. 2.4

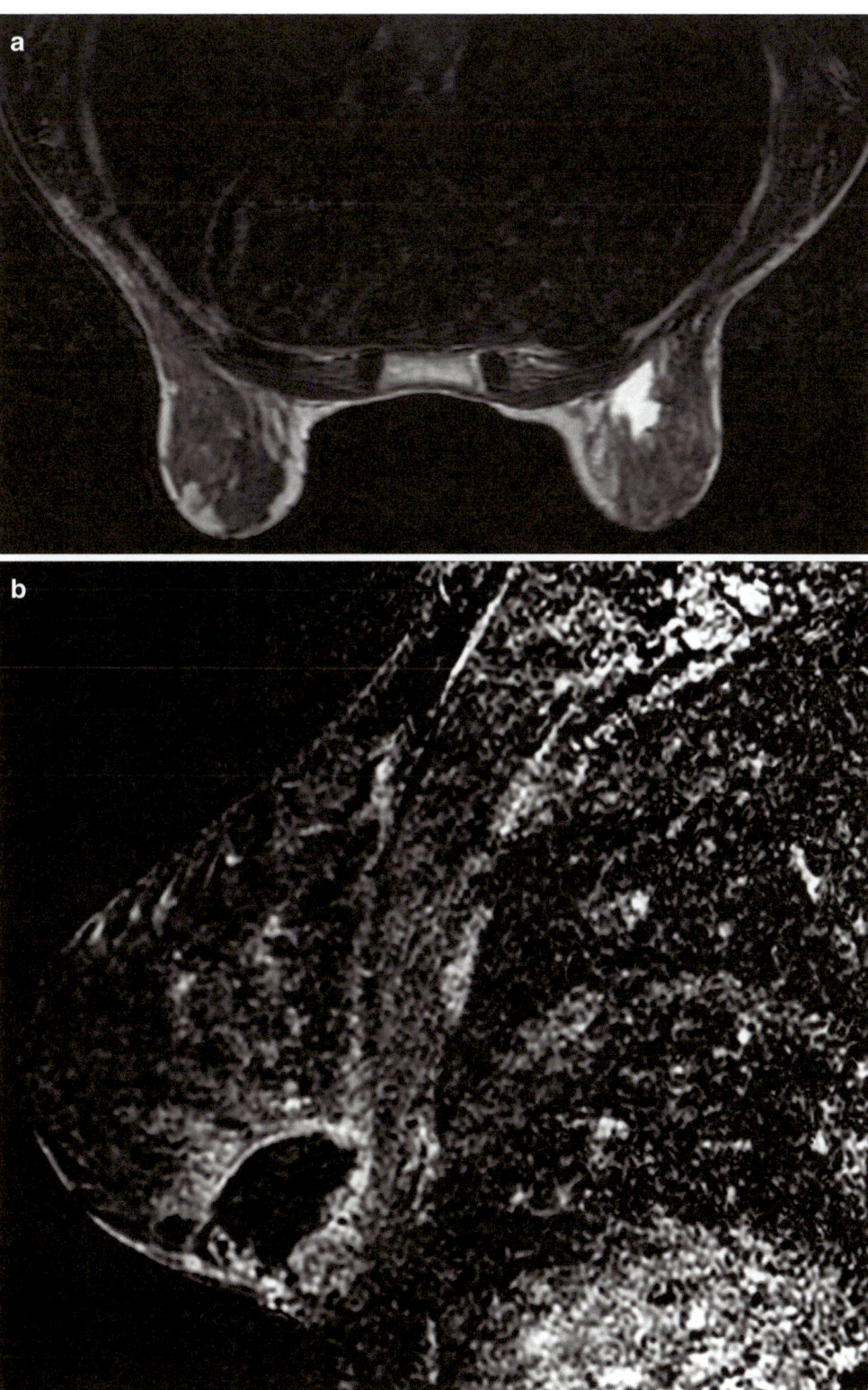

CASE 3
SIMPLE CYSTS

PATIENT HISTORY

A 52-year-old female for screening breast MRI.

RADIOLOGY FINDINGS

Fig. 2.1 (**a**) Sagittal T2-weighted image demonstrates multiple round and oval circumscribed high-signal-intensity masses in the breast. (**b**) Sagittal subtracted T1-weighted image demonstrates no enhancement of the masses.

BI-RADS ASSESSMENT

BI-RADS 2. Benign findings.

DIAGNOSIS

Simple cysts

DISCUSSION

- Simple cysts are the most common breast masses seen on MRI.
- Simple cysts are of low signal intensity or equal to adjacent fibroglandular tissue on T1-weighted images and of high signal intensity on T2-weighted images.
- If there is protein content in the fluid, the cyst may be intermediate to high signal on T1-weighted images.
- There is no enhancement on postcontrast imaging.
- There may be thin, peripheral rim enhancement if the cysts are inflamed.

REFERENCES

Berg WA, Birdwell RL, Gombos EC, et al. Diagnostic imaging breast. 1st ed. Salt Lake City: Amirsys; 2006. p. 48–51. Section IV 1.
Morris EA, Liberman L, editors. Breast MRI diagnosis and intervention. New York: Springer; 2005. p. 147–52.

Fig. 2.1

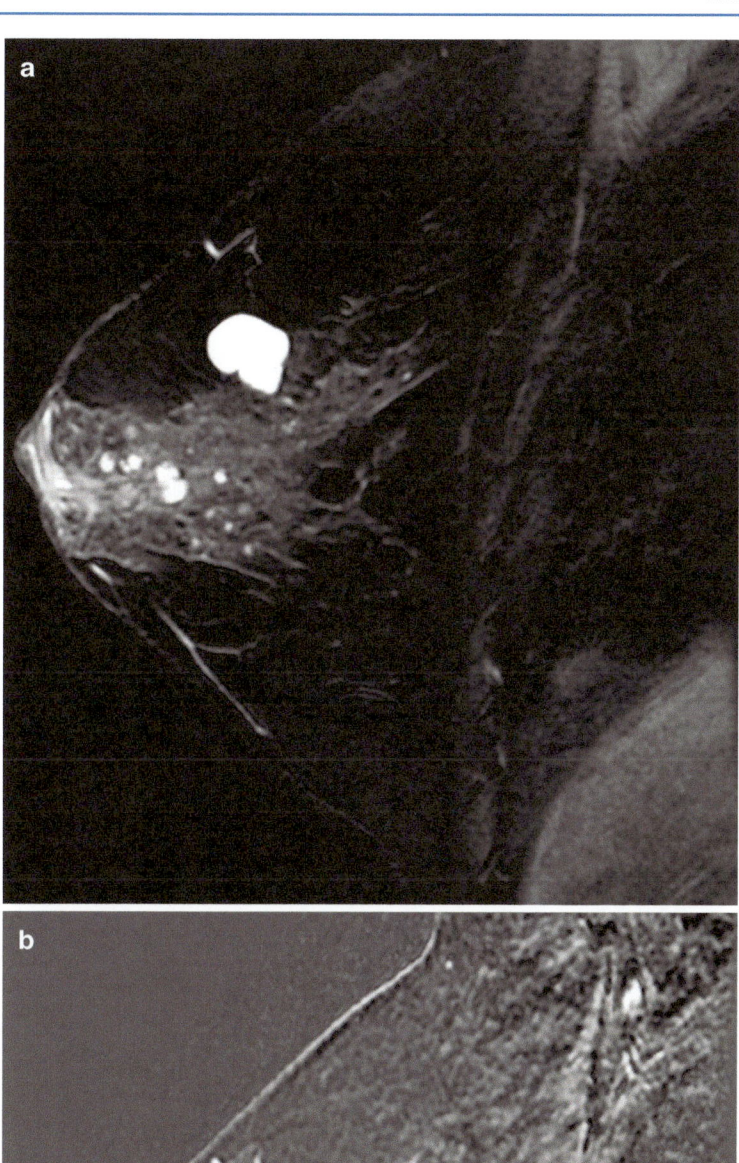

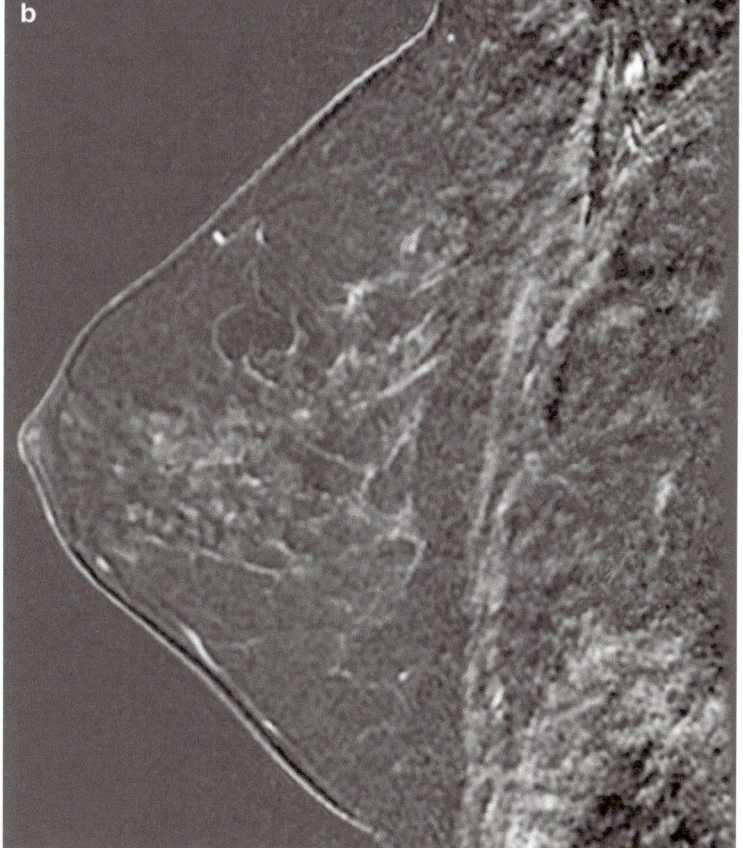

Case 4
Invasive Ductal Carcinoma (IDC) with Axillary Lymph Node Metastasis

Patient History

A 55-year-old female with a diagnosis of invasive ductal carcinoma. MRI for treatment planning.

Radiology Findings

Fig. 2.1 (**a**) Axial subtracted T1-weighted and (**b**) sagittal contrast-enhanced delayed T1-weighted images show an irregular spiculated rim-enhancing mass in the lower outer left breast at anterior depth.

Fig. 2.2 Sagittal T2-weighted image shows a low-signal spiculated mass in the lower left breast at anterior depth.

Fig. 2.3 Kinetic curve demonstrates washout kinetics (type III).

Fig. 2.4 (**a**) Axial subtracted T1-weighted and (**b**) sagittal contrast-enhanced delayed T1-weighted images show an enhancing oval mass with irregular margins in the upper outer left breast consistent with an enlarged lymph node.

BI-RADS Assessment

BI-RADS 6. Known biopsy-proven malignancy.

Diagnosis

Invasive ductal carcinoma (not otherwise specified) with axillary lymph node metastasis (IDC)

Discussion

- Eighty percent of breast cancers are ductal in origin.
- Up to 65 % of breast cancers diagnosed in the USA represent invasive ductal carcinoma, not otherwise specified.
- IDC most commonly presents as an enhancing mass (rim enhancement or irregular enhancement) with spiculated margins on MRI.
- Less commonly, IDC can be seen as non-mass-like enhancement or regional/diffuse enhancement on MRI.
- Most common kinetic curve with IDC is washout enhancement kinetics (type III).
- Secondary signs of malignancy such as skin thickening, nipple inversion, and lymphadenopathy can be seen on MRI.

References

Liberman L, Morris EA, Lee M, et al. Breast lesions detected on MR imaging: features and positive predictive value. AJR. 2002; 179:171–78.

Orel SG, Schnall MD. MR imaging of the breast for detection, diagnosis and staging of breast cancer. Radiology. 2001;220:13–30.

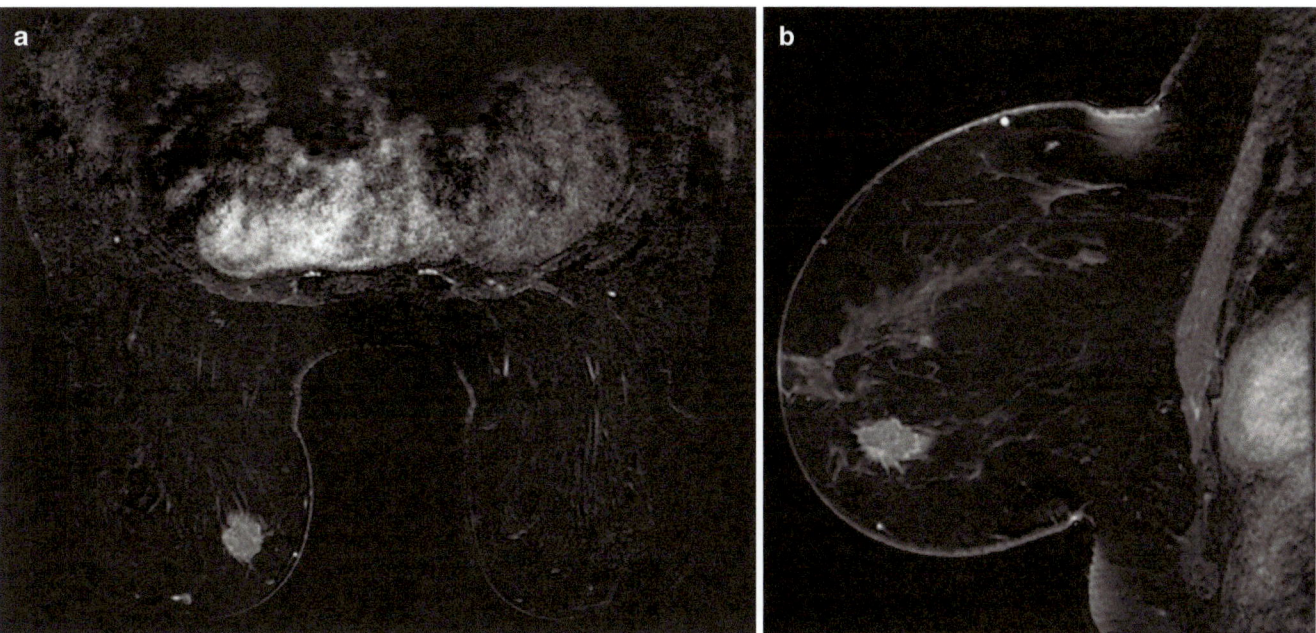

Fig. 2.1

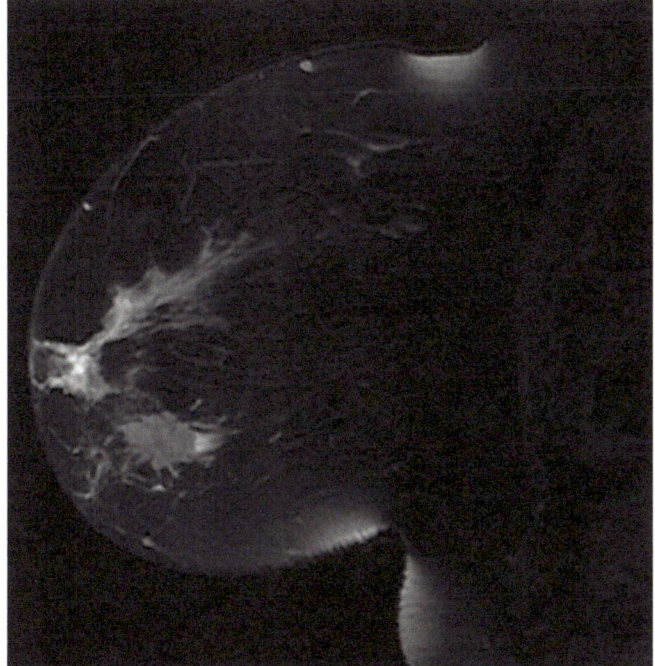

Fig. 2.2

Fig. 2.3

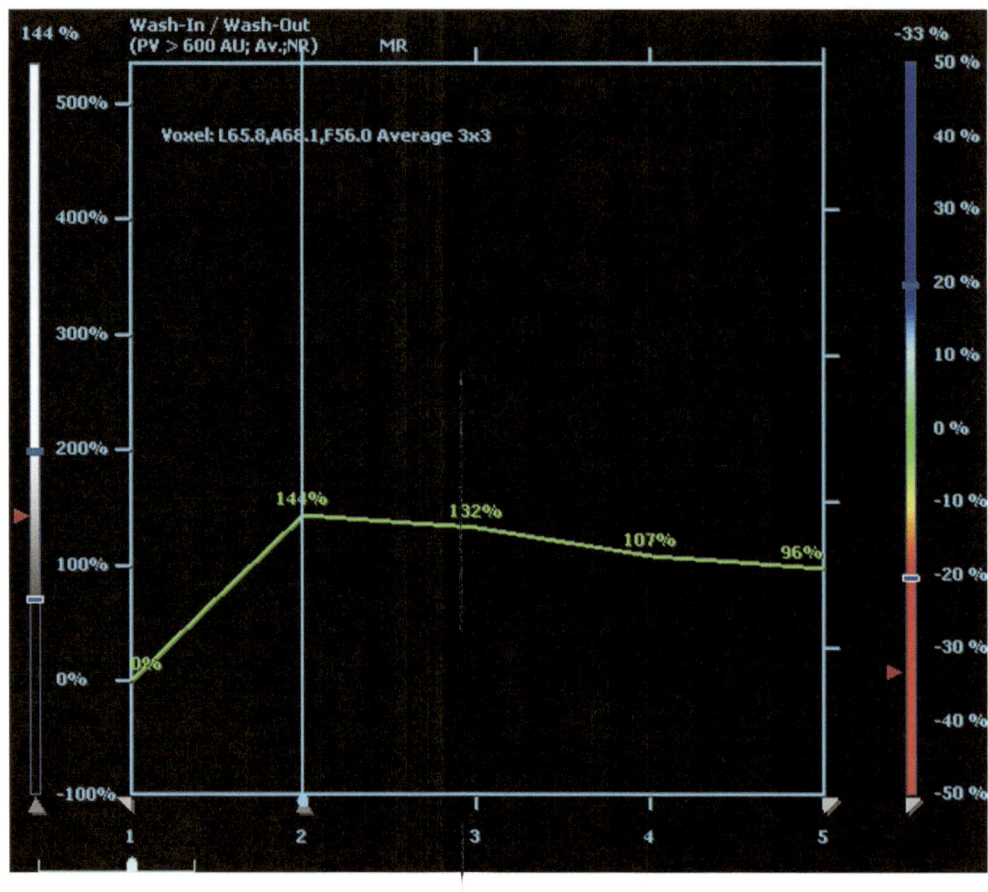

Fig. 2.4

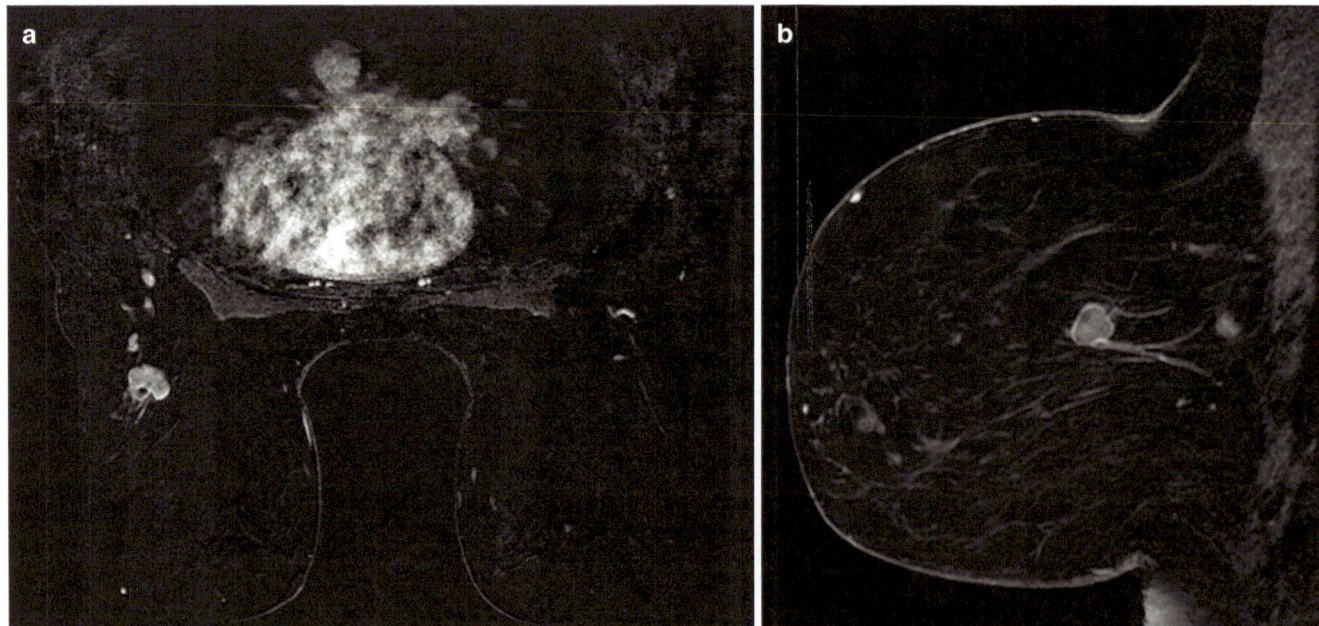

CASE 5
INTRACAPSULAR RUPTURE OF SILICONE BREAST IMPLANT

PATIENT HISTORY

A 55-year-old female for evaluation of implant rupture.

RADIOLOGY FINDINGS

Fig. 2.1 (**a**) Axial fast STIR water-suppressed T1-weighted and (**b**) sagittal fast STIR water-suppressed T1-weighted images show low-signal lines within a high-signal silicone implant in the right breast, referred to as the "linguine sign." The left breast silicone implant is intact.

Fig. 2.2 Axial fast STIR water-suppressed T1-weighted image from a different patient shows high signal trapped within a fold of the silicone implant in the right breast, referred to as the "inverted tear drop" or "keyhole sign".

BI-RADS ASSESSMENT

BI-RADS 2. Benign finding.

DIAGNOSIS

Intracapsular rupture of silicone breast implant

DISCUSSION

- Intracapsular rupture of a breast implant is defined as a disruption or tear of the implant shell in which silicone gel moves outside of the implant shell but stays within the fibrous capsule.

- Intracapsular rupture occurs more commonly than extracapsular rupture.
- MRI is highly sensitive and specific in diagnosing extracapsular and intracapsular implant rupture.
- The following continuum all represent signs of intracapsular rupture:
  - A gel leak can cause small amounts of silicone to leak out of the shell and become trapped within folds of the implant. This is often referred to as the "inverted tear drop sign," the "noose sign," or the "keyhole sign."
  - A "subcapsular line sign" is due to silicone leakage between the implant and fibrous capsule.
  - The "linguine sign" is caused by folding and collapsing of the implant shell on itself due to leakage of the silicone outside of the shell while the fibrous capsule remains intact. The low-signal lines of the implant shell are seen against the high-signal silicone.
- A rupture or tear of a saline implant is identified clinically, and therefore, imaging is not necessary to make the diagnosis.

REFERENCES

Deangelis GA, Lange EE, Miller LR, Morgan RF. MR imaging of breast implants. Radiographics. 1994;14:783–94.

Everson LI, Parantainen H, Detlie T, et al. Diagnosis of breast implant rupture: imaging findings and relative efficacies of imaging techniques. AJR. 1994;163:57–60.

Morris EA, Liberman L, editors. Breast MRI diagnosis and intervention. New York: Springer; 2005. p. 239–49.

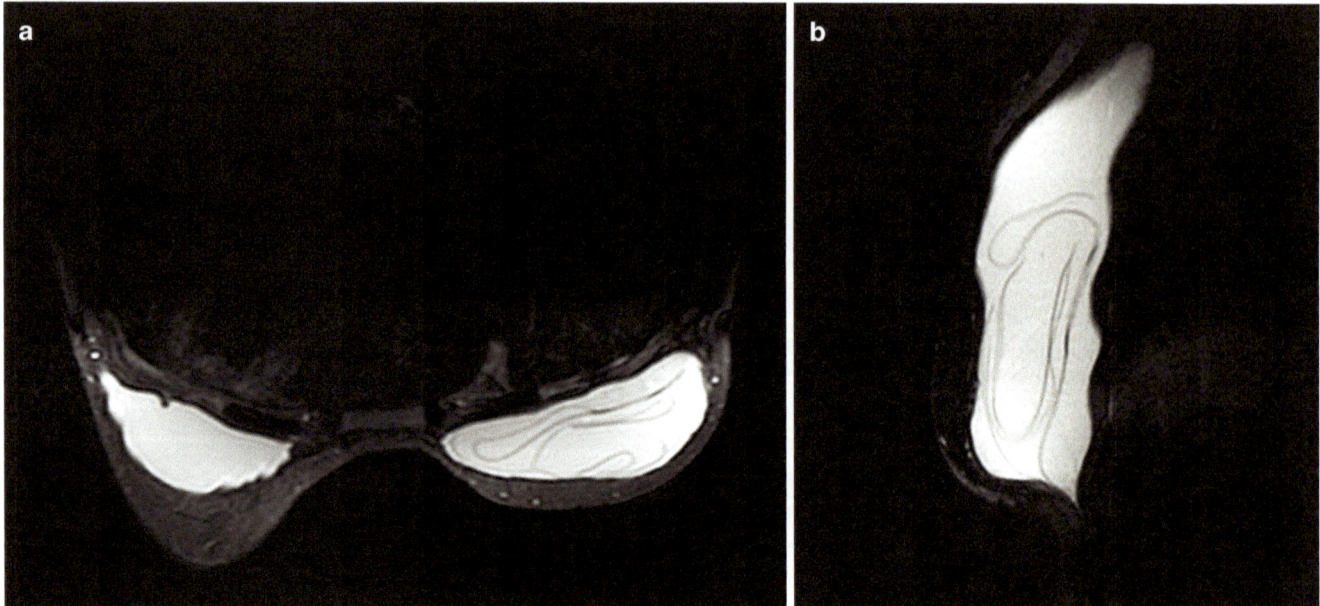

Fig. 2.1

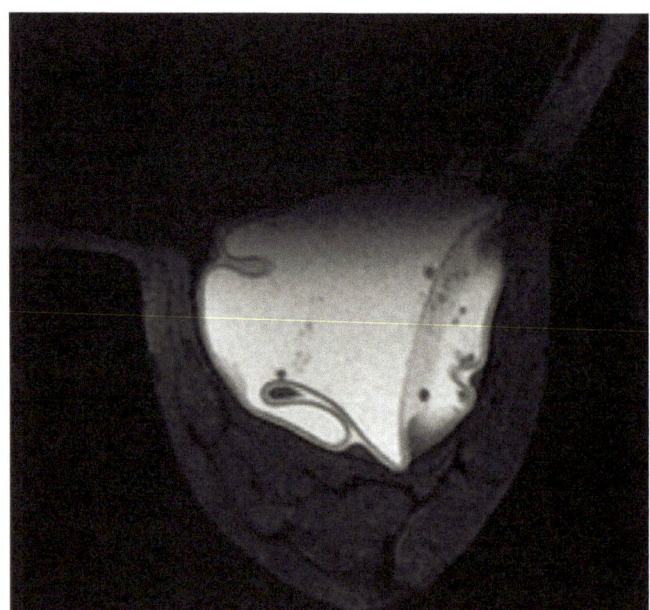

Fig. 2.2

CASE 6
EXTRACAPSULAR RUPTURE OF SILICONE BREAST IMPLANT

PATIENT HISTORY

A 55-year-old female for evaluation of implant rupture.

RADIOLOGY FINDINGS

Fig. 2.1 (**a**) Axial fast STIR water-suppressed T1-weighted and (**b–d**) sagittal fast STIR water-suppressed T1-weighted images show high signal adjacent to and outside the fibrous capsule.

BI-RADS ASSESSMENT

BI-RADS 2. Benign finding.

DIAGNOSIS

Extracapsular rupture of silicone breast implant

DISCUSSION

- Extracapsular rupture is defined as a rupture of the implant shell and fibrous capsule where the silicone occurs outside of the fibrous capsule. Silicone is seen in adjacent breast tissue.

- MRI is highly sensitive and specific in diagnosing extracapsular and intracapsular implant rupture.
- Extracapsular rupture is often caused by a strong external force such as trauma from a motor vehicle accident or closed capsulotomy (manual compression to break up a capsule causing pain).
- Migration of silicone from implant rupture can be seen within the adjacent breast tissue, intraductal, transdermal, and in the axillary lymph nodes.
- Extracapsular rupture on MRI (best seen on water-suppressed images) is seen as free silicone, which is outside of the implant shell and fibrous capsule.

REFERENCES

Caskey CI, Berg WA, Hamper UM, Sheth S, Chang BW, Anderson ND. Imaging spectrum of extracapsular silicone: correlation of ultrasound, MR imaging, mammographic and histopathologic findings. Radiographics. 1999;19:S39–51.

Everson LI, Parantainen H, Detlie T, et al. Diagnosis of breast implant rupture: imaging findings and relative efficacies of imaging techniques. AJR. 1994;163:57–60.

Morris EA, Liberman L, editors. Breast MRI diagnosis and intervention. New York: Springer; 2005. p. 239–49.

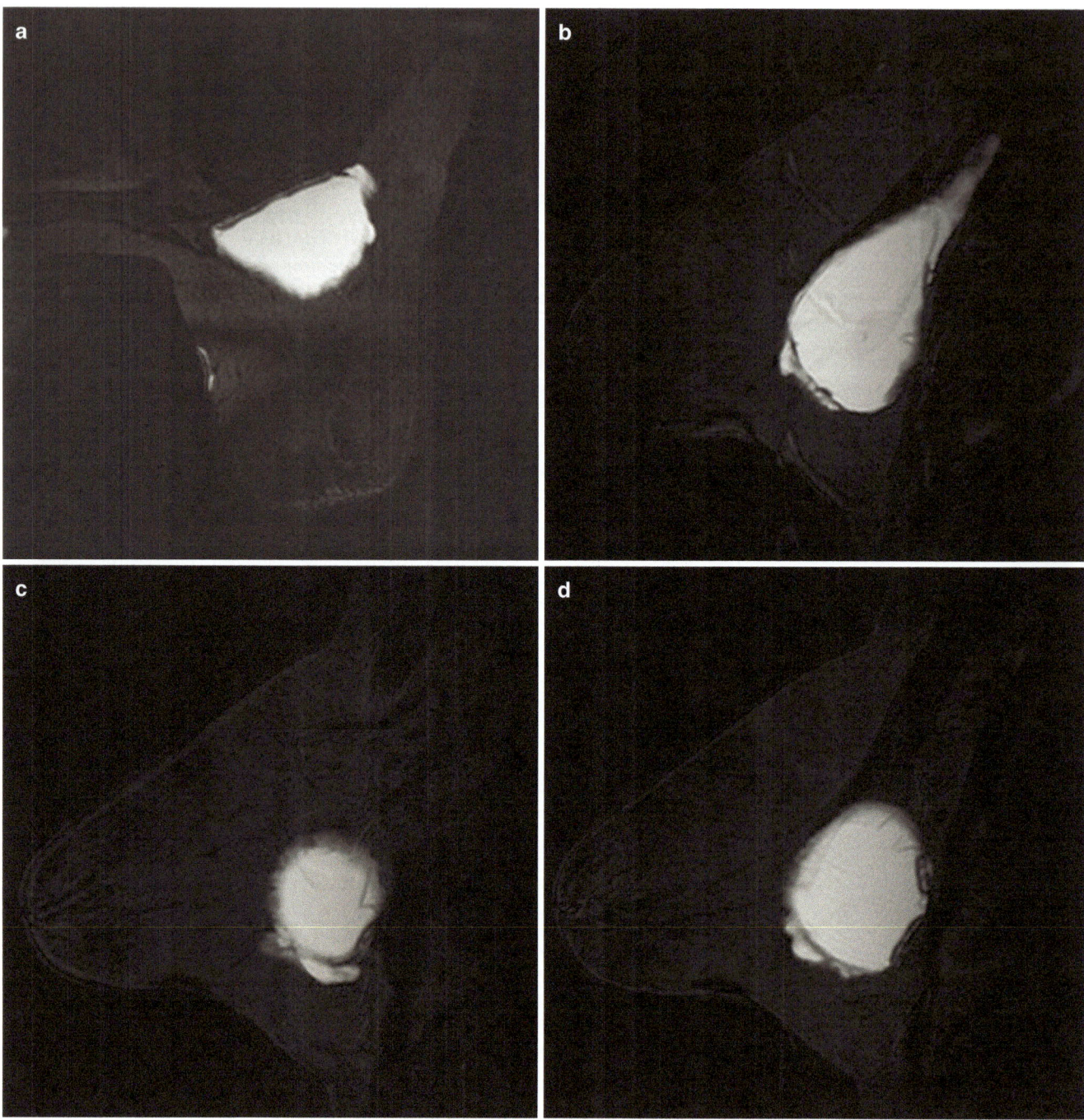

Fig. 2.1

CASE 7
FIBROADENOMA

PATIENT HISTORY

A 46-year-old female with a strong family history of breast cancer. BRCA1 gene carrier.

RADIOLOGY FINDINGS

Fig. 2.1 (**a**) Sagittal T1-weighted image demonstrates an oval low-signal-intensity mass in the upper breast at anterior depth. (**b**) Sagittal subtracted T1-weighted image demonstrates the mass in the upper breast to be homogeneously enhancing.

Fig. 2.2 Sagittal fat-suppressed T2-weighted image in a different patient demonstrates a mass in the retroareolar plane at middle depth to be high signal relative to adjacent tissue. A cyst is seen in the lower breast.

Fig. 2.3 Kinetic curve demonstrates plateau enhancement (type II).

BI-RADS ASSESSMENT

BI-RADS 2. Benign finding (following diagnostic workup and biopsy).

DIAGNOSIS

Fibroadenoma

DISCUSSION

- Most common benign breast mass.
- More common in young women.
- Fibroadenomas contain epithelial and stromal elements.
- In younger women, fibroadenomas contain greater amount of epithelial elements than stromal elements. In postmenopausal women, fibroadenomas contain greater amount of stromal elements.
- Signal intensity and contrast enhancement depend on fluid content in the mass.
- Fibroadenomas are of low signal on T1-weighted images.
- Myxoid fibroadenomas are high signal on T2-weighted images and have homogeneous enhancement.
- As the fibroadenomas become less cellular and more sclerotic, enhancement decreases.
- Nonenhancing internal septations are diagnostic of fibroadenomas.
- Kinetic curve is persistent or plateau.

REFERENCES

Hochman MG, Orel SG, Powell CM, Schnall MD, Reynolds CA, White LN. Fibroadenomas: variety of MR appearances with radiologic – histopathologic correlation. Radiology. 1997;204:123–29.

Morris EA, Liberman L, editors. Breast MRI Diagnosis and Intervention. New York: Springer; 2005. p. 141.

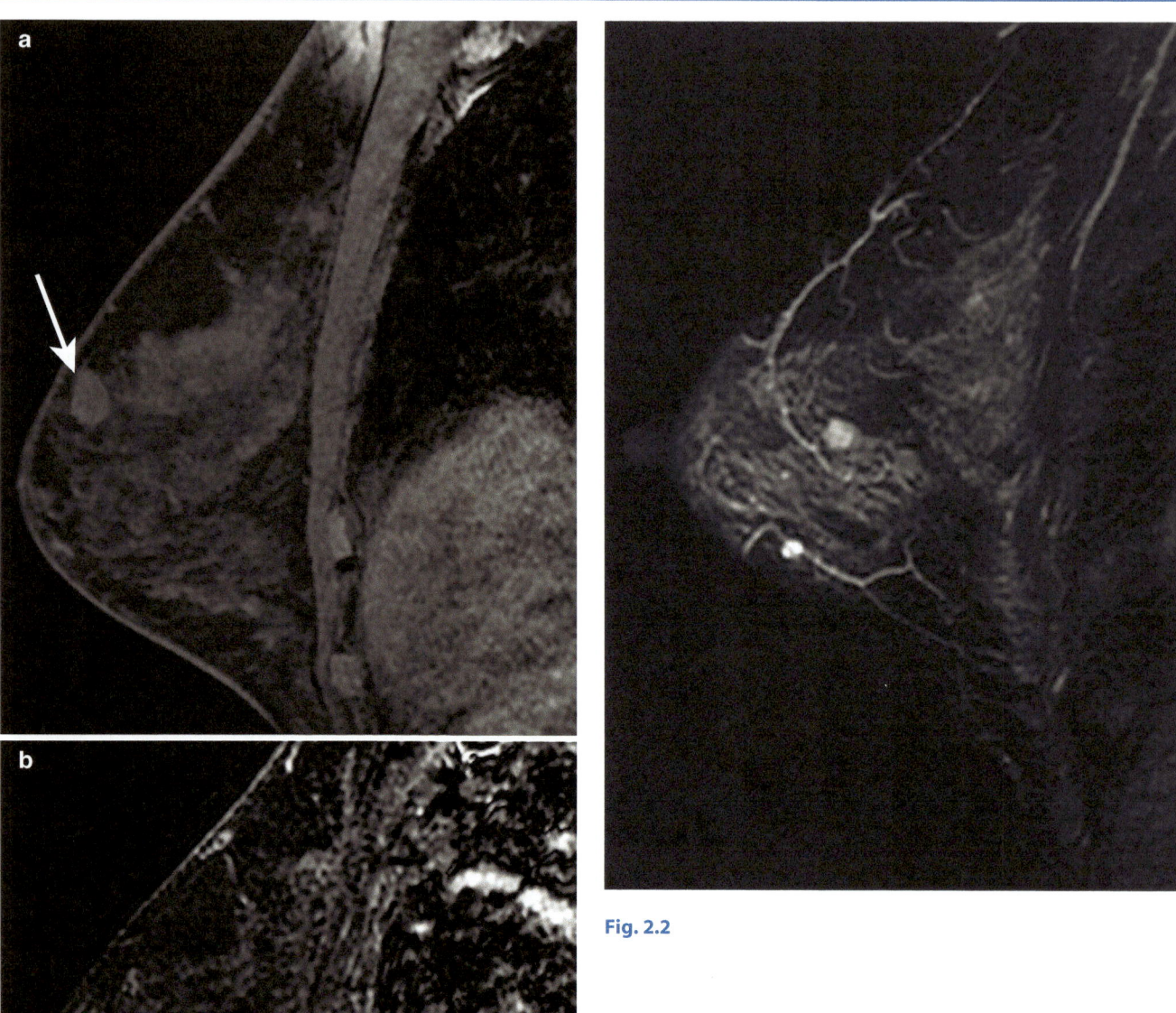

Fig. 2.2

Fig. 2.1

Fig. 2.3

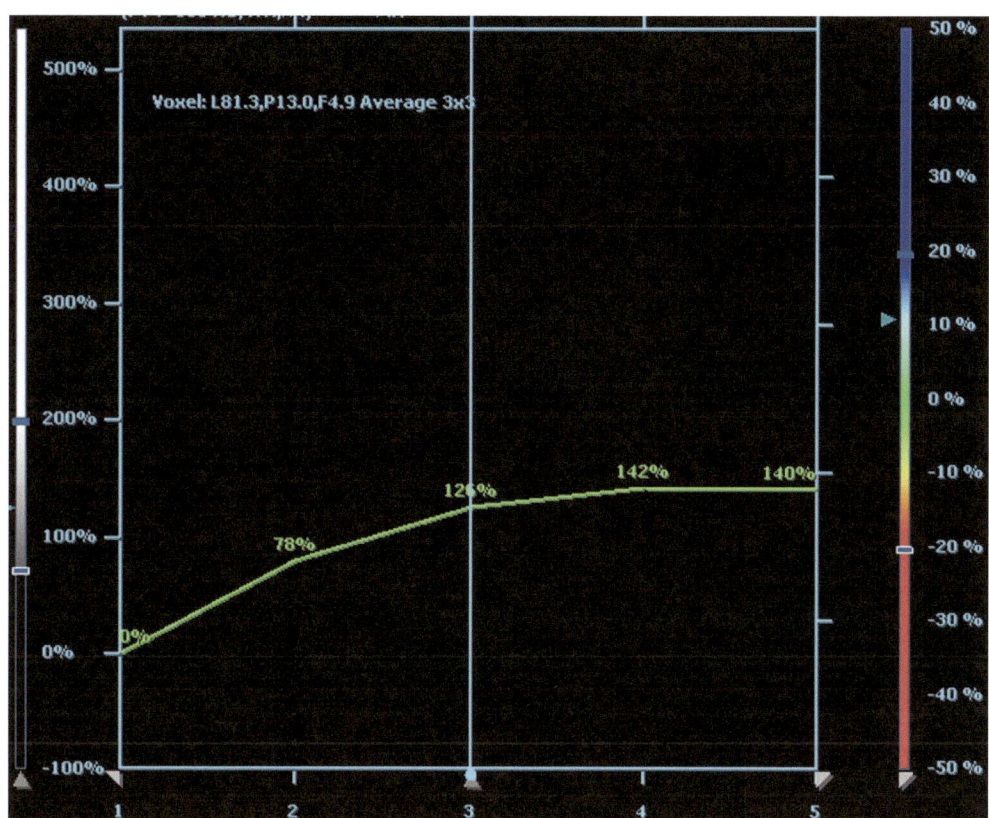

Case 8
Inflammatory Breast Carcinoma (IBC)

Patient History

A 35-year-old female with diagnosis of inflammatory breast carcinoma. MRI for treatment planning.

Radiology Findings

Fig. 2.1 Axial (**a**) contrast-enhanced delayed T1-weighted and (**b**) sagittal subtracted T1-weighted images show non-mass-like enhancement extending from the nipple to the central right breast in the retroareolar plane. There is abnormal enhancement of the nipple and skin.
Fig. 2.2 Axial nonfat-suppressed T1-weighted image shows low signal in the skin and extending from the nipple to the central right breast in the retroareolar plane.
Fig. 2.3 Sagittal T2-weighted image shows high signal in the skin and the retroareolar breast.

BI-RADS Assessment

BI-RADS 6. Known biopsy-proven malignancy.

Diagnosis

Inflammatory breast carcinoma (IBC)

Discussion

- Inflammatory breast carcinoma accounts for 1–4 % of breast cancers, with the average age of onset between 45 and 54 years of age.

- The pathologic feature that defines IBC is dermal lymphatic invasion, which is a diagnosis made by performing a skin-punch biopsy.
- IBC is an aggressive malignancy, which tends to metastasize at an early stage, with the median survival duration of 12–36 months.
- Clinically, can see skin edema (peau d'orange), skin erythema, palpable mass, breast enlargement, nipple retraction, and breast pain.
- IBC can be seen as an enhancing mass, multiple enhancing masses with irregular margins, or non-mass-like enhancement on MRI.
- Associated findings of IBC seen on MRI include the following:
  – Skin thickening with enhancement
  – Axillary and internal mammary lymphadenopathy
  – Nipple and pectoralis muscle invasion

References

Bilgren-Gunhan I, Ustun EE, Memis A. Inflammatory breast carcinoma: mammographic, sonographic, clinical and pathologic findings in 142 cases. Radiology. 2002;223:829–38.
Macura KJ, Ouwerkerk R, Jacobs MA, Bluemke DA. Patterns of enhancement on breast MR images: interpretation and imaging pitfalls. Radiographics. 2006;26:1719–34.
Yang WT, Le-Petross HT, Macapinlac H, et al. Inflammatory breast cancer: PET/CT, MRI, mammographic and sonographic findings. Breast Cancer Res Treat. 2008;109:417–26.

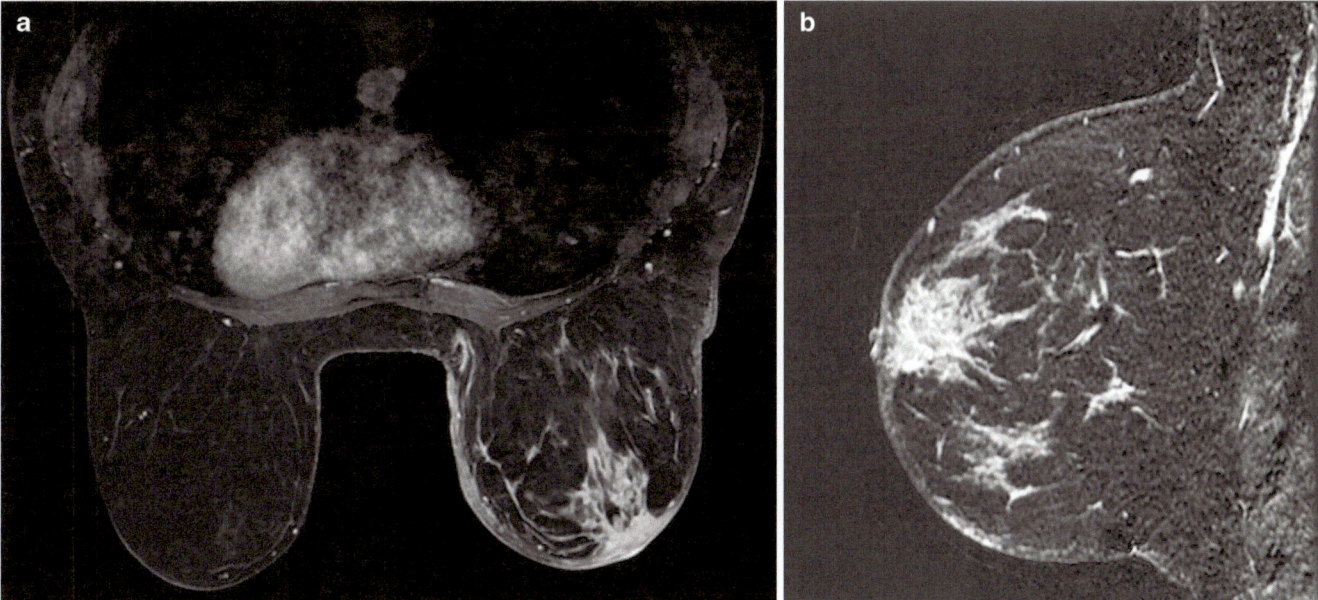

Fig. 2.1

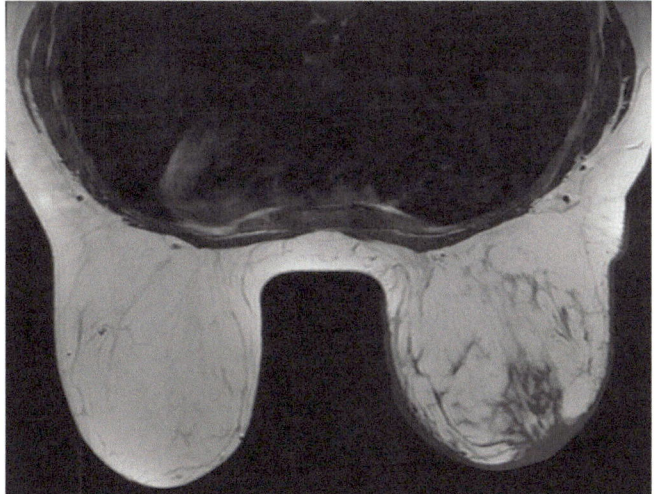

Fig. 2.2

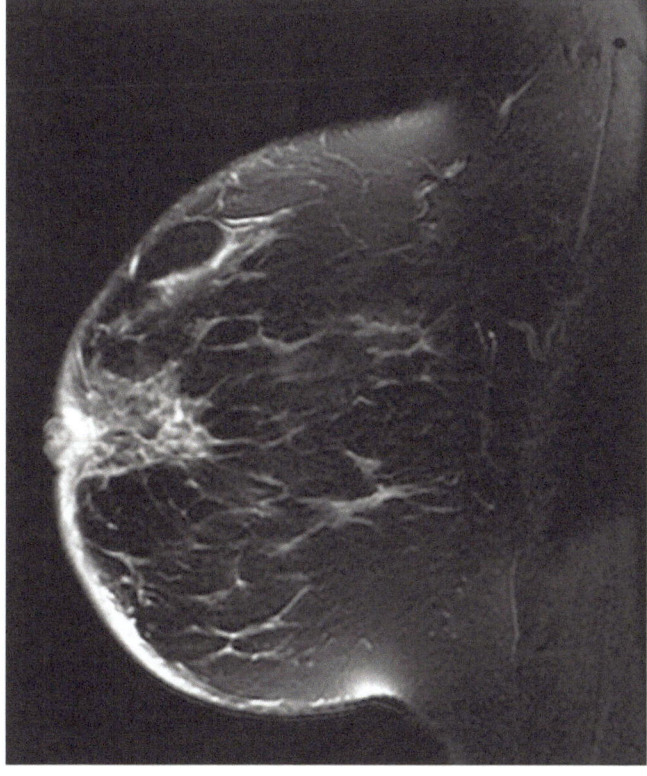

Fig. 2.3

CASE 9
PAPILLOMA

PATIENT HISTORY

A 45-year-old female with lifetime risk of breast cancer >20 %. Screening breast MRI.

RADIOLOGY FINDINGS

Fig. 2.1 Axial subtracted T1-weighted image demonstrates an enhancing mass with circumscribed margins in the retroareolar plane at middle depth. There is an adjacent enhancing tubular structure representing a dilated duct.
Fig. 2.2 Kinetic curve demonstrates plateau enhancement (type II) of the mass.
Fig. 2.3 Axial subtracted T1-weighted image in a different patient demonstrates an enhancing oval mass with circumscribed margins in the retroareolar plane at a middle depth.

BI-RADS ASSESSMENT

High-risk lesion.

DIAGNOSIS

Papilloma

DISCUSSION

- Papillomas seen on MRI tend to be associated with dilated ducts.
- Papillomas and associated dilated ducts are of low signal intensity on noncontrast T1-weighted images unless the duct fluid has increased protein or hemorrhage.
- On postcontrast T1-weighted images, papillomas enhance uniformly unless there are areas of sclerosis.
- Papillomas tend to be mammographically occult.
- May be solitary or multiple.
- Solitary papillomas are mostly central in location in a major duct.
- Multiple papillomas are mostly peripheral and can be bilateral.
- They arise from a terminal ductal lobular unit.
- When diagnosed by core needle biopsy, excision is generally recommended due to potential of upgrade to high-risk lesion or malignancy.

REFERENCES

Morris EA, Liberman L, editors. Breast MRI diagnosis and intervention. New York: Springer; 2005. p. 141–47.
Rovno HD, Siegelman ES, Reynolds C, Orell HG, Schnall MD. Solitary intraductal papilloma: findings at MR imaging and MR galactography. AJR. 1999;172:151–5.

Fig. 2.1

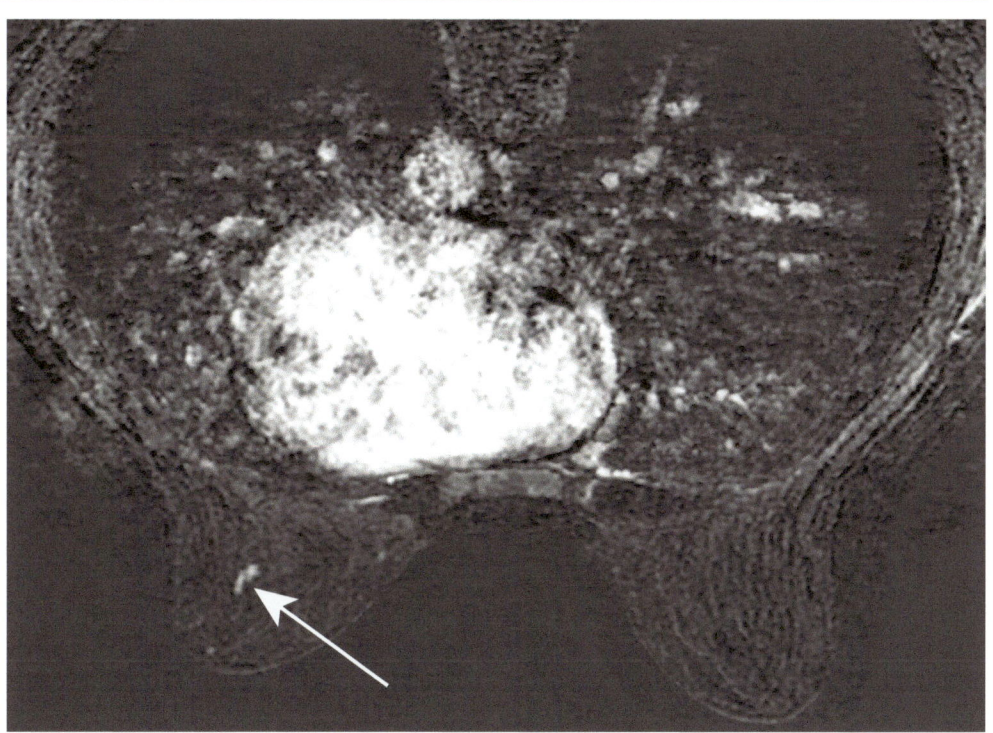

Fig. 2.2

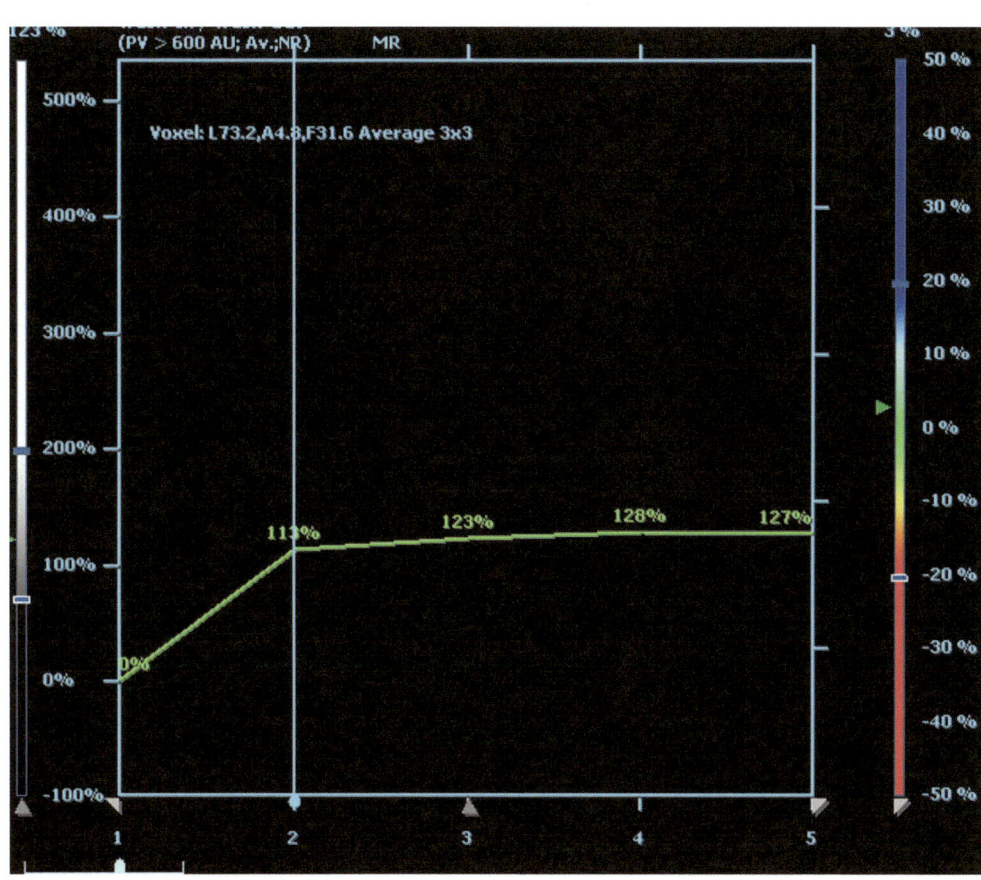

Fig. 2.3

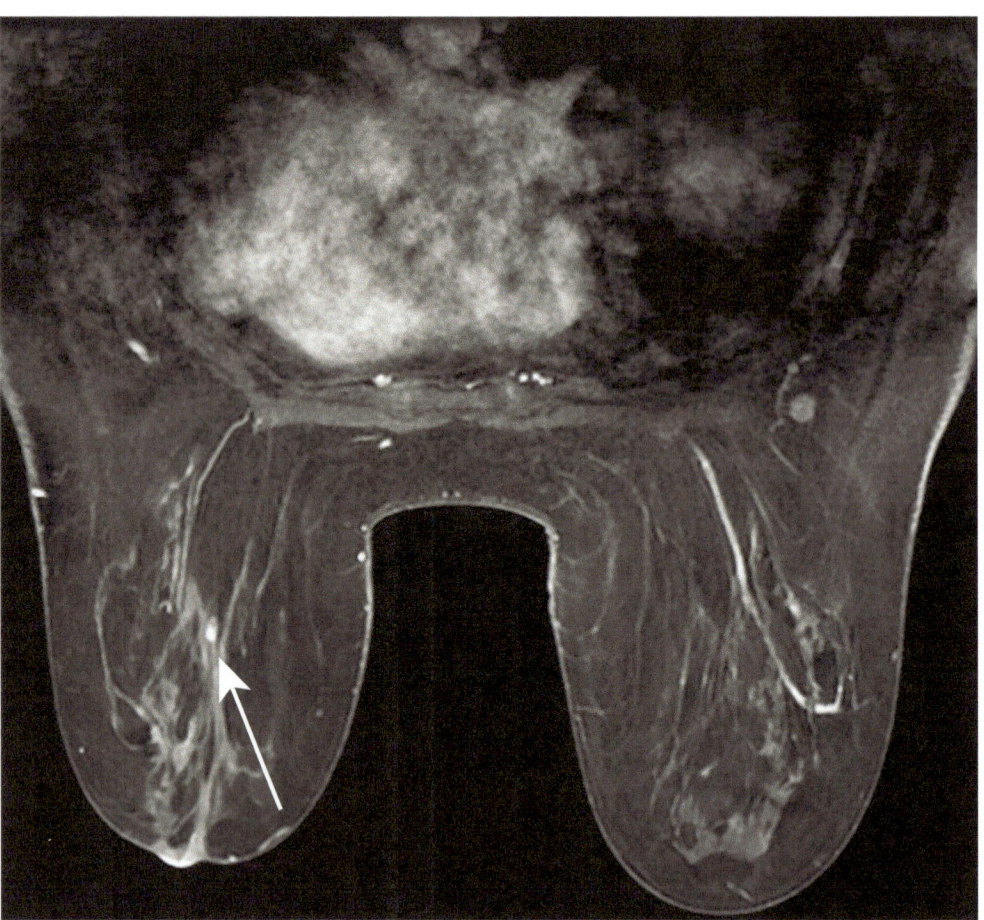

CASE 10
RECURRENCE AFTER MASTECTOMY

PATIENT HISTORY

A 54-year-old female with history of bilateral mastectomies and reconstruction with implants for breast MRI.

RADIOLOGY FINDINGS

Fig. 2.1 Sagittal T1-weighted image demonstrates an irregular high-signal-intensity mass in the upper breast adjacent to the capsule.

Fig. 2.2 Sagittal contrast-enhanced T1-weighted image demonstrates a heterogeneously enhancing mass in the upper breast. Kinetic curve (not shown) demonstrates plateau enhancement (type II).

BI-RADS ASSESSMENT

BI-RADS 4. Suspicious abnormality (following diagnostic workup, prior to biopsy).

DIAGNOSIS

Recurrence after mastectomy

DISCUSSION

- Recurrent breast carcinoma is defined as invasive or noninvasive cancer in a breast that has been treated for a prior cancer.

- Even though cancer recurrence rate in the postmastectomy breast is low because of the theoretical removal of all breast tissue, residual glandular breast tissue can remain after mastectomy with or without breast reconstruction.
- Cancer recurrence can occur within regional lymph nodes or within the reconstructed breast, with reported rates in the literature of between 5 and 15 %.
- Recurrence after mastectomy is usually always detected clinically.
- The purpose of breast MRI in mastectomy patients is to evaluate the chest wall in specific cases in which there is concern of chest wall recurrence.
- MRI is helpful in differentiating between tumor recurrence versus fat necrosis.
- Women who are BRCA gene carriers have a similar rate of recurrence when compared with normal-risk women.
- Postmastectomy recurrence is treated with radiation therapy.

REFERENCES

Berg WA, Birdwell RL, Gombos EC, et al. Diagnostic imaging breast. 1st ed. Salt Lake City: Amirsys; 2006. p. 54–7. Section IV.
Molleran VM, Mahoney M. Breast MRI. 1st ed. Philadelphia: Saunders; 2014. p. 132–3.

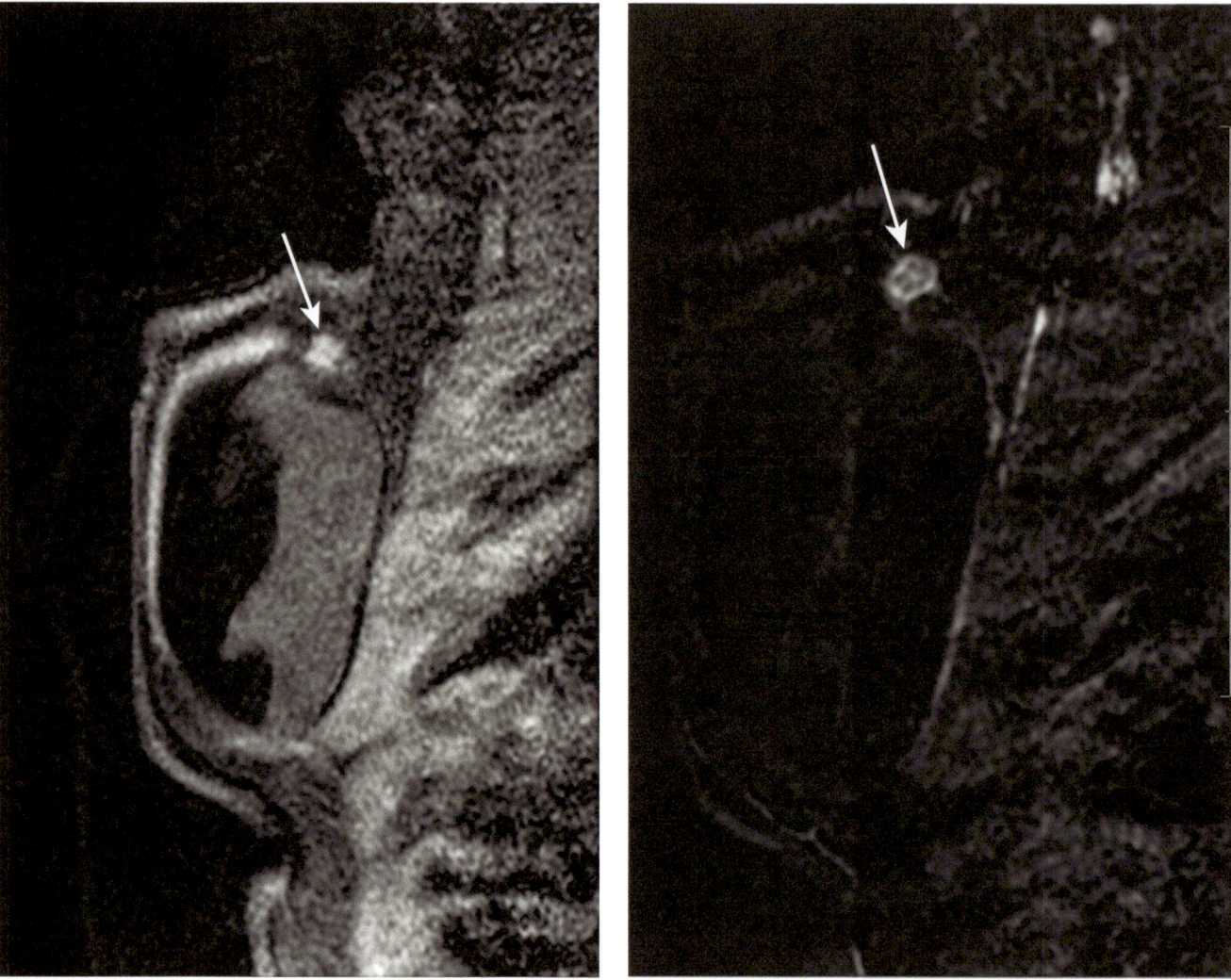

Fig. 2.1   Fig. 2.2

CASE 11
INVASIVE LOBULAR CARCINOMA (ILC) WITH AXILLARY LYMPH NODE METASTASIS

PATIENT HISTORY

A 50-year-old female with recent diagnosis of left invasive lobular carcinoma. MRI for treatment planning.

RADIOLOGY FINDINGS

Fig. 2.1 Axial (**a**) contrast-enhanced T1-weighted and (**b**) subtracted T1-weighted images show two adjacent heterogeneously enhancing irregular masses with spiculated margins in the left breast at middle depth.
Fig. 2.2 Sagittal contrast-enhanced delayed T1-weighted image demonstrates the larger of the two heterogeneously enhancing masses in the upper left breast at middle depth.
Fig. 2.3 Axial subtracted T1-weighted image shows an enlarged enhancing lymph node in the left axilla.

BI-RADS ASSESSMENT

BI-RADS 6. Known biopsy-proven malignancy.

DIAGNOSIS

Invasive lobular carcinoma (ILC) with axillary lymph node metastasis

DISCUSSION

- ILC accounts for 10–15 % of all invasive breast cancers, being the second most common breast cancer.
- Presentations of ILC on MRI include the following:
  - Ill-defined mass with spiculated margins
  - Enhancing architectural distortion
  - Single mass with surrounding multiple enhancing foci
  - Enhancing foci with interconnecting strands or regional or focal heterogeneous enhancement
  - No imaging findings (negative MRI)
- Unlike other invasive breast cancers that demonstrate rapid enhancement and washout, ILC has a tendency to demonstrate delayed maximal enhancement. Only the minority of ILC exhibit washout kinetics.

REFERENCES

Lopez JK, Bassett LW. ILC of the breast: spectrum of mammography, US and MRI imaging findings. Radiographics. 2009;29:165–76.
Qayyum A, Birdwell RL, Daniel BL. MRI imaging features of infiltrating lobular carcinoma of the breast: histopathologic correlation. AJR. 2002;178:1227–32.

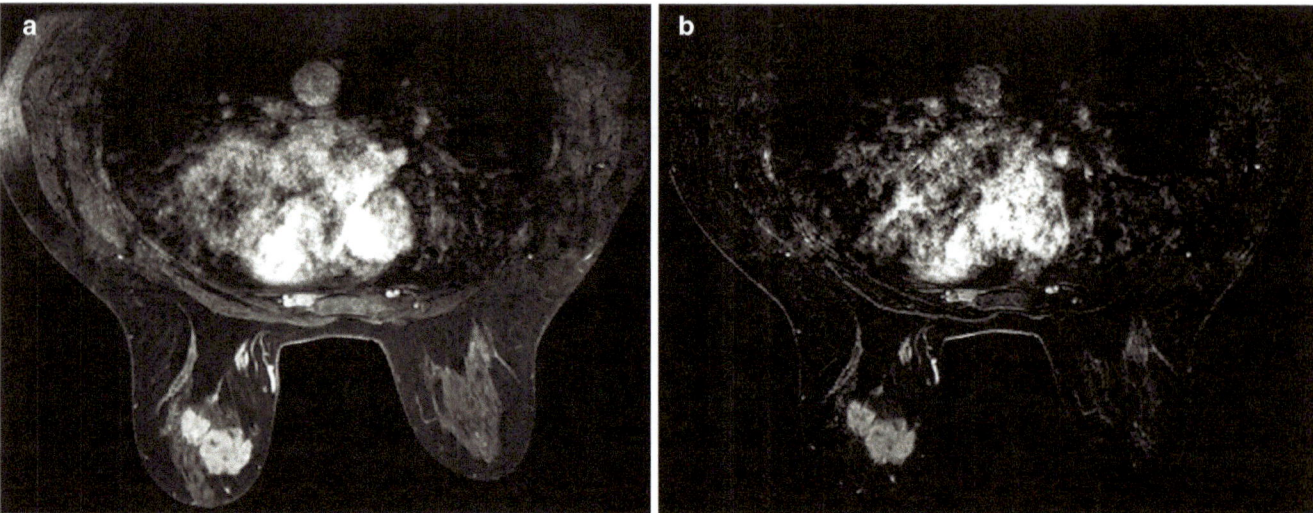

Fig. 2.1

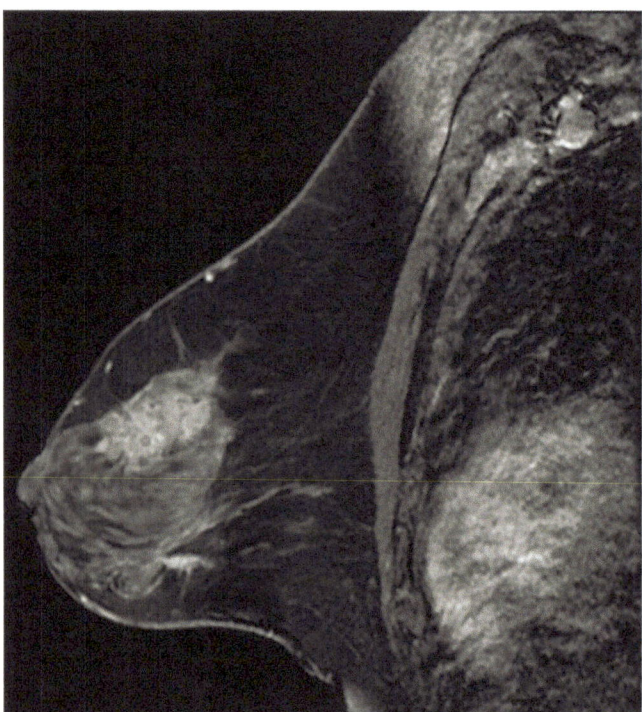

Fig. 2.2

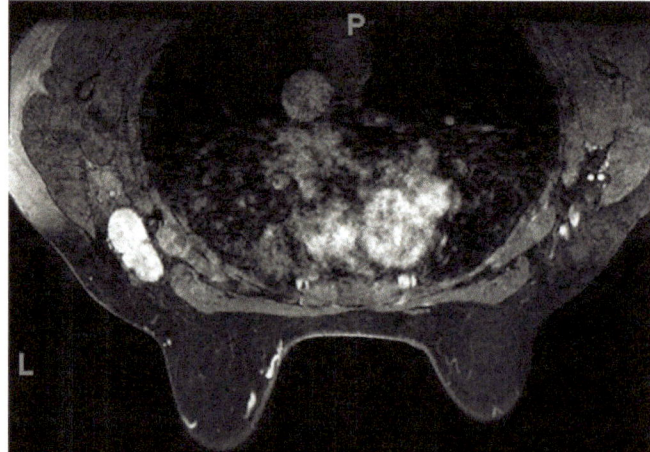

Fig. 2.3

CASE 12
BREAST CANCER WITH INVOLVEMENT OF THE PECTORALIS MUSCLE

PATIENT HISTORY

A 64-year-old female with a recent diagnosis of invasive lobular carcinoma of the right breast. MRI for treatment planning.

RADIOLOGY FINDINGS

Fig. 2.1 Axial (**a**, **b**) subtracted T1-weighted images show enhancement and thickening of the right pectoralis muscle.

BI-RADS ASSESSMENT

BI-RADS 6. Known biopsy-proven malignancy.

DIAGNOSIS

Breast cancer with involvement of the pectoralis muscle

DISCUSSION

- The definition of chest wall invasion by breast cancer is tumor infiltrating the ribs, intercostal muscles, and/or serratus anterior muscle.

- Tumor with chest wall invasion are classified as T4a, regardless of size. This results in a minimum TNM classification of at least IIIb disease.
- Mammography and ultrasound is usually limited in making a diagnosis of muscle or chest wall invasion.
- MRI is often used preoperatively to stage the extent of a recently biopsy-proven cancer, especially for patients considering breast conservation therapy.
- Enhancement of the pectoralis major muscle greater than normal physiologic enhancement is suggestive of pectoralis involvement of tumor.
- Loss of the fat planes or close proximity between the tumor and the pectoralis muscle are not reliable indicators of invasion.
- Tumors that invade the chest wall are typically preoperatively treated with chemotherapy and/or chest wall radiation, followed by more extensive surgery, including chest wall resection.
- When a tumor superficially invades the pectoralis muscle, a portion of the muscle may be resected, or when deep muscle invasive is present, a radical mastectomy with removal of the entire muscle may be required.

REFERENCES

Mandell J. Core radiology: a visual approach to diagnostic imaging. 1st ed. Cambridge: Cambridge University Press; 2013. p. 645.

Molleran VM, Mahoney M. Breast MRI. 1st ed. Philadelphia: Saunders; 2014. p. 108–9.

Morris EA, Schwartz LH, Drotman MB, et al. Evaluation of pectoralis major muscle in patients with posterior breast tumors on breast MR images: early experience. Radiology. 2000;214(1):67–72.

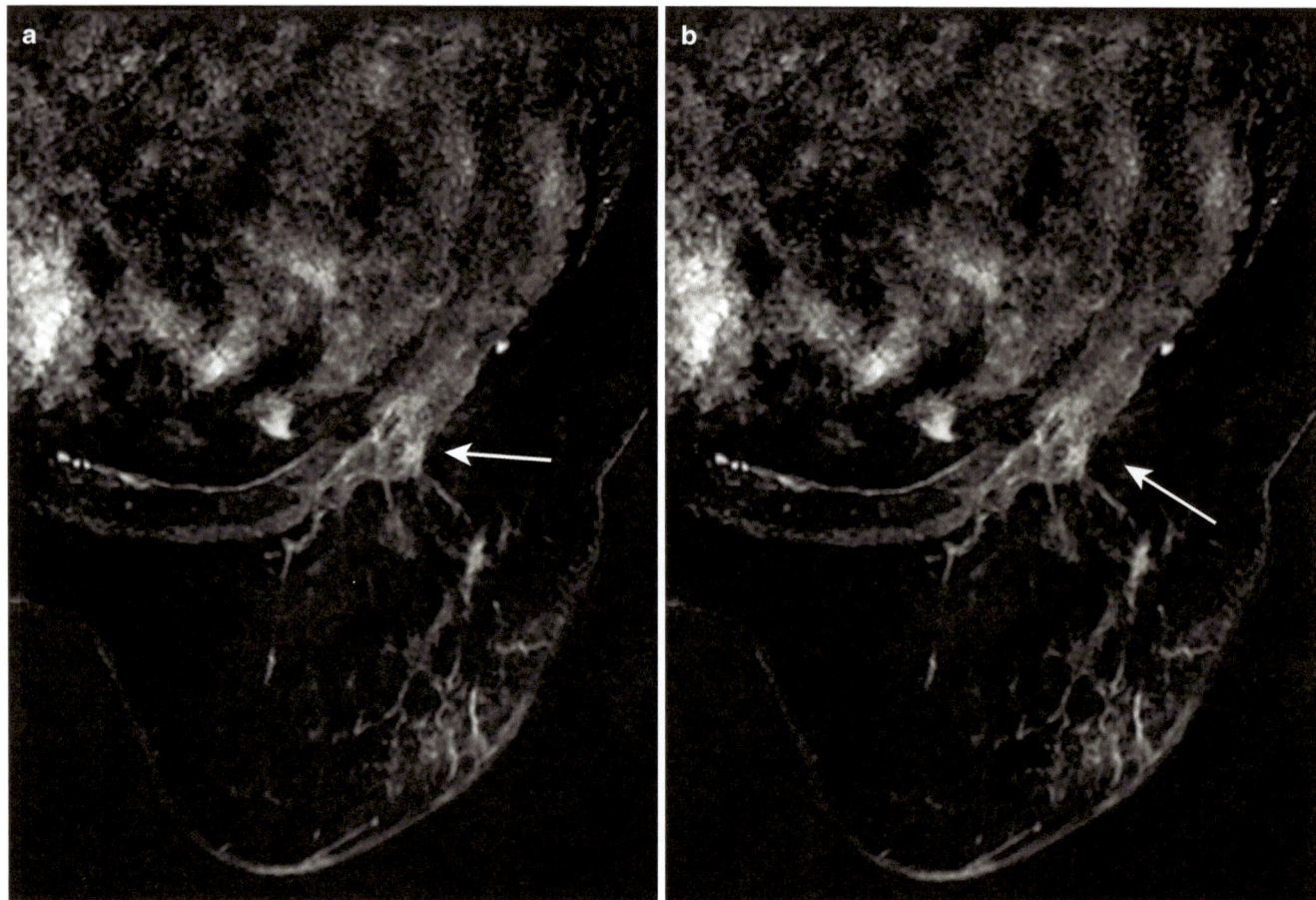

Fig. 2.1

CASE 13
DUCTAL CARCINOMA IN SITU, LOW GRADE (DCIS)

PATIENT HISTORY

A 73-year-old female with a diagnosis of left breast invasive ductal carcinoma. MRI for treatment planning.

RADIOLOGY FINDINGS

Fig. 2.1 Axial (**a**) contrast-enhanced and (**b**) subtracted T1-weighted images show clumped enhancement extending from the nipple to the middle depth of the right breast. Enhancing mass with irregular margins in the outer posterior left breast represents a biopsy-proven invasive ductal carcinoma.

Fig. 2.2 Sagittal T2-weighted image shows high signal in a ductal distribution extending from the nipple to the middle depth of the right breast.

Fig. 2.3 Sagittal contrast-enhanced delayed T1-weighted image shows clumped enhancement extending from the nipple to the middle depth of the right breast.

BI-RADS ASSESSMENT

BI-RADS 4. Suspicious abnormality (following diagnostic workup, prior to biopsy).

DIAGNOSIS

Ductal carcinoma in situ, low grade (DCIS)

DISCUSSION

- DCIS is a malignancy confined to the ducts of the breast.
- Preinvasive form of cancer.
- DCIS is responsible for up to 33 % of detected breast cancers, and 30–50 % of DCIS will progress to invasive cancer.
- Ninety percent of DCIS presents as calcifications on mammography.
- On MRI, DCIS is most commonly seen as clumped non-mass-like enhancement in a focal ductal, linear, segmental, or regional distribution.
- MRI allows for a more accurate assessment of the extent of the disease, which improves the treatment and prognosis.

REFERENCES

Morris EA, Liberman L, editors. Breast MRI diagnosis and intervention. New York: Springer; 2005. p. 164–66.

Raza S, Vallejo M, Chikarmane SA, Birdwell RL. Pure ductal carcinoma in situ: a range of MRI features. AJR. 2008;191:689–99.

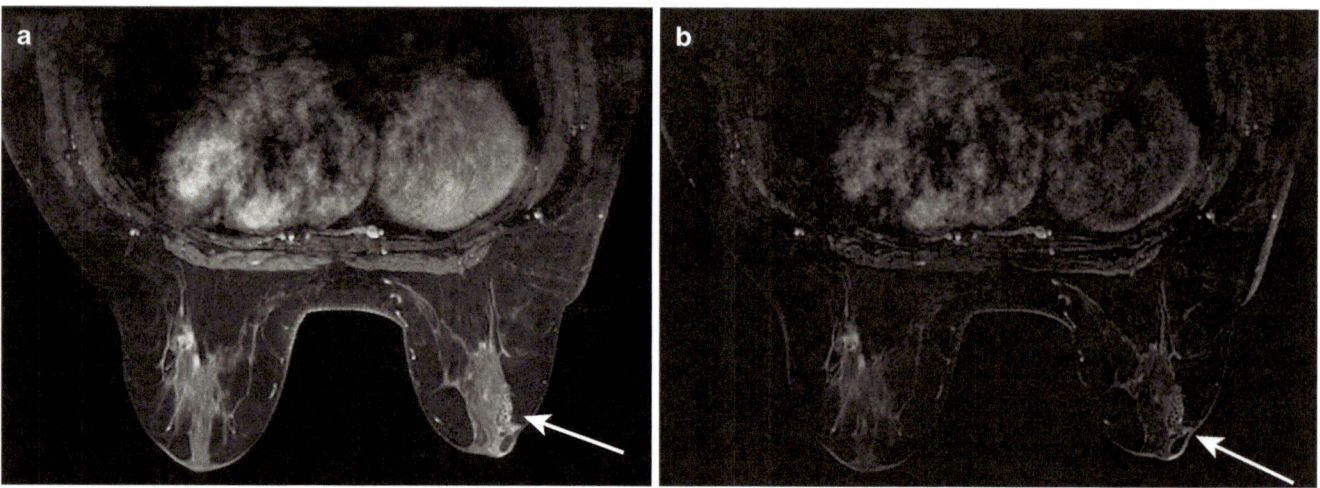

Fig. 2.1

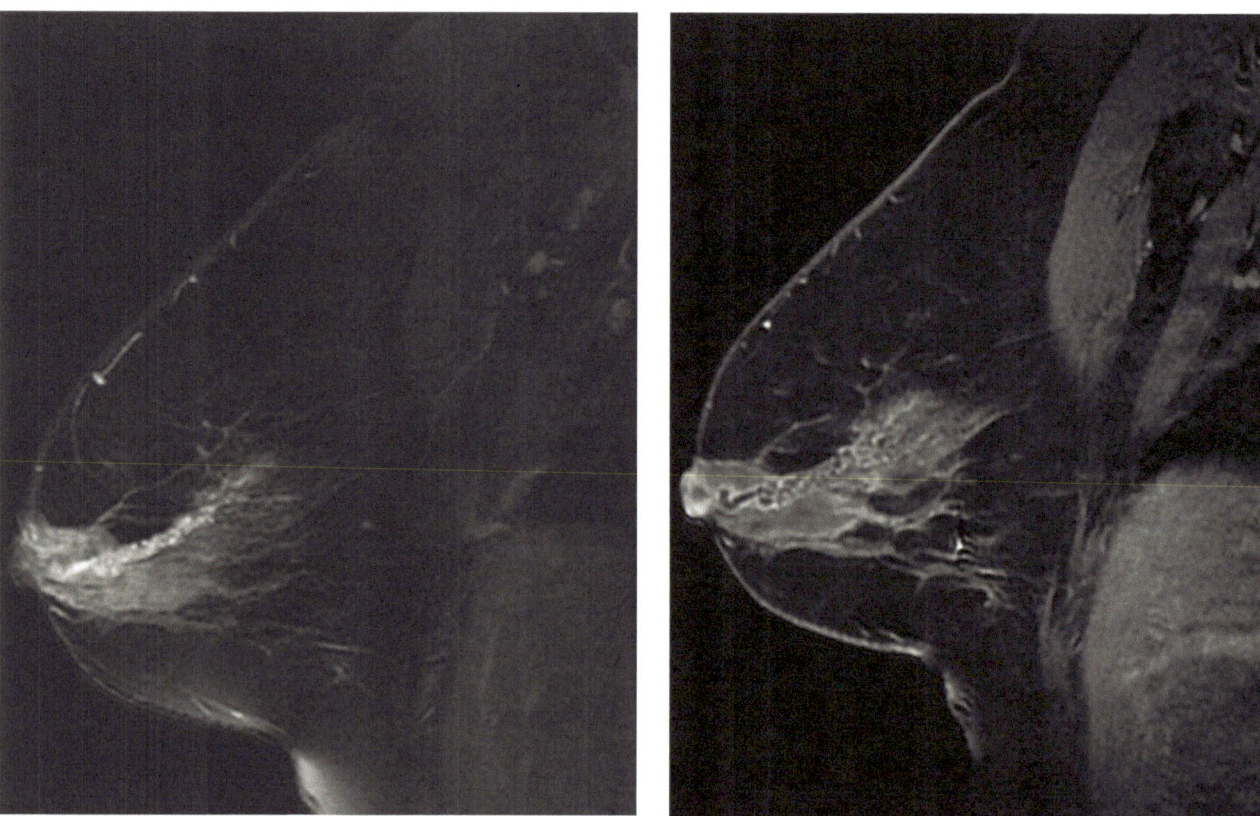

Fig. 2.2

Fig. 2.3

Appendix 1: Interventional Breast Procedures

MRI-Guided Wire Localization

Indication

BI-RADS 4 or 5 lesions detected only on MRI.

Procedure Steps
- Review prior MRI images.
- Obtain informed consent.
- Place the patient in the prone position in a dedicated breast coil within the magnet.
- Breast is placed in biopsy compression device (with a grid).
- Fiducial marker placed on skin at a slight distance from the expected lesion location (so fiducial marker does not obscure the lesion).
- Axial localizing sequence is obtained.
- Noncontrast sagittal T1-weighted sequence is obtained.
- Gadopentetate dimeglumine, 0.1 mmol/L/kg body weight, is injected intravenously as a rapid bolus.
- Immediately following contrast administration, sagittal fat-suppressed T1-weighted sequence is obtained.
- Images are reviewed.
- A cursor is placed over the lesion and X (horizontal) and Y (vertical) coordinates are determined based on the location of the fiducial marker and grid lines.
- Z (depth) coordinate is determined based on the depth from the skin surface.
- Depth in millimeters is calculated by multiplying the number of sagittal slices from the skin to the lesion and the slice thickness.
- No. of slices × slice thickness (in mm)
- Skin is cleansed and a local anesthetic is administered to the skin and deeper tissues.
- Skin incision is made with a scalpel.
- Needle guide is inserted into the grid.
- Needle is inserted to a depth of 5–10 mm deep to the lesion.
- Thickness of the needle guide is 20 mm.
- Therefore, the depth that the needle must be inserted is Z depth + needle guide thickness (20 mm) + depth of tip of wire beyond lesion (10 mm).
- Z depth + 20 mm + 10 mm
- Sagittal T1-weighted images are obtained to confirm needle location.
- Wire is inserted into the needle up to the mark. At this point, the wire tip is outside the needle.
- Needle is removed and wire is left in place.
- Wire position is confirmed with T1-weighted images.
- Postprocedure 2-view mammogram is obtained to show location of the wire.
- Specimen radiographs can be obtained, but usually the lesions are not visualized by mammography.

Reference
Morris EA, Liberman L, editors. Breast MRI diagnosis and intervention. 1st ed. New York: Springer; 2005. p. 284–9.

MRI-Guided Vacuum-Assisted Biopsy

Indication

BI-RADS 4 or 5 lesions detected on MRI imaging.

Procedure Steps
- Review prior MRI images.
- Obtain informed consent.
- Place the patient in the prone position in a dedicated breast coil within the magnet.
- Breast is placed in biopsy compression device (with a grid).
- Fiducial marker placed on skin at a slight distance from the expected lesion location (so that fiducial marker does not obscure the lesion).
- Axial localizing sequence is obtained.
- Noncontrast sagittal T1-weighted sequence is obtained.
- Gadopentetate dimeglumine, 0.1 mmol/L/kg body weight, is injected intravenously as a rapid bolus.
- Immediately following contrast administration, sagittal fat-suppressed T1-weighted sequence is obtained.
- Images are reviewed.
- A cursor is placed over the lesion and X (horizontal) and Y (vertical) coordinates are determined based on the location of the fiducial marker and grid lines.
- Z (depth) coordinate is determined based on the depth from the skin surface.

- Depth in millimeters is calculated by multiplying the number of sagittal slices from the skin to the lesion and the slice thickness.
- No. of slices × slice thickness (in mm)
- Skin is cleansed and a local anesthetic is administered to the skin and deeper tissues.
- Skin incision is made with a scalpel.
- Depth stop on the introducer is set at the determined depth.
- Stylet is put inside the introducer.
- Stylet and introducer are put in the needle guide, which is then placed in the grid.
- Stylet is advanced in the breast to the level of the depth stop.
- Stylet is removed and replaced with the obturator.
- MRI is obtained for confirmation of position; the obturator is removed and replaced with the biopsy device.
- Biopsy core samples are obtained.
- Biopsy device is removed and replaced with obturator.
- MRI for confirmation of lesion sampling.
- Titanium clip placed at biopsy site.
- Postprocedure 2-view mammogram obtained to document clip placement.

Reference
Morris EA, Liberman L, editors. Breast MRI diagnosis and intervention. 1st ed. New York: Springer; 2005. p. 302–10.

Mammography-Guided Wire Localization

Indication

- Excision of previously diagnosed cancer or high-risk lesion and localization of lesion not amenable to stereotactic or ultrasound guided biopsy.

Procedure Steps
- Obtain informed written consent.
- Determine approach by assessing shortest distance to the lesion on craniocaudal view (superior or inferior approach) or on lateral view (medial or lateral approach).
- Place breast in grid compression with opening of window placed over the skin of the determined approach (e.g., if taking a superior approach, the breast is placed in craniocaudal compression with the open grid window over the superior aspect of the breast).
- Imaging obtained to localize the lesion is within the window of the grid.
- X and Y coordinates of the lesion determined using the grid.
- Crosshairs are placed to form a target on the breast.
- Skin is cleansed and local anesthesia is used to anesthetize the skin and deeper tissue.
- The needle is advanced through the lesion, perpendicular to the skin at the determined target, allowing the crosshairs to be seen forming a cross over the hub of the needle.

- Image is obtained to assure the hub of the needle is seen over the lesion on the mammogram, thus assuring that the X and Y coordinate is accurate.
- The breast is taken out of compression and placed in orthogonal compression.
- An image is obtained in the orthogonal view to assess the depth of the needle, noting that the needle should traverse the lesion (the actual amount that the needle should traverse the lesion depends on the needle/wire system being used).
- The wire is placed through the hollow needle.
- Using the pinch–pull technique, the wire is held in place while the needle is removed from the breast.
- The hook of the wire is deployed within the breast once the needle is removed.
- The final image is obtained to document that the wire is through the lesion.
- The specimen is sent for radiograph to assure that the lesion is within the specimen and that the wire has been removed from the breast intact.

Reference
Kopans DB. Breast imaging. 2nd ed. Philadelphia: Lippincott Williams and Wilkins; 1998. p. 637–92.

Ultrasound-Guided Core Biopsy

Indication

Sonographically detected mass or axillary lymph node requiring a pathologic diagnosis.

Procedure Steps

- Obtain informed consent.
- Skin is cleansed and a local anesthetic is administered to the skin and deeper tissues.
- Insert a coaxial trocar corresponding to the biopsy device under ultrasound guidance with tip to the edge of the mass.
- Inner stylet of coaxial trocar removed. Biopsy device placed through coaxial trocar.
- Samples obtained of the mass.
- Stainless steel or titanium biopsy site marker placed in the mass through coaxial trocar.
- Postprocedure 2-view mammogram of the breast biopsied should be obtained to demonstrate clip placement.

References

Berg WB, Birdwell RB, Gombos EC, et al. Diagnostic imaging breast. 1st ed. Salt Lake City: Amirsys; 2006. Section V-2, p. 40–3.
Cardenosa G. Breast imaging companion. 3rd ed. Philadelphia: Lippincott Williams and Wilkins; 2008. p. 523–32.

Ultrasound-Guided Cyst Aspiration

Indication

- Symptomatic cysts or atypical features on ultrasound.
- Patient anxiety or request.
- Uncertainty of whether a hypoechoic mass represents a complicated cyst versus solid mass.

Procedure Steps

- Obtain informed consent.
- Skin is cleansed and a local anesthetic is administered to the skin and deeper tissues.
- A needle attached to a syringe is advanced into the cyst under ultrasound guidance.
- Cyst aspirated until no longer visualized.
- Bloody, clear, or mucoid fluid is sent to cytology.
- If fluid is sent to cytology, a microclip should be placed in the area of the cyst.
- All other fluids are discarded.
- If lesion is solid or partially solid, convert to an ultrasound-guided core needle biopsy.
- If a clip is placed, a postprocedure 2-view mammogram of the breast should be obtained to document clip placement.

References

Berg WA, Birdwell RL, Gombos EC, et al. Diagnostic imaging breast. 1st ed. Salt Lake City: Amirsys; 2006. Section V-2, p. 2–3.
Cardenosa G. Breast imaging companion. 3rd ed. Philadelphia: Lippincott Williams and Wilkins; 2008. p. 499–501.

Ultrasound-Guided Wire Localization

Indication

Excision of previously diagnosed cancer or high-risk lesion by prior core biopsy. Other indication is the localization of lesion that is best seen by ultrasound.

Procedure Steps
- Obtain informed written consent.
- Review prior ultrasound images.
- Skin is cleansed and local anesthesia is used to anesthetize the skin and deeper tissue.
- Choose the length of the needle by measuring the distance from the distal end of the lesion to the estimated skin entry +2 cm.
- A hollow needle is advanced through the lesion.
- Once the needle is placed through the lesion, a wire is advanced through the hollow needle.

- The wire tip should be just beyond the lesion.
- Using the pinch–pull technique, the wire is held in place while the needle is removed from the breast.
- The hook of the wire is deployed within the breast once the needle is removed.
- Make an "X" mark on the overlying skin with a permanent marker directly over the lesion. Depth from the mark to the lesion should be provided to the surgeon.
- Orthogonal mammograms are not necessary if the appropriate wire placement is documented on ultrasound.
- Specimen imaging is required. If the lesion is not seen mammographically, ultrasound imaging can be performed in a saline bath to demonstrate the lesion within the specimen.

References
Berg WB, Birdwell RB, Gombos EC, et al. Diagnostic imaging breast. 1st ed. Salt Lake City: Amirsys; 2006. Section V 2, p. 20–1.
Kopans DB. Breast imaging. 2nd ed. Philadelphia: Lippincott Williams and Wilkins; 1998. p. 637–92.

Galactography

Indication

Single-duct spontaneous bloody, serous, or clear nipple discharge.

Procedure Steps

- Obtain informed consent.
- Breast placed on the magnification stand (or the patient placed in the supine position) with gooseneck light positioned to illuminate the nipple.
- Nipple is cleansed.
- Duct opening is identified by squeezing the nipple to express a small drop of nipple discharge.
- The cannula is connected to the tubing and syringe containing 1–3 mL of Optiray contrast.
- A blunt (27 or 30 gauge), straight, or right-angled cannula, connected to tubing and a contrast filled syringe, is inserted into the duct opening.
- The cannula is taped in place to the patient's breast.
- Contrast is injected slowly into the duct until the patient feels fullness in her breast or there is reflux of contrast from the duct.

  - Special attention is paid not to inject air into the duct, as it can mimic a filling defect on the mammogram.
  - If resistance occurs while injecting, it may be the result of the cannula being placed against the wall of the duct or extravasation of contrast outside of the duct. Stop injection and reposition cannula.

- Once contrast has been injected, a magnification craniocaudal and lateral view is obtained.
- Images are assessed for a filling defect within the duct or abrupt termination of the duct. Both findings will require biopsy.
- Galactography can assess for a mass within or compromising a duct, but cannot differentiate benign or malignant etiology.

References

Fajardo LL, Jackson VP, Hunter TB. Interventional procedures in diseases of the breast: needle biopsy, pneumocystography and galactography. AJR. 1992;158:1231–8.

Kopans DB. Breast imaging. 2nd ed. Philadelphia: Lippincott Williams and Wilkins; 1998. p. 703–4.

Stereotactic-Guided Vacuum-Assisted Biopsy

Indication

Nonpalpable, mammographically detected BI-RADS 4 or 5 lesions that are not amenable to ultrasound-guided core needle biopsy.

Procedure Steps
- Obtain informed written consent.
- Breast should be suspended through the opening of the stereotactic table, with the breast positioned in compression against the image receptor plate.
- Stereotactic images should be obtained ($+15°$ and $-15°$).
- Lesion should be targeted on stereotactic images.
- Skin is cleansed and the local anesthetic is administered to the skin and deeper tissues.

- A small incision is made in the skin with a scalpel.
- The probe/needle should be advanced to the prefire position with stereotactic images obtained to verify the position of the probe/needle.
- The probe/needle should be "fired" with stereotactic images obtained to verify the position of the probe/needle.
- Biopsy core samples should be obtained. The number of samples varies with the size of the probe/needle.
- Specimen radiograph should be obtained to verify calcifications in core samples. This is optional for noncalcified masses.
- Stainless steel or titanium clip should be placed at the biopsy site through the hollow probe.
- Postprocedure two-view mammogram of the biopsied breast should be obtained to demonstrate clip placement.

Reference
Berg WA, Birdwell RL, Gombos EC, et al. Diagnostic imaging breast. 1st ed. Salt Lake City: Amirsys; 2006. Section IV 2, p. 28–9.

Appendix 2: High-Yield Facts

BI-RADS lexicon mnemonic for mass shape (*For mammography, ultrasound, and MRI*)	"*RIO*" *R*ound *I*rregular *O*val
BI-RADS lexicon mnemonic for mass margins (*For mammography ONLY*)	"*COMIS*" *C*ircumscribed *O*bscured *M*icrolobulated *I*ndistinct *S*piculated

BI-RADS lexicon mnemonic for mass margins
(*For ultrasound ONLY*)
	Circumscribed
	OR
	Not circumscribed ("*AIMS*")
	    *A*ngular
	    *I*ndistinct
	    *M*icrolobulated
	    *S*piculated

BI-RADS lexicon mnemonic for mass margins
(*For MRI ONLY*)
	Circumscribed
	OR
	Not circumscribed ("*IS*")
	    *I*rregular
	    *S*piculated

ACS Recommendations for Breast MRI Screening as an Adjunct to Mammography

- Recommend annual MRI screening (based on evidence).
  - BRCA mutation.
  - First-degree relative of *BRCA* carrier, but untested.
  - Lifetime risk 20–25 % or greater, as defined by BRCAPRO or other models that are largely dependent on family history.
- Recommend annual MRI screening (based on expert consensus opinion).
  - Radiation to chest between age 10 and 30 years.
  - Li–Fraumeni syndrome and first-degree relatives with breast cancer diagnosis.
  - Cowden and Bannayan–Riley–Ruvalcaba syndromes and first-degree relatives.
- Insufficient evidence to recommend for or against MRI screening.
  - Lifetime risk 15–20 %, as defined by BRCAPRO or other models that are largely dependent on family history.

- Lobular carcinoma in situ (LCIS) or atypical lobular hyperplasia (ALH).
  - Atypical ductal hyperplasia (ADH).
  - Heterogeneously or extremely dense breast on mammography.
  - Women with a personal history of breast cancer, including ductal carcinoma in situ (DCIS).
- Recommend against MRI screening (based on expert consensus opinion).
  - Women at <15 % lifetime risk

Breast Lesion Triangulation Mnemonic

- *M*uffins (Medial) *R*ise and *L*ead (Lateral) *F*alls.
  - If a lesion is only seen on the CC view, obtain a lateral view.
    - If the lesion is located medially on the CC view, it will be more superior in the lateral view when compared with that in the MLO view.
    - If the lesion is located laterally on the CC view, it will be more inferior in the lateral view when compared with that in the MLO view.

Mammography Findings That Can Be Categorized by BI-RADS 3 (Short-Term Follow-Up)

- Findings must be seen on a baseline mammogram or a mammogram without comparison studies available.
- Cluster of calcifications on spot-magnification views that are round or oval.
- Solid nonpalpable noncalcified mass with round or oval shape and circumscribed margins.
- Nonpalpable focal asymmetry seen on two views with concave margins and interposed fat.
- Miscellaneous findings:
  - Single dilated duct
  - Architectural distortion at known biopsy site without dense central mass
  - Multiple similar lesions of intermediate suspicion

Differential Diagnosis of Bilateral Axillary Lymphadenopathy

- Lymphoma
- Leukemia
- SLE
- Sarcoidosis
- Rheumatoid arthritis
- Mixed connective tissue
- HIV
- Granulomatous disease
- Drug reaction (Dilantin)

Differential Diagnosis of Unilateral Axillary Lymphadenopathy

- Primary breast cancer with ipsilateral axillary lymphadenopathy spread
- Granulomatous disease
- Infection (mastitis)
- Extracapsular silicone leak

Differential Diagnosis of a Filling Defect on Galactography

- Papilloma
- Intraductal papillary carcinoma
- Blood clot
- Inspissated material
- Air bubble

Differential Diagnosis of a Spiculated Mass on Mammography

- Cancer
- Radial scar
- Postbiopsy scar
- Fat necrosis
- Sclerosing adenosis
- Abscess
- Hematoma
- Granular cell tumor

Differential Diagnosis of Skin Thickening (>2.5 mm)

- Inflammatory breast cancer
- Postsurgical
- Postradiation
- Cardiac failure
- Mastitis
- Renal failure
- Hypoalbuminemia
- Thrombophlebitis of the breast (Mondor's disease)
- Thrombosis in the subclavian vein or SVC (SVC syndrome)

Differential Diagnosis of Increased Breast Density

- Estrogen replacement
- Weight loss
- Inflammatory breast cancer
- Mastitis
- Postradiation
- Trauma
- Lymphatic obstruction
- Congestive heart failure
- Renal failure
- Postsurgical

Causes of Gynecomastia

- Idiopathic (most common)
- Drugs
- Estrogen excess (exogenous estrogen administration, testicular tumor, or adrenocortical tumor)
- Male breast cancer
- Hypogonadism (Klinefelter syndrome or pituitary insufficiency)
- Hyperthyroidism
- Liver failure and cirrhosis

Drugs That Cause Gynecomastia

- Marijuana
- Estrogen
- Cimetidine
- Spironolactone
- Phenothiazides
- Amphetamines
- Digitalis

US Features of a Malignant Lesion

- Spiculation
- Angular margins
- Hypoechogenicity
- Acoustic shadowing
- Branch pattern
- Extension into a duct
- Microlobulation
- Not parallel
- Calcifications

US Features of a Benign Lesion

- Hyperechoic
- Parallel
- Macrolobulation
- Thin pseudocapsule
- Acoustic enhancement

Differential Diagnosis of a Hyperechoic Mass

- Acute hemorrhage
- Acute hematoma
- Focal fibrosis
- Hemangioma
- Angiolipoma
- Spindle cell lipoma
- Malignancy

Tumors That Commonly Metastasize to the Breast

- Contralateral breast cancer
- Melanoma
- Lung cancer
- Lymphoma
- Leukemia

Enhancement Kinetic Curves on Breast MRI (Fig. A.1)

- Type I: persistent; typically benign
- Type II: plateau; indeterminate
- Type III: washout; suspicious

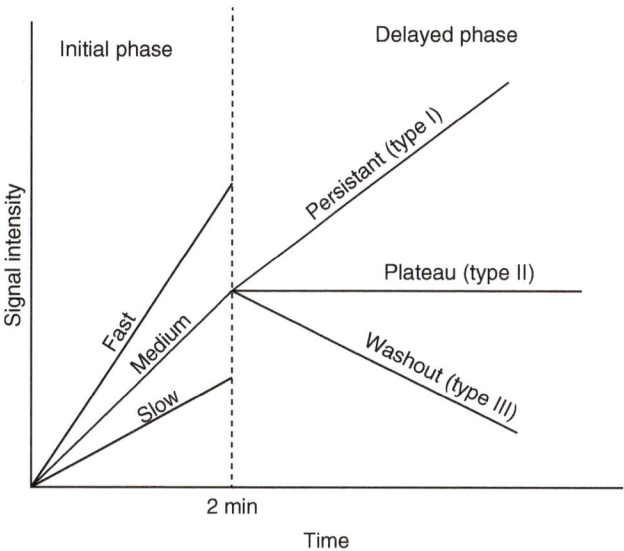

Fig. A.1

High-Risk Lesions at Core Needle Biopsy That Require Excision (*Controversial)

- ADH
- ALH*
- LCIS*
- Papilloma*
- Radial scar

Diagnosis That Increase the Lifetime Risk of Developing Breast Cancer

- ADH
- LCIS
- ALH
- Radial scar

Normal Double-Lumen Silicone Breast Implant (Fig. A.2)

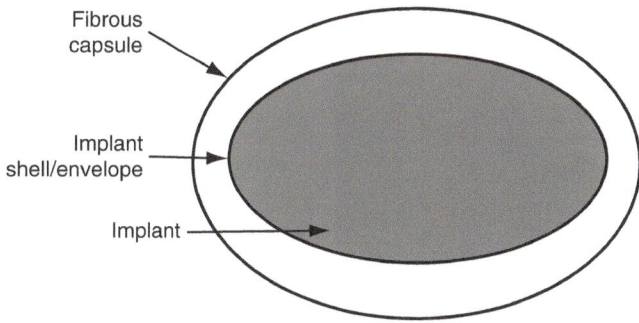

Fig. A.2

Capsular Contracture of a Silicone Implant (Fig. A.3)

Capsular contracture results when normal scar tissue forms a capsule around the breast implant and tightens and/or squeezes the breast implant. This may occur over several months to years and can result in changes in breast shape, sensation of hardness of the breast, or breast pain due to contracture of the implant.

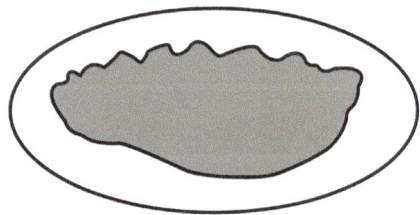

Fig. A.3

Radial Folds of a Silicone Implant (Fig. A. 4)

Infolding of the implant shell, termed radial folds, can be a normal finding seen in silicone implants. This should not be confused with implant rupture.

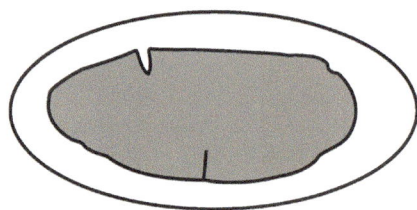

Fig. A.4

Intracapsular Rupture of Silicone
Implant (Fig. A.5a, b)

Rupture of the implant shell walls results in lines within the implant that have a "stepladder" appearance on ultrasound and "linguine" sign on MRI (Fig. A.5a).

   or

   A small intracapsular leak with silicone gel on the surface of the shell creates a "subcapsular line" sign (Fig. A.5b).

   "Inverted teardrop" or "keyhole" sign of a silicone implant (Fig. A.6).

   "Inverted tear drop" sign or "keyhole" sign is when silicone is within a radial fold.

   It is a nonspecific finding that may be seen with a focal intracapsular rupture or extensive gel bleed.

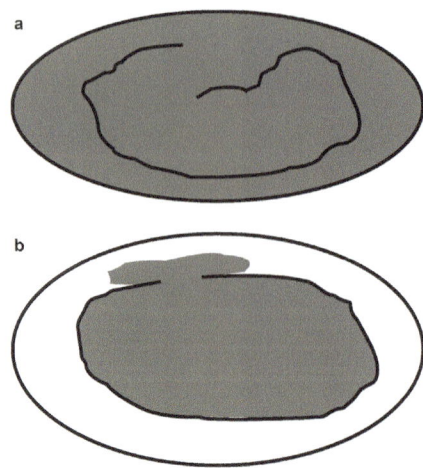

Fig. A.5

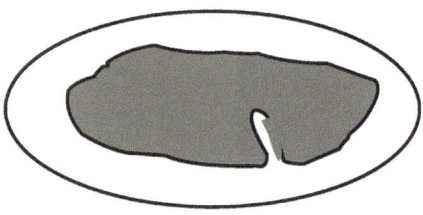

Fig. A.6

Findings Seen in Implant Rupture

- Saline implant – implant collapse
- Silicone implant:
  - Intracapsular rupture: US shows a "stepladder" appearance. MRI shows a "linguine sign." No mammographic findings seen.
  - Extracapsular – high density seen on mammography if silicone gel is within the tissues. Silicone may be seen in lymph nodes.
  - Ultrasound shows a "snowstorm" appearance (extreme echogenicity with extensive shadowing).

References

American College of Radiology (ACR) BI-RADS® Atlas. ACR BI-RADS® Atlas. 5th ed. Reston: American College of Radiology; 2013.

Gay SP, Woodcock RJ Jr. Radiology recall. 2nd ed. Philadelphia: Lippincott William & Wilkins; 2008. p. 537–75.

Saslow D, Boetes C, Burke W, et al. American Cancer Society Guidelines for breast screening with MRI as an adjunct to mammography. J Clin. 2007;57:75–89.

Sickles EA. Periodic mammographic follow-up of probably benign lesions: results in 3,184 consecutive cases. Radiology. 1991; 179:463–8.

Weissleder R, Wittenberg J, Harisinghani MG, Chen JW. Primer of diagnostic imaging. 4th ed. Mosby, Elsevier; 2007. p. 729–60.

Appendix 3: BI-RADS Key Facts

ACR BI-RADS® Atlas Fifth Edition
QUICK REFERENCE

ACR — AMERICAN COLLEGE OF RADIOLOGY — QUALITY IS OUR IMAGE

MAMMOGRAPHY

Breast composition		a. The breasts are almost entirely fatty
		b. There are scattered areas of fibroglandular density
		c. The breasts are heterogeneously dense, which may obscure small masses
		d. The breasts are extremely dense, which lowers the sensitivity of mammography
Masses	Shape	Oval
		Round
		Irregular
	Margin	Circumscribed
		Obscured
		Microlobulated
		Indistinct
		Spiculated
	Density	High density
		Equal density
		Low density
		Fat-containing
Calcifications	Typically benign	Skin
		Vascular
		Coarse or "popcorn-like"
		Large rod-like
		Round
		Rim
		Dystrophic
		Milk of calcium
		Suture
	Suspicious morphology	Amorphous
		Coarse heterogeneous
		Fine pleomorphic
		Fine linear or fine-linear branching
	Distribution	Diffuse
		Regional
		Grouped
		Linear
		Segmental
Architectural distortion		
Asymmetries	Asymmetry	
	Global asymmetry	
	Focal asymmetry	
	Developing asymmetry	
Intramammary lymph node		
Skin lesion		
Solitary dilated duct		
Associated features	Skin retraction	
	Nipple retraction	
	Skin thickening	
	Trabecular thickening	
	Axillary adenopathy	
	Architectural distortion	
	Calcifications	
Location of lesion	Laterality	
	Quadrant and clock face	
	Depth	
	Distance from the nipple	

ULTRASOUND

Tissue composition (screening only)		a. Homogeneous background echotexture – fat
		b. Homogeneous background echotexture – fibroglandular
		c. Heterogeneous background echotexture
Masses	Shape	Oval
		Round
		Irregular
	Orientation	Parallel
		Not parallel
	Margin	Circumscribed
		Not circumscribed
		- Indistinct
		- Angular
		- Microlobulated
		- Spiculated
	Echo pattern	Anechoic
		Hyperechoic
		Complex cystic and solid
		Hypoechoic
		Isoechoic
		Heterogeneous
	Posterior features	No posterior features
		Enhancement
		Shadowing
		Combined pattern
Calcifications		Calcifications in a mass
		Calcifications outside of a mass
		Intraductal calcifications
Associated features		Architectural distortion
		Duct changes
	Skin changes	Skin thickening
		Skin retraction
	Edema	
	Vascularity	Absent
		Internal vascularity
		Vessels in rim
	Elasticity assessment	Soft
		Intermediate
		Hard
Special cases		Simple cyst
		Clustered microcysts
		Complicated cyst
		Mass in or on skin
		Foreign body including implants
		Lymph nodes – intramammary
		Lymph nodes – axillary
	Vascular abnormalities	AVMs (arteriovenous malformations/pseudoaneurysms)
		Mondor disease
		Postsurgical fluid collection
		Fat necrosis

MAGNETIC RESONANCE IMAGING

Amount of fibroglandular tissue (FGT)	a. Almost entirely fat b. Scattered fibroglandular tissue c. Heterogeneous fibroglandular tissue d. Extreme fibroglandular tissue		Associated features	Nipple retraction	
				Nipple invasion	
				Skin retraction	
				Skin thickening	
Background parenchymal enhancement (BPE)	Level	Minimal		Skin invasion	Direct invasion
		Mild			Inflammatory cancer
		Moderate		Axillary adenopathy	
		Marked		Pectoralis muscle invasion	
	Symmetric or asymmetric	Symmetric		Chest wall invasion	
		Asymmetric		Architectural distortion	
Focus			Fat containing lesions	Lymph nodes	Normal
Masses	Shape	Oval			Abnormal
		Round		Fat necrosis	
		Irregular		Hamartoma	
	Margin	Circumscribed		Postoperative seroma/hematoma with fat	

		Not circumscribed
		   - Irregular
		   - Spiculated
			Location of lesion	Location	

				Depth	
	Internal enhancement characteristics	Homogeneous	Kinetic curve assessment Signal intensity (SI)/time curve description	Initial phase	Slow
		Heterogeneous			Medium
		Rim enhancement			Fast
		Dark internal septations		Delayed phase	Persistent
					Plateau
					Washout
Non-mass enhancement (NME)	Distribution	Focal	Implants	Implant material and lumen type	Saline

		Linear			Silicone
					   - Intact
					   - Ruptured

		Segmental			
		Regional			Other implant material
		Multiple regions			Lumen type
		Diffuse		Implant location	Retroglandular
	Internal enhancement patterns	Homogeneous			Retropectoral
		Heterogeneous		Abnormal implant contour	Focal bulge
		Clumped		Intracapsular silicone findings	Radial folds
		Clustered ring			Subcapsular line
Intramammary lymph node					Keyhole sign (teardrop, noose)
Skin lesion					Linguine sign
Non-enhancing findings	Ductal precontrast high signal on T1W		Extracapsular silicone	Breast	
	Cyst				
	Postoperative collections (hematoma/seroma)			Lymph nodes	
	Post-therapy skin thickening and trabecular thickening		Water droplets		
	Non-enhancing mass		Peri-implant fluid		
	Architectural distortion				
	Signal void from foreign bodies, clips, etc.				

BI-RADS® ASSESSMENT CATEGORIES

Category 0: **Mammography:** Incomplete – Need Additional Imaging Evaluation and/or Prior Mammograms for Comparison
Ultrasound & MRI: Incomplete – Need Additional Imaging Evaluation

Category 1: Negative

Category 2: Benign

Category 3: Probably Benign

Category 4: Suspicious | Mammography & Ultrasound: | Category 4A: Low suspicion for malignancy
Category 4B: Moderate suspicion for malignancy
Category 4C: High suspicion for malignancy

Category 5: Highly Suggestive of Malignancy

Category 6: Known Biopsy-Proven Malignancy

For the complete Atlas, visit **acr.org/birads**

Statistical Terms and Their Definitions

Term	Definition
True-positive (TP)	Tissue diagnosis of cancer within 1 year after a positive examination. BI-RADS 3 category assessments made at screening examination are considered positive examinations
True-negative (TN)	No known tissue diagnosis of cancer within 1 year of a negative examination (BI-RADS categories 1 or 2 for screening; BI-RADS categories 1,2, or 3 for diagnostic)
False-negative (FN)	Tissue diagnosis of cancer within 1 year of a negative examination (BI-RADS categories 1 or 2 for screening; BI-RADS categories 1, 2, or 3 for diagnostic)
False-positive 1 (FP$_1$)	No known tissue diagnosis of cancer within 1 year of a positive mammogram. Includes BI-RADS category 3 assessments made at screening
False-positive 2 (FP$_2$)	No known tissue diagnosis of cancer within 1 year after recommendation for tissue diagnosis or surgical consultation on the basis of a positive examination (BI-RADS category 4 or 5)
False-positive 3 (FP$_3$)	Concordant benign breast tissue diagnosis (or discordant benign breast tissue and no known diagnosis of cancer) within 1 year after recommendation of the basis of a positive examination (BI-RADS category 4 or 5).
Positive predictive value 1 (PPV$_1$) (abnormal finding at screening)	The percentage of all screening examinations (BI-RADS categories 0, 3, 4, and 5) that result in a tissue diagnosis of cancer within 1 year $PPV_1 = TP/(number\ of\ positive\ screening\ examinations) = TP/(TP + FP_1)$
Positive predictive value 2 (PPV$_2$) (biopsy recommended)	The percentage of all diagnostic (or rarely, screening) examinations recommended for tissue diagnosis or surgical consultation (BI-RADS categories 4 and 5) that result in a tissue diagnosis of cancer within 1 year $PPV_2 = TP/(number\ of\ screening\ or\ diagnostic\ examinations\ recommended\ for\ tissue\ diagnosis) = TP/(TP + FP_2)$
Positive predictive value 3 (PPV$_3$) (biopsy performed)	The percentage of all known biopsies done as a result of positive diagnostic examinations (BI-RADS categories 4 and 5) that resulted in a tissue diagnosis of cancer within 1 year. Also known as biopsy yield of malignancy or the positive biopsy rate (PBR) $PPV_3 = TP/(number\ of\ biopsies) = TP/(TP + FP_3)$
Sensitivity	The probability of interpreting an examination as positive when cancer exists. Calculated as the number of positive examinations for which there was tissue diagnosis of cancer within 1 year of imaging examination, divided by all cancers present in the population examined in the same time period $Sensitivity = TP/(TP + FN)$
Specificity	The probability of interpreting an examination as negative when cancer does not exist. Calculated as the number of negative examinations for which there is no tissue diagnosis of cancer within 1 year of examination, divided by all the examinations for which there is no tissue diagnosis of cancer within the same time period
Cancer detection rate	The number of cancers detected at imaging per 1,000 patients examined
Abnormal interpretation rate (also known as recall rate)	Percentage of examinations interpreted as positive. For screening, positive examinations usually involve BI-RADS categories 0 assessments for mammography and (for auditing purposes) breast US, but BI-RADS categories 4 and 5 for breast MRI. This also includes BI-RADS 3 category assessments made at screening for all imaging modalities. For diagnostic imaging, positive examinations involved BI-RADS category 4 and 5 assessments $Abnormal\ interpretation\ rate = (positive\ examinations)/(all\ examinations)$

Source: These Statistical Terms are based on material from the Follow-up and Outcome monitoring section of the ACR BI-RADS® Atlas – 5th Edition

Cancer detection rate (per 1,000)	≥2.5
Abnormal interpretation (recall) rate	5–2 %
PPV$_1$	3–8 %
PPV$_2$	20–40 %
Sensitivity (if measurable)	≥75 %
Specificity (if measureable)	88–99 %

Source: Sickles EA and D'Orsi CJ. American College of Radiology (ACR) BI-RADS® Atlas (2013) ACR BI-RADS® Follow-up and Outcome Monitoring 2013. p 29, with permission

	Workup of abnormal screening	Palpable lump
Cancer detection rate (per 1,000)	≥20	≥40
Abnormal interpretation (recall) rate	8–25 %	10–25 %
PPV$_2$	15–40 %	25–50 %
PPV$_3$	20–45 %	30–55 %
Sensitivity (if measurable)	≥80 %	≥85 %
Specificity (if measureable)	80–95 %	83–95 %

Source: Sickles EA and D'Orsi CJ. American College of Radiology (ACR) BI-RADS® Atlas (2013) ACR BI-RADS® Follow-up and Outcome Monitoring 2013. p 29, with permission

Index

Lipoma
  BI-RADS assessment, 59
  breast architecture, 59
  diagnosis, 59
  patient history, 59
  radiology findings, 59, 60
Lobular carcinoma in situ (LCIS)
  analysis, 77
  BI-RADS assessment, 77
  diagnosis, 77
  patient history, 77
  radiology findings, 77, 78
Lymphadenopathy, 206
Lymphoma
  analysis, 31
  BI-RADS assessment, 31
  diagnosis, 31
  patient history, 31
  radiology findings, 31–33

M
Magnetic resonance imaging (MRI) artifacts
  diagnosis, 196
  inhomogeneous fat saturation artifact, 196
  motion artifact, 196
  patient history, 196
  phase wrap, 196
  radiology findings, 196–199
  silicone saturation artifact, 196
  susceptibility artifacts, 196
Malignancy, 218
Mammographic artifacts
  analysis, 2
  diagnosis, 2
  patient history, 2
  radiology findings
    chin artifact, 2, 4
    deodorant and hair artifact, 2, 5
    motion artifact, 2, 5
    ventricular peritoneal shunt
      catheter, 2–4
Mastitis
  BI-RADS assessment, 39
  diagnosis, 39
  patient history, 39
  radiology findings, 39–41
  skin-punch biopsy, 39
  Staphylococcus aureus and Streptococcus, 39
Medullary carcinoma
  analysis, 74
  BI-RADS assessment, 74
  diagnosis, 74
  patient history, 74
  radiology findings, 74–76
Micropapillary carcinoma
  BI-RADS assessment, 152
  diagnosis, 152
  mammography, 152
  MRI, 152
  patient history, 152
  radiology findings, 152, 153
  sonography, 152
Milk of calcium
  BI-RADS assessment, 29
  calcium-oxalate calcifications, 29
  diagnosis, 29

  patient history, 29
  radiology findings, 29, 30
Mondor's disease
  BI-RADS assessment, 105
  diagnosis, 105
  mammogram and ultrasound, 105
  patient history, 105
  radiology findings, 105–107
  thrombophlebitis, 105
Motion artifact, 196
MRI artifacts. *See* Magnetic resonance
      imaging (MRI) artifacts
Mucinous carcinoma
  BI-RADS assessment, 138
  diagnosis, 138
  MRI, 138
  mucin, 138
  patient history, 138
  radiology findings, 138–140
Multiple, bilateral circumscribed masses
  analysis, 44
  BI-RADS assessment, 44
  diagnosis, 44
  patient history, 44
  radiology findings, 44, 45

N
Neurofibromatosis type I (NF I)
  BI-RADS assessment, 42
  diagnosis, 42
  neoplasms, 42
  patient history, 42
  radiology findings, 42, 43
  von Recklinghausen's disease, 42
Nipple inversion, 206
Nonpuerperal abscess
  BI-RADS assessment, 163
  diagnosis, 163
  differential diagnosis, 163
  patient history, 163
  radiology findings, 163–164
  risk factors, 163
  symptoms, 163
  systemic antibiotics, 163
Noose sign, 209

O
Oil cyst
  BI-RADS assessment, 123
  diagnosis, 123
  patient history, 123
  radiology findings, 123, 124
  steatocystoma multiplex, 123
  surgery, accidental trauma and
      radiation therapy, 123

P
Paget's disease
  BI-RADS assessment, 36
  diagnosis, 36
  nipple–areolar complex, 36
  patient history, 36
  radiology findings, 36–38
  skin thickening and heterogeneity, 36